Practical Electrophysiology, Second Edition

Todd J. Cohen, M.D., F.A.C.C., F.H.R.S.

Editor-in-Chief Emeritus, *EP Lab Digest*

Associate Professor of Medicine at SUNY Stony Brook

Director of Electrophysiology,

Director of Advanced EP Technology and Innovations,

Director of the Pacemaker-Arrhythmia Center,

Winthrop University Hospital, Mineola, NY

Practical Electrophysiology, Second Edition

HMP Communications, LLC
83 General Warren Boulevard
Suite 100
Malvern, PA 19355
Tel. 800-237-7285
www.hmpcommunications.com

Chairman/CEO: Jeff Hennessy
Group Publisher: Jeff Martin
Managing Editor: Jodie Elrod
Creative Director: Vic Geanopulos
Art Director: Karen Copestakes

ISBN 0-9706514-5-7

Table of Contents

Dedication

Dedicated to my dear father,
Edward George Cohen,
September 24, 1927 – March 23, 2004

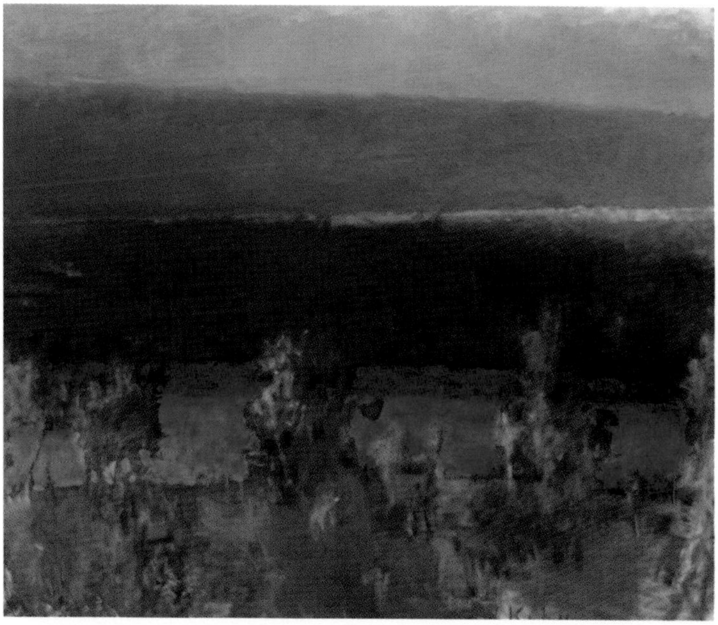

Palisades, 1991, oil on canvas © Wolf Kahn/Licensed by VAGA, New York, NY

In appreciation:

Melvin M. Scheinman, MD

Douglas Beinborn, MA, RN

Jeff Martin,
Vice President and Group Publisher, Cardiovascular Division,
HMP Communications

Jodie Elrod,
Editor, *Practical Electrophysiology* (First and Second Editions), and
Managing Editor, *EP Lab Digest*

Vic Geanopulos,
Creative Director, HMP Communications

Karen Copestakes,
Art Director, HMP Communications

Overview

Over the past three years since publishing the first edition of *Practical Electrophysiology*, several advances have occurred in this dynamic field. First, generally accepted guidelines for implanting devices such as pacemakers and implantable defibrillators have expanded. This includes the application of biventricular implants. For example, if a patient has severe LV dysfunction and will be frequently pacing and only has mild congestive heart failure, a biventricular device may be considered acceptable according to the more recent guidelines. Second, guidelines have been established for atrial fibrillation ablation. These guidelines include failure of at least one antiarrhythmic drug and the necessity to test lines of block (a definitive endpoint for the procedure). Third, a further understanding on how to manage device recalls has continued, which includes a more open communication between device manufacturers, the U.S. Food and Drug Administration, electrophysiologists and their patients. Finally, the application of robotics to electrophysiology and in particular, catheter ablation procedures, has provided a new method in which the operator can avoid direct radiation exposure during long and complicated procedures.

I have appreciated all of the feedback that we have received from the readers of this book. I sincerely hope that you enjoy the second edition of *Practical Electrophysiology*. In this second edition, the guidelines for catheter ablation and device implantation have all been updated. The EP catheters and implantable devices themselves have also been updated. Advances continue to be made with respect to hereditary conditions, with new genes now specified in a special table. A new chapter has been added regarding basic and advanced life support thanks to Douglas Beinborn, MA, RN from the Mayo Clinic. A chapter on lead extraction is also included. Test questions have been added after Parts 1, 2, and 3 to help review the materials. Overall, this book has been particularly useful as core curricula for cardiology fellows who rotate in electrophysiology and as an essential tool for ancillary staff in the electrophysiology laboratory, as well as the vendors related to electrophysiology products.

— *Todd J. Cohen, M.D., F.A.C.C., F.H.R.S.*

Medical Disclaimers

1. This publication is written and intended for health care professionals only. It is not written or intended for a general or non-professional audience. ANY READER WHO IS NOT A HEALTH CARE PROFESSIONAL SHOULD ALWAYS CONSULT WITH A PHYSICIAN OR OTHER COMPETENT HEALTH CARE PROFESSIONAL BEFORE UNDERGOING ANY MEDICAL TREATMENT, PROCEDURE OR THERAPY, INCLUDING BUT NOT LIMITED TO THOSE DISCUSSED IN THIS PUBLICATION OR OTHERWISE.

2. The authors, editors and publisher have endeavored to provide information that is accurate and in accord with accepted medical standards, all as of the date of publication. However, medical knowledge is constantly changing due to research and clinical experience, and as a result, the state of the art of medical treatments, procedures and therapies are constantly changing. Accordingly, the authors, editors and publisher specifically give no assurance that the information presented in this publication is accurate and complete in every respect, or that it is current beyond the publication date.

3. Patient experience and response to any medical treatment, procedure or therapy is never consistent. Accordingly, the authors, editors and publisher specifically give no assurance that any treatment, procedure or therapy discussed in this publication will always have the anticipated outcome.

4. The authors, editors and publishers shall have no obligation to update the information presented in this publication.

5. Health care professionals should always consult current literature before recommending or administering any medical treatment, procedure or therapy, especially (but not limited to) new, experimental or infrequently-used treatments, procedures and therapies. In the case of treatments, procedures and therapies involving drugs or devices, health care professionals should always consult the manufacturer's latest product information and recommendations, as well as independent studies.

6. THE AUTHORS, EDITOR AND PUBLISHER SHALL HAVE NO LIABILITY AND NO RESPONSIBILITY TO ANY PERSON OR ENTITY WITH RESPECT TO ANY LOSS OR DAMAGE CAUSED, OR ALLEGED TO BE CAUSED, DIRECTLY OR INDIRECTLY, BY THE USE OF ANY INFORMATION PRESENTED IN THIS PUBLICATION.

Foreword

Melvin M. Scheinman, M.D.

I am indeed pleased with the updated second edition of this unique book. Dr. Todd Cohen is an experienced cardiac electrophysiologist who shares his wide experience with the reader in a readily understandable format.

As I previously stated in the Foreword of the previous edition of *Practical Electrophysiology*, the primary audience of this book is for nurses and technicians who are interested in the field of cardiac electrophysiology. This book is important in that it not only describes the nuts and bolts of working in an electrophysiology lab, but also is an excellent review of all electrophysiology. The author very nicely evolves a story that starts with the recording of the surface ECG to the installation of complex devices and ablation procedures. This text is unique in that there is extensive discussion of the underlying pathophysiology (*i.e.*, syncope, congestive heart failure, arrhythmias, etc.) that result in the performance of electrophysiologic procedures.

The text will also serve to be of interest to hospital personnel responsible for the administrative oversight of cardiac electrophysiology programs. It provides a simple overview of a cardiac electrophysiology program and has a very practical chapter devoted to the electrophysiology team. This particular chapter contains very sage advice for the administration of these types of units.

The readers will be most appreciative of the fact that great pains were taken to make the text up-to-date. There is relevant discussion of all the major recent studies that form the backbone for procedures in the electrophysiology laboratory. These include the rationale and description of device implants as well as a description of the complex mapping devices that are currently used in the electrophysiology laboratory. The author nicely brings the reader up-to-date with a current and easily readable text.

In summary, I feel indebted to Dr. Cohen for a superb effort. I believe this text will serve as a trailblazer for much needed texts that are specifically designed for cardiac electrophysiology lab personnel. Dr. Cohen doesn't "talk down" to his audience; in fact, providing the rationale for cardiac electrophysiology referral in a clear, simple and concise manner is a real advance. This text should also be of interest to medical students or clinicians who wish to gain further insights into the field of cardiac electrophysiology.

— *Melvin M. Scheinman, M.D.*

Part 1

INTRODUCTION TO ELECTROPHYSIOLOGY

Chapter 1

The History of Electrophysiology

In 1895, Willem Einthoven described the waves recorded from his invention, the string galvanometer. His PQRST diagram is remarkably similar to the P, QRS, and T waves currently used daily by cardiologists everywhere for interpretation of a standard electrocardiogram (ECG). Therefore, it may appear that little has changed with respect to the image, principles, and nomenclature of a standard ECG tracing over the past century. However, tremendous changes have been made in the method of ECG recordings. For instance, there is no longer a need to immerse limbs in saline; precordial and unipolar electrodes have been developed, and digital/computerized recording systems have been implemented. Similar advancements have also been made in our understanding of electrical signals recorded from within the heart (intracardiac recordings) since the recording of the first His bundle. During the past half-century, we have witnessed the development of cardiopulmonary resuscitation, transthoracic cardioversion and defibrillation, and the advent of implantable devices (pacemakers, defibrillators, loop recorders, and biventricular devices). Innovations in catheter ablation have resulted in a very high success rate for most reentrant and focal supraventricular tachycardias and certain ventricular tachycardias. Even atrial fibrillation can be successfully managed in many circumstances via pulmonary vein isolation procedures and left atrial ablations. These procedures can be performed percutaneously with an ablation catheter.

In 1884, the first graphic documentation of ventricular fibrillation was performed by M. Hoffa. Shortly thereafter, in 1888, Augustus

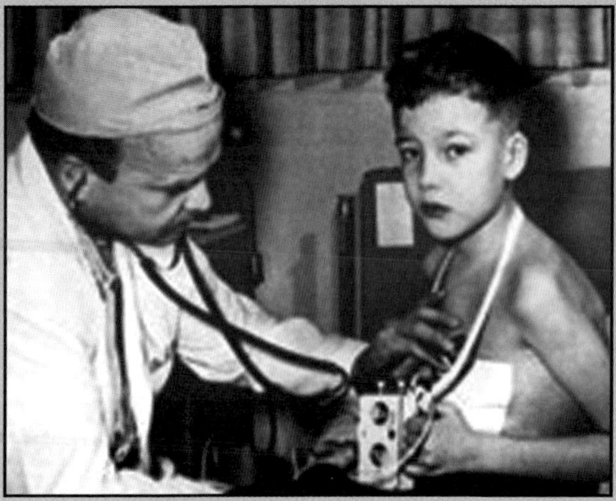

Figure 1.1: Dr. C. Walton Lillehei with a child who received one of the early Medtronic external pacemakers (Reproduced with permission of Medtronic, Inc., Minneapolis, MN).

Desiré Waller introduced his findings on electromotive properties of the human heart. Waller presented his dog with each paw in a pan of saline, from which the electrical potentials were recorded, and termed these electrical currents "electrograms." John A. McWilliam published his findings, "Electrical Stimulation of the Heart in Man," in 1889; in them he stated that "in certain forms of cardiac arrest there appears to be a possibility of restoring by artificial means the rhythmic beat."

In 1905, N. Floresco introduced "stimulating pincers" to measure the electric current on the blood glucose level. S. Tawara established the link between approaches to the AV node, the His bundle and the Purkinje fibers, discovered the left and right bundle branches and identified the Purkinje fibers as their termination; he then conceptualized these components as the specialized conduction system of the heart in 1906. Tawara's anatomic conclusions and physiological hypotheses provided the theoretical basis for Einthoven's interpretation of the electrocardiogram. Shortly thereafter, in 1924, W. Mobitz introduced the classification of heart blocks as type I and type II using an electrocardiogram. In 1929, Forssmann published the first "catheterization of the right heart" by performing the catheterization on himself.

The year 1932 brought about the invention of the first artificial pacemaker, by Albert S. Hyman. The device was operated by a hand crank and a spring motor, which turned a magneto (DC-current generator) to supply the electricity. Following Hyman, Claude Beck invented the Beck defibrillator in 1947. In 1957, Earl Bakken developed a wearable, external, battery-driven pacemaker (figure 1.1). Rune Elmqvist first tried to pace with an implantable pacemaker in 1958. The implantable pulse generator was powered by two rechargeable nickel-cadmium batteries, each delivering 50 microampere-hours; it had to be recharged once a week for 12 hours. Additionally, in July 1958, the transvenous catheter electrode was introduced, with fluoroscopy, via the basilic vein into the right ventricular outflow tract.

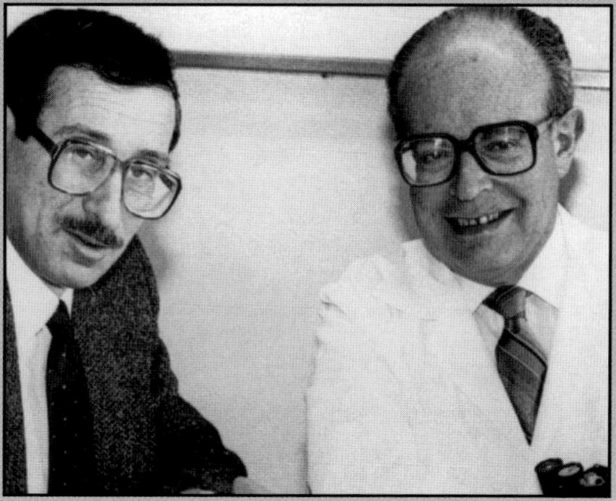

Figure 1.2: Drs. Morton Mower and Michel Mirowski were the inventors of the first implantable cardioverter-defibrillator. (Image courtesy of the Mirowski family and used with permission from the Mirowski Foundation.)

On May 19, 1959, the first insertion of a transvenous lead via cephalic vein cut-down was performed on a 67-year-old man. The battery-operated device had the capability of sensing spontaneous cardiac activity of variation in output and stimulation rate. A permanently attached cable delivered output to the electrodes.

In Uruguay in 1960, Orestes Fiandara and Roberto Rubio implanted the first permanent pacemaker in a human being. This unit was a pulse generator sutured to the left ventricular surface. The device showed an increased tolerance to exercise, and its use was a cure for the recurrence of Adams-Stokes episodes. The first pacemaker implantation in Germany soon followed in 1961. Two years later an implantable, synchronous cardiac pacemaker for long-term correction of complete heart block was performed, supported with intracardiac electrograms recording the performance of the pacemaker during normal sinus rhythm and atrial arrhythmias. Subsequently, dual-chamber and rate-responsive pacemakers made these devices physiologic.

In the late 1960s, Dr. Michel Mirowski conceived of a similar device to treat ventricular fibrillation. In the 1970s, Dr. Mirowski and Dr. Morton Mower collaborated on the development of the first implantable defibrillator (figure 1.2). The first-generation device required open-heart surgery and a long postoperative course. The first patient (from California) was brought to Johns Hopkins University and received the implant by surgeon Levi Watkins.

Transvenous and dual-chamber implantable defibrillators were subsequently developed. With further manufacturing sophistication, implantable cardioverter-defibrillators have become smaller and easier to implant. Currently, most implants are performed by cardiologists (electrophysiologists) and not by thoracic or cardiovascular surgeons.

The late 1990s and early 2000s were marked by the completion of prophylactic implantable defibrillator trials. The Multicenter Automatic Defibrillator Implantation Trials (MADIT and MADIT II)

Table 1.1: Key Events in the History of Electrophysiology

1884	Hoffa performs first graphic documentation of ventricular fibrillation
1888	Waller presents properties of the human heart as an electrical organ
1889	McWilliam publishes "Electrical Stimulation of the Heart in Man"
1895	Einthoven publishes report on string galvanometer (electrocardiograph machine)
1905	Floresco introduced "stimulating pincers"
1906	Tawara conceptualizes the conduction system of the heart
1924	Mobitz introduces classification of heart blocks as type I and type II
1929	Forssmann reports on the first heart catheterization, which he performed on himself
1932	Hyman invents the artificial pacemaker
1940	Wolff-Parkinson-White (WPW) syndrome first diagnosed
1947	Beck defibrillator invented and tried
1957	Bakken develops wearable, external, battery-driven pacemaker
1958	Elmqvist tries to pace with an implantable pacemaker
1959	First insertion of a "heart regulator"
1963	Hodgkin and Huxley describe cellular currents
1969	First recording of the His bundle
1980	First implantable cardioverter-defibrillator (ICD) implanted in a person
1982	Scheinman describes five patients with refractory supraventricular tachycardia in which DC shocks were delivered (first catheter ablation)
1985	FDA approves ICDs; first radiofrequency catheter ablation
1988	Tiered therapy for ICDs and pacing for atrial fibrillation suppression introduced
1989	Transvenous leads and biphasic waveform technology introduced
1991	Neher and Sakman receive Nobel Prize for inventing the patch-clamping method for detecting single-channel currents
1994	Haïssaguerre performed atrial fibrillation ablation
1996	The first Multicenter Automatic Defibrillator Implantation Trial (MADIT); steroid-eluting leads and increased diagnostic and memory capacity in ICDs
1997-1998	Dual-chamber ICDs and nonfluoroscopic 3-D mapping introduced; further reduction of ICD size; Antiarrhythmics Versus Implantable Defibrillators (AVID), Cardiac Arrest Survival Hamburg (CASH), and Canadian Implantable Defibrillator Study (CIDS) trials
1999	Atrial tachyarrhythmia therapies; Multicenter Unsustained Tachycardia Trial (MUSTT)
2000	ICDs with cardiac resynchronization
2002	Multicenter Automatic Defibrillator Implantation Trial II (MADIT II)
2003	Comparison of Medical Therapy, Pacing, and Defibrillation in Heart Failure (COMPANION) trial
2005	Sudden Cardiac Death in Heart Failure Trial (SCD-HeFT) published; Medicare approves MADIT II and SCD-HeFT indications for ICDs
2006	Fluid monitoring via transthoracic impedance included in ICD (as well as biventricular ICD)
2007	Robotic system utilizing steerable sheath to perform remote catheter manipulation receives FDA clearance
2007	ICD lead recall prompts additional consensus guidelines regarding recall management
2008	Utility of low profile catheter robotics system utilizing standard catheters and sheaths demonstrated in animal model
2008	Remote monitoring of implantable devices included in pacemakers and defibrillators
2009	Dronedarone recommended for approval by FDA advisory committee to treat non-permanent atrial fibrillation

demonstrated that prophylactic defibrillator placement in patients with coronary artery disease can help improve mortality prior to hemodynamically significant events. In addition, the Sudden Cardiac Death in Heart Failure Trial (SCD-HeFT) broadened the application of defibrillators to patients with mild to moderate congestive heart failure (New York Heart Association Class II or Class III), with ischemic and nonischemic cardiomyopathy, and a left ventricular ejection fraction less than 36 percent.

Finally, innovations in device technology led to the development of a biventricular implantable cardioverter-defibrillator that can resynchronize the heart in patients with drug-refractory congestive heart failure. Several clinical trials have demonstrated the benefit of these devices in drug-refractory congestive heart failure (New York Heart Association Class III and Class IV) with ejection fractions less than 36 percent and a wide QRS complex (greater than 120 milliseconds [msec]). The COMPANION trial demonstrated that biventricular implantable defibrillators can improve both mortality and rehospitalization rates in these patients. Future devices will possibly have four-chamber capability with multiple sensors to provide physiologic-based therapy.

Concurrent with advances in implantable devices came a better understanding of the mechanism of arrhythmias as well as the genetics of hereditary conditions. In the 1960s, Hodgkin and Huxley developed a model of cellular currents to describe the action potential. In the 1970s, Neher and Sakman developed a patch-clamping method for detecting single-channel currents and a clearer understanding of ionic currents became evident. In addition, specific genes were isolated which were responsible for hereditary conditions such as hypertrophic cardiomyopathy, long QT syndrome, arrhythmogenic right ventricular cardiomyopathy/dysplasia, and Brugada syndrome.

The development of catheter ablation has taken a parallel course to that of device development. Prior to 1982, ablation of the atrioventricular (AV) junction to achieve therapeutic AV block could be accomplished only by direct dissection of the AV junction during open-heart surgery, with surgical mortality rates as high as 10 percent. In 1982, Melvin Scheinman and colleagues described five patients with refractory supraventricular tachycardia (SVT) in which DC shocks were delivered to an electrode catheter positioned near the His bundle (AV junction), which produced complete heart block that successfully controlled the tachycardia. DC energy was then applied to the ablation of reentrant supraventricular tachycardia, such as AV-node reentrant tachycardia and Wolff-Parkinson-White syndrome.

The DC ablation registry for SVT identified a higher risk of sudden cardiac death in these patients, presumably due to the baro-trauma of the intracardiac DC energy delivery. In 1985, Stephen Huang employed a more controllable radiofrequency energy delivered to a large-tip electrode. The technique has evolved into a highly successful and effective method for treating the majority of supraventricular tachycardia types. With most tachycardias (except atrial fibrillation), a greater than 90 percent success (cure) rate can be achieved with minimal adverse effects.

In 1994, M. Haïssaguerre and colleagues described catheter ablation of atrial fibrillation. Their team subsequently identified potentials from the pulmonary veins that initiated atrial fibrillation. More recently, Carlo Pappone developed an anatomically-based method of isolating the pulmonary veins using three-dimensional mapping and a circular mapping catheter. Subsequent refinement of this technique has streamlined catheter ablation of atrial fibrillation.

In the late 1990s and early 2000s, applying three-dimensional mapping to catheter ablation has helped to define the anatomy of the endocardium and its structures and to record the electrical activity in a rapid and meaningful fashion to facilitate catheter ablation. Cooled-tip radiofrequency catheter ablation, large-tip high-energy radiofrequency catheter ablation, and cryotherapy were subsequently added to the armamentarium of electrophysiologists.

The application of robotics to catheter ablation procedures has helped minimize radiation exposure to the operator during more complex procedures. Magnetic catheter navigation and robotic manipulation using a steerable sheath have both yielded positive results, and electrophysiology acceptance of these procedures continues to grow. The challenges to overall acceptance include the complexity of the equipment that is currently available as well as their capital expense.

In the past few years, electrophysiology has seen the development of generally accepted guidelines for atrial fibrillation ablation and the expansion of implantable device guidelines (please see the specific chapters that discuss each of these areas). Remote monitoring of implantable devices has improved dramatically from simple transtelephonic monitoring of pacemakers to remote interrogations of both pacemakers and implantable defibrillators (including biventricular devices). This monitoring includes, in some instances, the fluid status of the patient as exhibited by weight gain of the patient, or a change in transthoracic impedance, which can be recorded in some implantable defibrillators.

In summary, device and catheter ablation developments have followed a similar path. Each modality has helped control and/or cure the vast majority of cardiac arrhythmias. Atrial fibrillation management remains a frontier for refinement in both arenas.

Chapter 2

Cardiac Anatomy and the Electrical Conduction System

Extending throughout the human body is a complex circulatory system comprised of veins and arteries, which circulates blood in order to replenish tissues and vital organs with oxygen and nutrients. The main component of this system is the heart (or myocardium), which functions as the circulatory engine pumping blood (composed of red blood cells containing hemoglobin to carry oxygen, white blood cells to fight infections and platelets to help with clotting) throughout the body. The heart has many components that must work effectively in order to optimize cardiovascular performance.

The sac surrounding the heart is called the pericardium. The parietal pericardium is the outermost layer. It is secured in the thoracic cavity between the lungs and fused to the diaphragm's central tendon. It is also attached to the back of the sternum, or breastbone, by the superior and inferior sternopericardiac ligaments. The visceral pericardium is the innermost layer of the pericardium. It is a layer of tissue that is closely adhered to the heart. The pericardial space is the middle layer between the parietal and visceral pericardia. It is composed of a fluid that serves as a lubricant so that the heart can move without friction. Figure 2.1 shows the layers of the heart.

The myocardium is the muscle layer of the heart. It is composed of cardiac muscle cells (myocytes), which are one-third smaller than

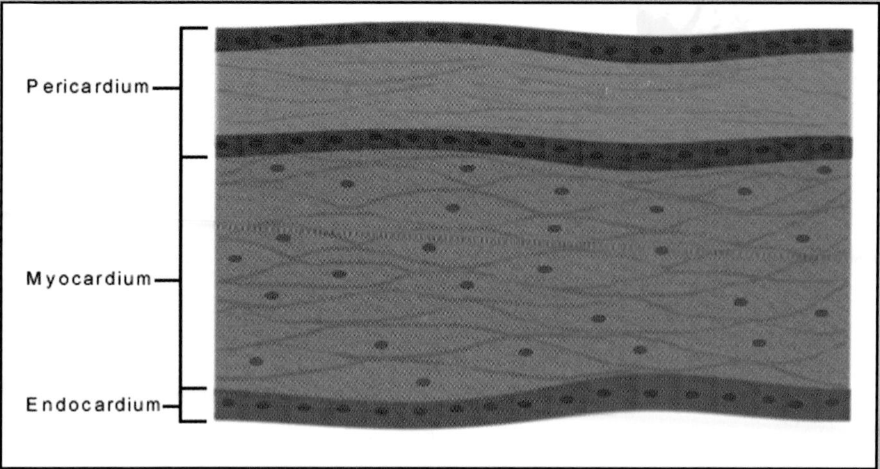

Figure 2.1: The three layers of the heart: the pericardium, the myocardium, and the endocardium. The pericardium's three layers can be seen as well. The myocardium is the cardiac muscle composed of slightly striated muscle cells. The endocardium is the inner layer made of tightly packed endothelial cells.

somatic muscle cells and are not as striated. Within the heart there are at least two types of myocardial muscle fibers: those of the atria (upper chambers) and those of the ventricles (lower chambers). The innermost layer of the heart is called the endocardium. The endocardium is a tissue layer made of closely packed endothelial cells that provide a smooth surface for blood flow.

The human myocardium is an efficient organ, configured to separate oxygenated and deoxygenated blood. The septum separates the left and right sides of the atrium and ventricle. Each side of the heart consists of an atrium and a ventricle. The atrium's principle function is blood transport (receiving blood flow and efficiently delivering it to the ventricle). Appropriate atrial contraction and timing is essential in order to maximize the blood flow from the heart (cardiac output). Externally, the separation of these chambers is evident by grooves on the surface of the heart. The groove separating the atria and the ventricles is called the coronary sulcus (also called the atrioventicular, or AV groove). The two atria are separated by the interatrial groove, and the two ventricles are separated by the anterior longitudinal sulcus and the posterior longitudinal sulcus. The anterior and posterior longitudinal sulci join together at the incisura apicis cordis, a notch near the apex of the heart. Figure 2.2 depicts the heart valves and their characteristics.

Inside the heart, valves are present which separate each chamber as well as their respective outflow artery. These valves must open and close properly in order to ensure complete blood transference. Each valve is composed of flaps (leaflets or cusps). The atrioventricular valves are attached to chordae tendineae, fibrous strands that attach to papillary muscles on the ventricular walls. When the

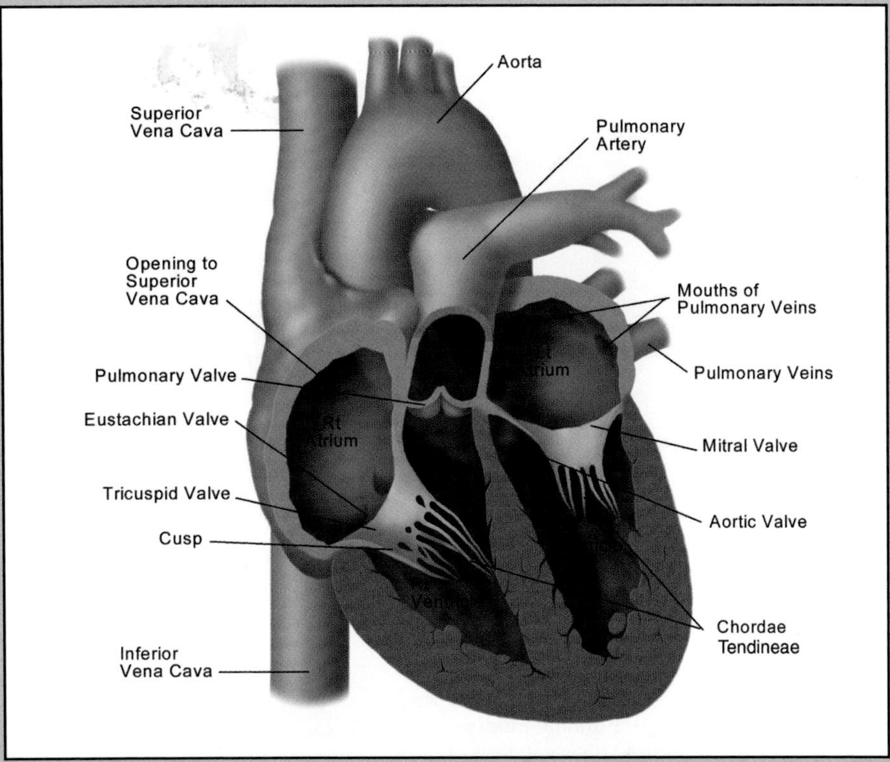

Figure 2.2: The heart and its major components. The atrioventricular valves, tricuspid and mitral, are shown with their respective leaflets and chordae tendineae, which attach to the papillary muscles. There are also the semilunar valves, pulmonary and aortic, separating the ventricles and their connecting arteries. In each atrium one can see the mouths of the veins that deliver blood into the chambers and their respective valves or lack thereof.

ventricle contracts, so do the papillary muscles, which apply pressure to the fibrous strands and keep the valves closed.

The right-sided atrioventricular valve, the tricuspid valve, is composed of three leaflets: anterior, medial, and posterior. The atrioventricular valve on the left side, known as the mitral valve, is composed of an anterior and posterior leaflet. The valves separating the ventricles and the great arteries are semilunar valves. The semilunar valve separating the right ventricle and the pulmonary artery is the pulmonic valve. The valve separating the left ventricle and the aorta is the aortic valve.

The superior and inferior vena cavae and coronary sinus deliver blood into the right atrium. Unlike the superior vena cava, which has no valve, the inferior vena cava has an eustachian valve, which is a semilunar extension of the atrial lining membrane. The coronary sinus vein may have a thebesian valve, a semicircular fold of the atrial lining membrane that might prohibit easy

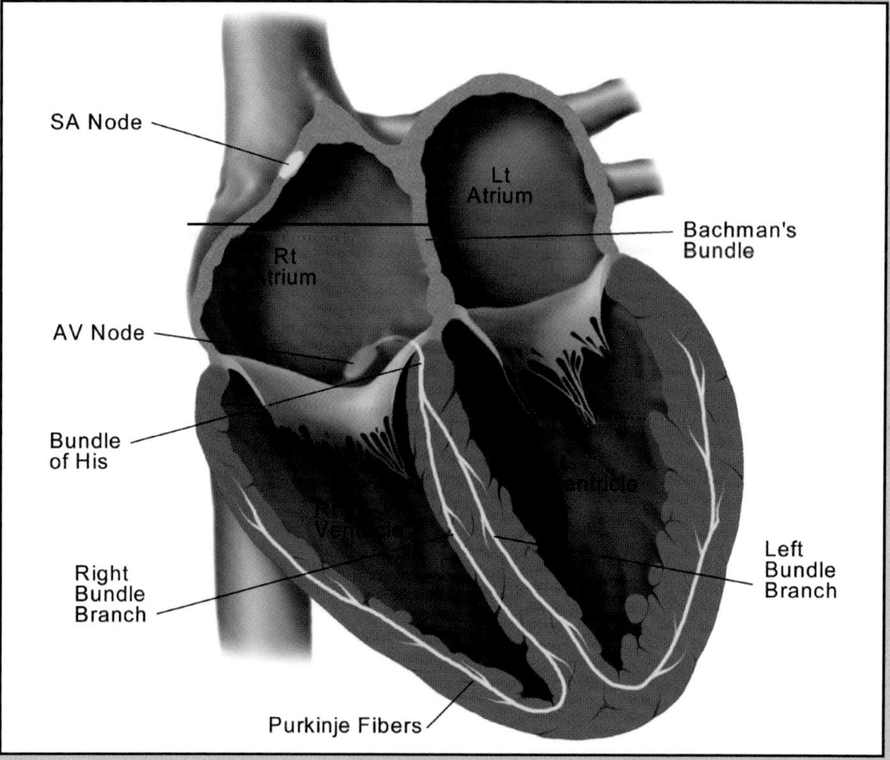

Figure 2.3: The main parts in the electrical conduction system of the heart and the flow of the electrical current. The SA node, the AV node, and the His bundle can be seen in the upper part of the heart, and the bundle branches and the Purkinje fibers in the lower part of the heart.

catheter access into the coronary sinus. The pulmonary veins in the left atrium do not have valves.

Deoxygenated blood from the upper body enters the right atria through the superior vena cava. Deoxygenated blood from the lower body spills into the right atria via the inferior vena cava. Once blood passes through the right atrium and ventricle, it is pumped through the pulmonary artery into the lungs. In the lungs, blood is oxygenated and carbon dioxide is removed; then the blood returns via the pulmonary veins to the left atrium. After passing through the left ventricle, it is pumped throughout the body via the aorta.

The heart has its own coronary arterial and venous system. These systems parallel one another. The coronary arteries originate from the aorta. The right coronary artery arises from the right coronary sinus and branches into the posterior lateral branch and/or posterior descending artery (when dominant) in approximately 75 percent of patients. This vessel typically supplies blood to the sinoatrial (SA) and atrioventricular (AV) nodes. The left coronary artery arises from the left aortic coronary cusp, initially as

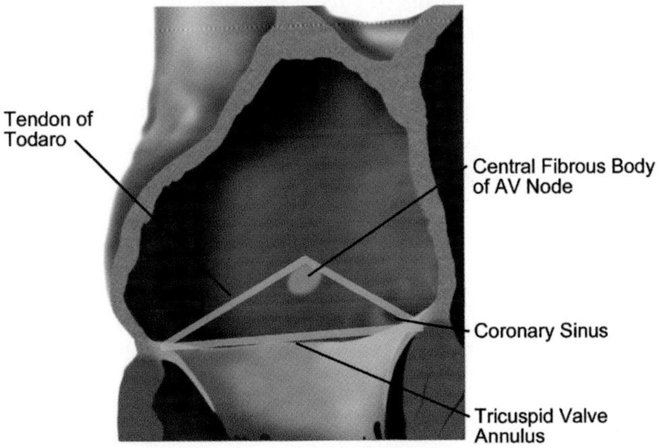

Figure 2.4: Shows a schematic of the triangle of Koch.

the left main coronary artery, which divides into the left anterior descending coronary artery and left circumflex branch. The coronary sinus vein drains deoxygenated blood from the myocardium into the right atrium; it is an epicardial structure with branches which extend to the left atrium and ventricle (potential targets for multisite pacing and cardiac resynchronization; see Chapter 27). (Traditional pacing consists of right atrial and ventricular pacing.) Figure 2.3 shows the pathway of the electrical conduction and its various components.

The electrical conduction system of the heart is responsible for the proper synchronized contractions of the atria and ventricles. Conduction starts at the SA node, the pacemaker of the heart. The spindle-shape SA node is composed of nodal and transitional cells. It lies at the junction of the superior vena cava and the right atrium, one millimeter below the surface of the heart. Interatrial conduction (right to left atrium) is facilitated via Bachman's bundle located in the interatrial septum. Electrical conduction will not pass the coronary sulcus, because normally no specialized conduction system is present. Normally all atrial conduction is filtered through the AV node.

The AV node lies beneath the atrial endocardium, superior and anterior to the coronary sinus ostium. This structure provides a delay in conduction between the atria and the ventricles in order to ensure complete ventricular filling. The AV node's distal end is connected to the His bundle. From the His bundle, two pathways emerge: the left and right bundle branches. These branches travel down the septum into the left and right ventricles, respectively, and ramify into Purkinje fibers that reach the ventricular endocardium. The Purkinje fibers are responsible for delivering electrical current in order to initiate ventricular contraction.

An important anatomical landmark for mapping and catheter ablation is the triangle of Koch, which lies in the lower part of the right atrium. The sides of this triangle are important for identifying the septal component of the AV node. Anatomic landmarks of the triangle consist of 1) the tendon of Todaro, 2) the coronary sinus ostium, and 3) the tricuspid valve septal leaflet. Figure 2.4 shows a schematic of the triangle of Koch. Note the apex of the triangle is where the central fibrous body of the AV node is located (near the AV junction or fast pathway of the AV node). The coronary sinus ostium is near posteroseptal accessory pathways, or below where the slow pathway of the AV node is located.

Chapter 3

The Cardiac Action Potential

The cardiac action potential is the recording of the changes of electrical potential over time recorded from inside a cardiac myocyte (heart muscle cell). The action potential is due to the flow of electrolytes through the plasma membrane changing the voltage across the cell. The inside of the myocyte changes its electrical potential with the inflow and outflow of electrolytes through ion channels. These ion channels serve as gates that open and close, thereby controlling the ionic flow. The gates respond to changes in the membrane potential (differences in voltage).

The potassium, sodium and calcium channels are ion channels that allow for inscription of the action potential. The potassium channels have a single voltage-sensitive gate that is closed in the resting state and opens slowly in response to depolarization. The sodium channels have two voltage-sensitive gates: a gate that is closed in the resting state and opens quickly in response to depolarization, and a gate that is open in the resting state, called the "inactivation gate", which closes slowly in response to depolarization. As the cell is depolarized, threshold for opening the L-type calcium (Ca++) channel is achieved, which is responsible for the plateau of the action potential. When a certain threshold potential is reached, the potassium ions (K+) dribble out of the cell, while the sodium ions (Na+) pour into the cell, which causes the rapid influx of Na+ relative to the efflux of K+. The result, an increase in voltage by about 15 millivolts (mV) to 20 mV, is called the overshoot of the action potential. Figure 3.1 shows a simplistic schematic of a myocyte and its ionic channels (only Na+ and K+ illustrated).

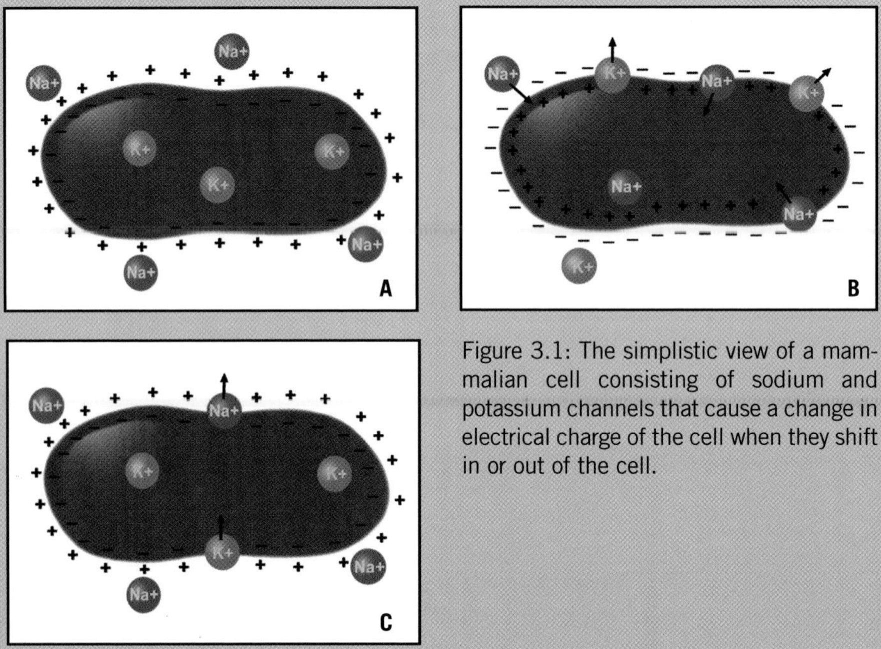

Figure 3.1: The simplistic view of a mammalian cell consisting of sodium and potassium channels that cause a change in electrical charge of the cell when they shift in or out of the cell.

Cardiac cells are excitable cells. When excitable cells are stimulated fittingly, the gates of the ion channels open and close in a sequential, stereotyped manner. One can view the action potential as consisting of three components: depolarization, repolarization, and resting. However, it is classically divided into phases 0, 1, 2, 3, and 4 (figure 3.2).

Potassium (K+) conductance is high at rest and is the chief determinant of resting potential (*i.e.*, electrostatic forces counterbalance the K+ gradient). In some instances and in certain tissue, such as SA and AV nodal tissue, the resting phase continues to rise until a certain threshold triggers the action potential. This characteristic is called spontaneous phase 4 depolarization.

When a stimulus excites the cell, some of the sodium channels open, allowing some Na+ ions to rush into the cell, causing a decrease in the membrane potential. When the threshold potential is reached, the additional Na+ gates open, initiating a rapid depolarization phase of the action potential. This rapid action potential upstroke is due to the opening of voltage-sensitive Na+ channels carrying an inward Na+ current (I_{Na}). In the SA and AV nodes, a similar phenomenon is due to analogous Ca++ currents (I_{Ca}). The Na+ pours into the cell, so that the interior of the cell becomes more positive than it was in the resting phase, causing a rapid decrease in membrane potential (phase 0) with an overshoot to +25 mV.

Phase 1 is early rapid repolarization, and is partly due to inactivation of I_{Na} and activation of a transient outward current (I_{to}). The peak action potential generally reaches a positive magnitude of less than +30mV. The depolarization of one cardiac cell tends to cause all adjacent cells to

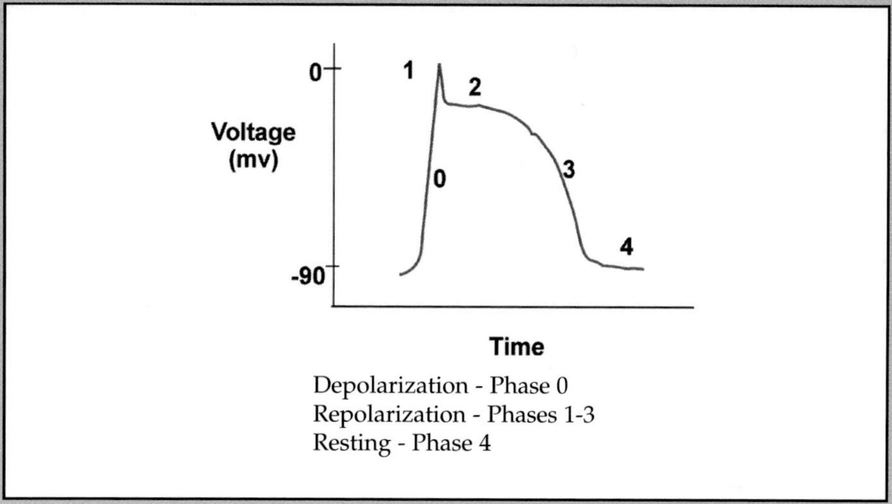

Figure 3.2: The typical electrical activity of the cell. The graph is divided into phases, each representing an electrical state of the cell. The phases have been separated into three general sections (depolarization, repolarization, and resting) that encompass the electrical activity of the cell at the time.

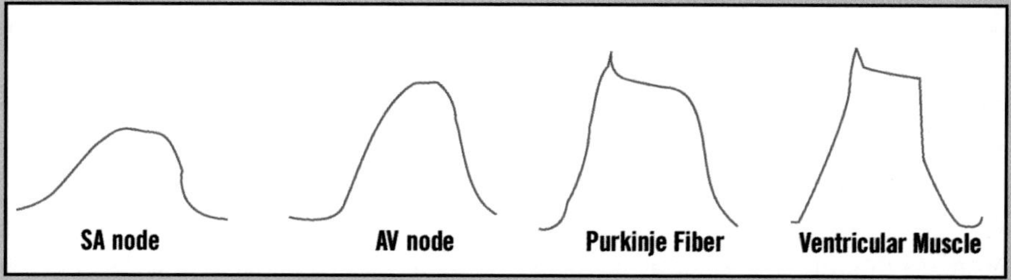

Figure 3.3: The cardiac action potentials of different cells of the heart's electrical system including the SA node, the AV node, Purkinje fibers, and ventricular muscle.

depolarize, creating a wave of depolarization (electric current) across the heart. Sequentially, inactivation gates close the Na+ channels, and K+ channels open slowly, allowing potassium ions to exit the cell slowly (phase 2). During this phase there is a decrease in conductance to most ions. Slow I_{Ca} channels stay open and provide some inward current counteracting repolarization. The plateau viewed during phase 2 seems to suspend and extend the repolarization phase. It is unique to cardiac cells.

In phase 3 there is a final rapid repolarization. This is the result of activation of outward K+ currents and the inactivation of slow inward Ca++ and Na+ currents. The period of time from the end of phase 1 to the end of phase 3 is known as repolarization. At the end of repolarization, both gates of the sodium channels are closed, but the potassium gates remain open because of their

Table 3.1: Properties of Transmembrane Potentials in Mammalian Hearts

	Sinus Nodal Cell	AV Nodal Cell	Purkinje Fiber	Ventricular Muscle Cell
Resting Potential (mV)	-50 to -60	-60 to -70	-90 to -95	-80 to -90
Action Potential Amplitude (mV)	60 to 70	70 to 80	120	110 to 120
Overshoot (mV)	0 to 10	5 to 15	30	30
Duration (msec)	100 to 300	100 to 300	300 to 500	200 to 300

propensity to close slowly and return to the phase 4 resting potential.

The phase 4 activity that again leads to a spontaneous depolarization is called automaticity. In some cardiac cells, a leakage of ions across the membrane causes a gradual decrease in membrane potential, leading to threshold potential and a depolarizing current.

The contour of the action potential varies with the different cells in the specialized conduction system (figure 3.3). The shape of the action potential is a determinant of the conduction velocity, the refractory period, and the automaticity of cardiac tissue, and thus directly affects cardiac rhythms. The action potentials that differ the most from atrial, ventricular, or Purkinje fibers are those of the SA node and the AV node.

The slow depolarization in the SA and AV nodes occurs because these tissues lack the sodium channels that contribute extensively to the rapid depolarization phase seen in other cardiac tissues. Instead, SA and AV nodal tissues are thought to rely extensively on the slow calcium channels for depolarization (table 3.1).

Chapter 4

Electrocardiograms

The electrocardiogram, or ECG, is a graphic representation of the electrical activity from the heart. The standard 12-lead ECG (figure 4.1) is a recording of electrodes placed on all four limbs and across the precordium (or chest) of the patient.

There are certain medical indications for recording an ECG. Guidelines have been published by the American College of Cardiology and the American Heart Association Task Force on clinical privileges in cardiology. An electrocardiogram is appropriate in the following instances:

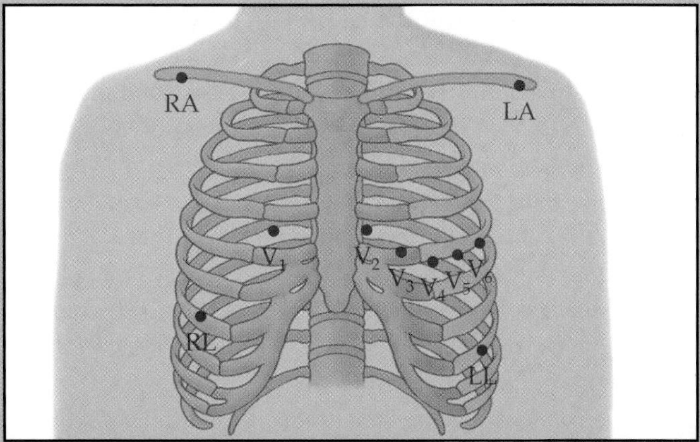

Figure 4.1: The standard locations of a 12-lead electrocardiogram. This is a vector representation of the electrical potential generated from the myocardium as recorded across the body surface. LA stands for left arm; LL, left leg; RA, right arm; RL, right leg; V1-V6, precordial leads.

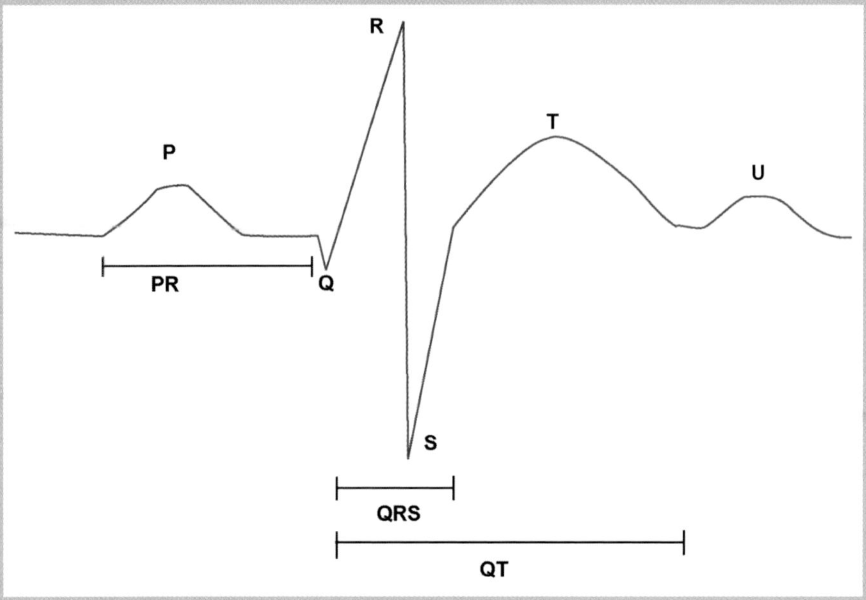

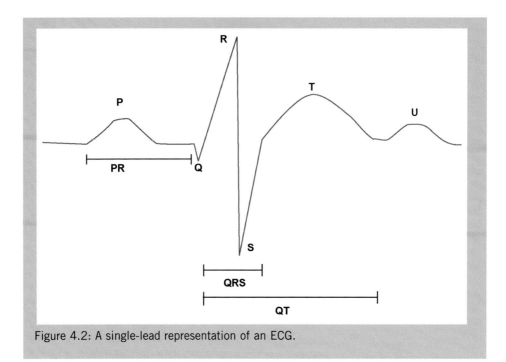

Figure 4.2: A single-lead representation of an ECG.

1) in patients suspected of having heart disease.
2) to assess the results of therapy on a patient.
3) in patients (usually over the age of 40) who are at risk for myocardial infarction and/or heart failure due to hypercholesterolemia, diabetes, obesity, smoking, hypertension, or family history.
4) for people in stressful and high-risk occupations, such as pilots, who are required to have an ECG to ensure that health problems do not affect their job performance.
5) to assess the optimal preoperative status of a patient, and to assess whether there are any postoperative complications.
6) to assess the cardiac effects of systemic diseases or conditions such as renal failure, diabetic acidosis, hypokalemia, and electrolyte abnormalities, and to assess the potential cardiotoxic effects of drugs.

Figure 4.2 shows a single-lead representation of an ECG. The P wave reflects atrial depolarization. Sinus node activity is silent.

The QRS complex represents the depolarization of the ventricles. The Q wave is the first negative deflection, the R wave is the first positive deflection, and the S wave is the second negative deflection. In patients who have a bundle-branch block pattern, which is a widened QRS complex, an R prime (R′) complex following the S wave signifies block in the right bundle branch.

The final wave is usually the T wave, which represents ventricular repolarization. In general, the QT interval is representative of ventricular repolarization. It is prolonged in certain conditions such as hereditary long QT syndrome, in which the patient is at risk for polymorphic ventricular tachycardia

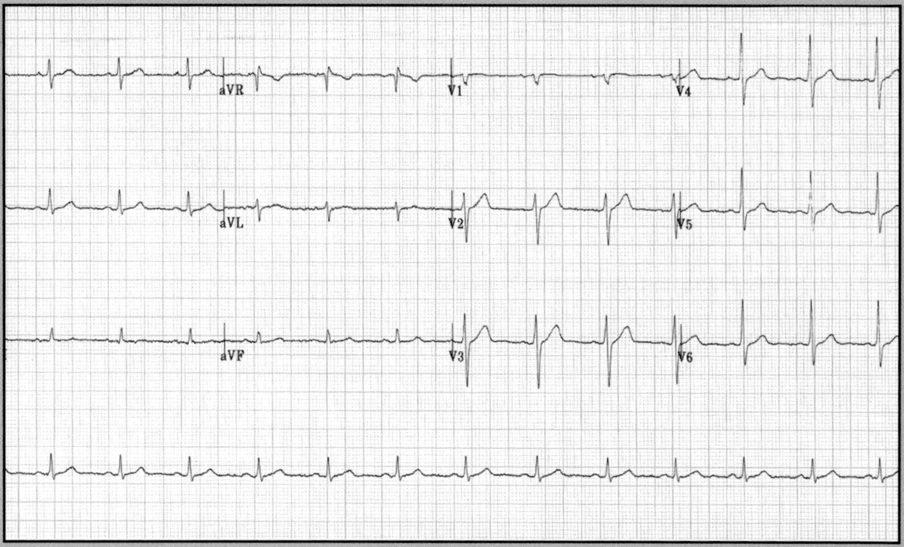

Figure 4.3: A standard 12-lead electrocardiogram.

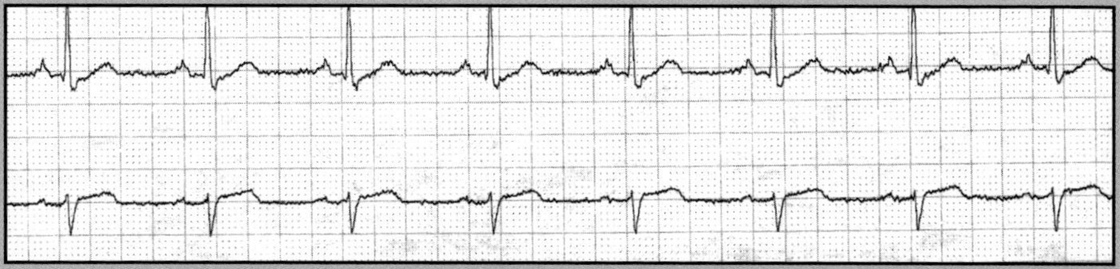

Figure 4.4: A tracing of normal sinus rhythm.

and ventricular fibrillation (torsades de pointes). Some drugs (class IA antiarrhythmic drugs such as procainamide and quinidine, along with certain antihistamines and antibiotics) may prolong the QT interval as well. The QT interval varies with the heart rate. It can be corrected (QTc) by the Bazett's formula, which is QT divided by the square root of the R-to-R interval.

The PR interval is indicative of AV conduction. Delay in AV conduction may occur at or below the AV node. If the PR interval is delayed—greater than 200 msec in duration—the patient usually has AV nodal disease, but may have additional infranodal delay. In addition, QRS duration greater than 120 msec usually represents an intraventricular conduction delay suggestive of a bundle-branch block pattern. These delays may be due to other abnormalities such as left ventricular hypertrophy as a result of long-standing hypertension or electrolyte abnormalities such as hypokalemia. Furthermore, a QT interval greater than 450 msec may represent a congenital, electrolyte-, or drug-related repolarization abnormality. See table 4.1 for more information about the normal baseline interval measurements.

Table 4.1: Normal Baseline Interval Measurements

Interval	Measurement	Normal Range (msec)
Surface ECG		
PR Interval	Onset of P wave to onset of QRS complex	120 to 200
QRS Duration	Onset of QRS complex to end of QRS complex	80 to 110
QT Interval	Onset of QRS complex to end of T wave	250 to 400
Corrected QT	Divide QT interval by the square root of R-to-R interval	< 450 males < 470 females

In addition to the waves described above, a U wave (an upward bump after the T wave) may be present. The normal U wave is usually recorded in V2-V4 and is less than 25 percent of the amplitude of the preceding T wave. It may become prominent in hypokalemia, severe ischemia, or digitalis toxicity.

Figure 4.3 is a standard 12-lead electrocardiogram. Leads I, II, and III are standard limb lead electrodes. There are indirect limb leads called aVR, aVL, and aVF. The precordial leads (V1–V6) are very useful at showing electrical activity that may occur across the ventricles, which are projected on the chest wall as unipolar signals. Occasionally a mirror image of these electrodes across the chest may be placed on the right side in order to better record right-sided activity (such as a right ventricular myocardial infarction).

Figure 4.4 shows a tracing of normal sinus rhythm. This is typically at a heart rate of 60 to 100 beats per minute. The heart rate in figure 4.4 is between 60 and 75 beats per minute. This is calculated by counting the number of big boxes, each of which represents 200 msec, with smaller boxes representing 40 msec in duration (ECG paper speed of 25 mm/sec). Figure 4.5 shows standard ECG paper and an illustrated tracing demonstrating a simple method to determine heart rate. One can count the number of boxes between QRS complexes to determine the heart rate. If the time between QRS complexes were one big box, the heart rate would be 300 beats per minute. If the beats span two big boxes, the heart rate would equal 150 beats per minute; three big boxes, 100 beats per minute; four big boxes, 75 beats per minute; five big boxes, 60 beats per minute; and six big boxes, 50 beats per minute.

Keeping this in mind, one can quickly distinguish a tachycardia from a bradycardia. In general, tachycardias are identified with heart rates above 100 beats per minute. Bradycardias are defined with heart rates below 60 beats per minute. In figure 4.6, we can see a sinus bradycardia present. The heart rate in this tracing is 50 beats per minute. As one can see in the

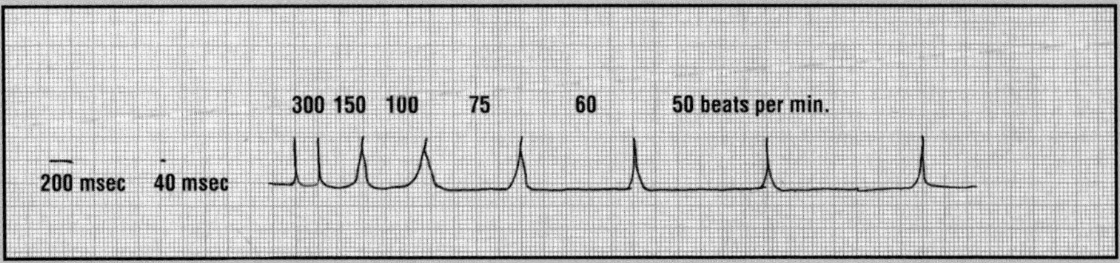

Figure 4.5: An easy method to determine heart rate is by counting the big boxes between QRS complexes. If one box separates 2 complexes, the rate is 300 beats per minute; 2 boxes, 150 beats per minute; 3 boxes, 100 beats per minute; 4 boxes, 75 beats per minute; 5 boxes, 60 beats per minute; and 6 boxes, 50 beats per minute. Alternatively, 60,000 can be divided by the time between complexes (in msec) in order to give the heart rate in beats per minute.

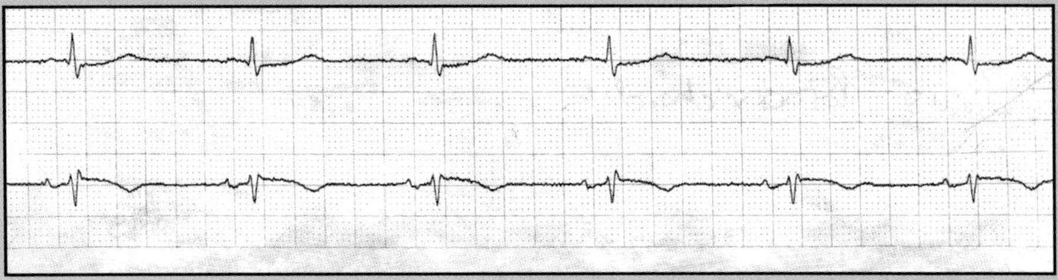

Figure 4.6: Sinus bradycardia.

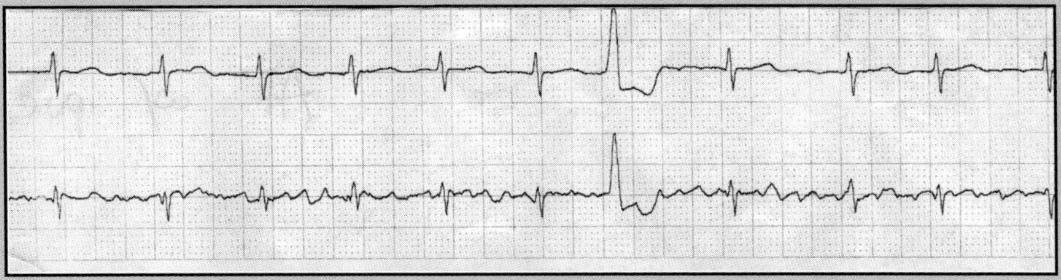

Figure 4.7: A case of atrial fibrillation. There are no discrete P waves, but chaotic atrial activity is seen between the QRS complexes.

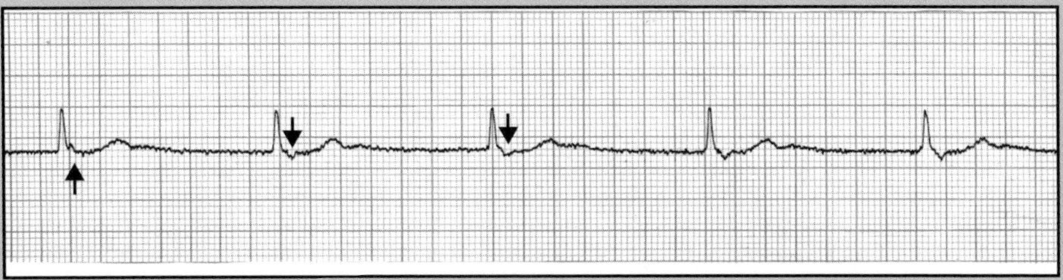

Figure 4.8: An ECG tracing with no P waves preceding the QRS complexes. P waves are present following the QRS complex (see arrow). The QRS complexes are narrowed, suggestive of a junctional bradycardia. The first QRS is followed by an upright P wave (probably sinus in origin).

strips of sinus rhythm, there is a P wave in front of every QRS.

In the case of atrial fibrillation (figure 4.7), there are no discrete P waves, but a chaotic atrial activity is recorded. In addition, during the tracing, there is a wide complex beat, which is either a ventricular premature contraction or an aberrantly conducted beat from the atrium. This occurs when a premature beat is conducted down one of the bundles and finds the other bundle refractory (unwilling to accept conduction).

Figure 4.8 shows an ECG tracing with no P waves preceding the QRS complexes. P waves are present (and inverted) following the QRS complex after the last 4 complexes. The QRS complexes are narrowed, suggestive of a junctional bradycardia.

There are many detailed textbooks that are much more comprehensive in describing the variety of cardiac arrhythmias. These textbooks are useful in diagnosis and interpretation of a 12-lead electrocardiogram. For the electrophysiology laboratory practitioner, courses are available through the American College of Cardiology and the Heart Rhythm Society. In addition, many hospitals offer courses and training sessions for critical care nurses.

Chapter 5

Basic and Advanced Cardiac Life Support

Guest Writer: Doug Beinborn, MA, RN

Basic life support (BLS) and advance cardiac life support (ACLS) should be part of the required training for personnel working in the electrophysiology laboratory. The goal of resuscitation is to support and restore effective oxygenation, ventilation, and circulation while maintaining intact neurologic function. Recertification is required every two years to maintain these skills and to obtain the clinical updates that have been incorporated into these programs. Everyone in the United States should be trained in the skills of BLS. Sudden cardiac arrest (SCA) is the leading cause of death in the United States, Canada, and Europe. It is estimated that 3,000,000 lives are claimed worldwide each year. There are approximately 450,000 SCA events per year in the United States. This equates to 1,200 events per day, 50 each hour, and one every 80 seconds. The number of deaths associated with SCA is greater than the mortality rates of stroke, lung cancer, breast cancer, and AIDS combined. SCA is 95 percent fatal in the United States, and 80 percent of these events occur at home.

BLS Training

The training associated with BLS covers many different emergency care aspects. BLS educates individuals to learn the skills for delivering cardiopulmonary resuscitation (CPR) to all ages. CPR consists of four main components, which are known as the ABCD's: airway, breathing, circulation, and defibrillation.

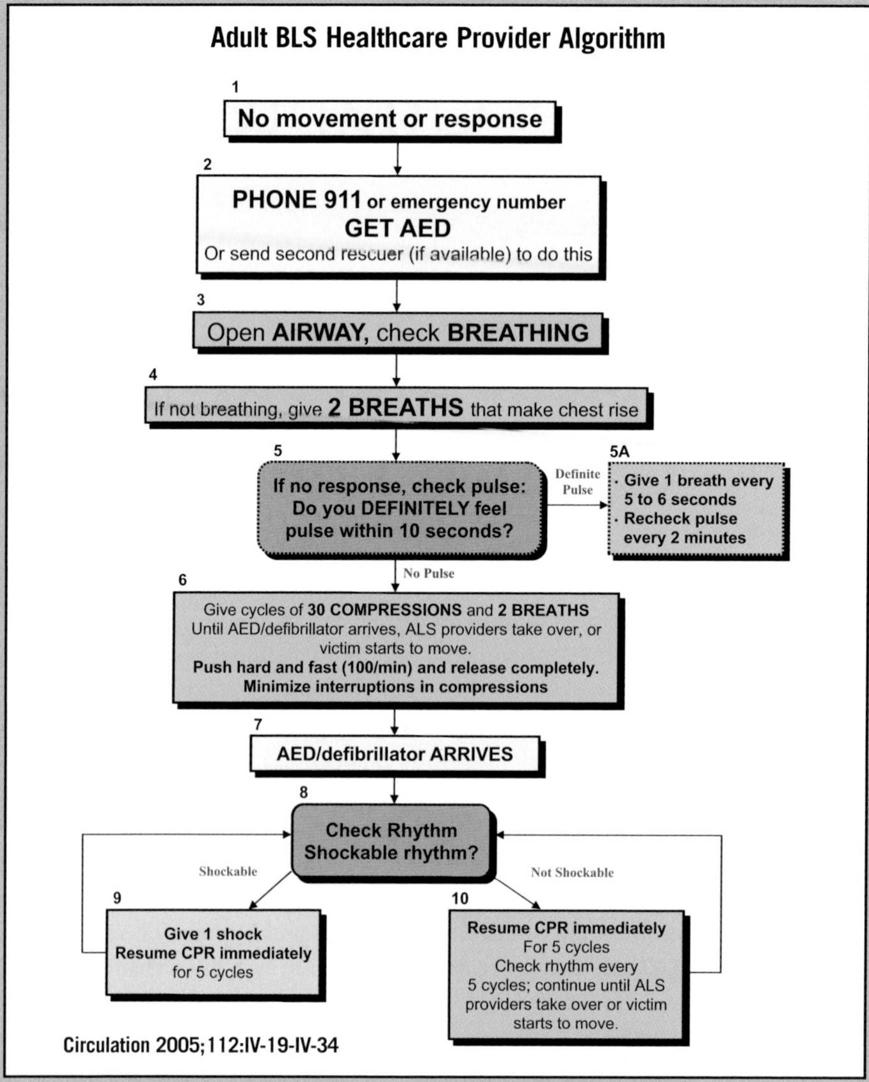

Figure 5.1: Adult BLS Healthcare Provider Algorithm (reprinted with permission from: ECC Committee, Subcommittees and Task Forces of the American Heart Association. 2005 American Heart Association Guidelines for Cardiopulmonary Resuscitation and Emergency Cardiovascular Care. *Circulation* 2005 Dec 13;112[Suppl I]:IV-19-IV-34).

During BLS training, participants learn how to operate automatic external defibrillators (AEDs). Airway management, including how to relieve choking victims, is also covered.

Quality CPR improves a victim's chances of survival. The four critical concepts for providing quality CPR include:

1. Push hard and push fast, with compressions at a rate of 100 per minute.

Table 5.1: The H's and T's of Cardiac Arrest

H's:	T's:
Hypovolemia	Toxins
Hypoxia	Tamponade (cardiac)
Hydrogen ion (acidosis)	Tension pneumothorax
Hyper-/hypokalemia	Thrombosis (coronary and pulmonary)
Hypoglycemia	Trauma
Hypothermia	

2. Allow for full chest recoil after each compression.
3. Minimize interruptions in chest compressions (interruptions should be no longer than 10 seconds).
4. Avoid hyperventilation.

The adult BLS algorithm is shown in figure 5.1. If no movement or response is elicited from the victim, the responder(s) need to activate 911, the emergency number in your institution, and to alert colleagues who are in close proximity. It is imperative to obtain an AED or defibrillator as a first step in the treatment of the unresponsive victim.

ACLS Overview

The ACLS course is designed for healthcare providers who either direct or participate in the resuscitation of a patient in the hospital or community setting. The course requires active participation of the students in order to enhance one's skills with arrest and peri-arrest patients through simulated cases. The course objectives of ACLS include:

1. Recognize and initiate early management of peri-arrest conditions that may result in cardiac arrest or complicate resuscitation outcomes.
2. Demonstrate proficiency in providing BLS care, including prioritizing chest compressions and integrating AED use.
3. Manage cardiac arrest until return of spontaneous circulation, termination of resuscitation, or transfer of care.
4. Identify and treat ischemic chest pain and expedite the care of patients with acute coronary syndromes.
5. Recognize other life-threatening clinical situations, such as stroke, and provide effective initial care and transfer to reduce disability and death.
6. Demonstrate effective communication as a member or leader of a resuscitation team, and recognize the impact of team dynamics on overall team performance.

Causes of Cardiac Arrest

During CPR, contributing factors for the arrest need to be reviewed in order to aid in the treatment of the patient. Contributing factors include the H's and T's (table 5.1). Remembering and reviewing these potential causes may reverse arrest due to appropriate treatment and intervention.

H's:

- *Hypovolemia:* This is associated with narrow complex tachycardia. The patient's history may indicate hypovolemia with the physical examination revealing flat neck veins. The recommended treatment is volume infusion, which may include crystalloid solution or packed red blood cells if associated with anemia.

- *Hypoxia:* Signs of hypoxia include hypoventilation, apnea, and bradycardia. It is physically associated with cyanosis with impaired arterial blood gases (ABGs) and the inability to maintain a proper airway. The treatment includes oxygenation, ventilation, and intubation.
- *Hydrogen ion acidosis:* With hydrogen ion acidosis, the ECG reveals smaller amplitude QRS complexes. The patient's history may include a history of diabetes and/or renal failure. The treatment may include sodium bicarbonate and hyperventilation.
- *Hyperkalemia:* With hyperkalemia, the ECG characteristics show evidence of widened QRS complex associated with peaked and high T waves and smaller P waves. The patient's history may include renal failure, diabetes, and recent dialysis. The treatment of hyperkalemia may include infusion of sodium bicarbonate, glucose with insulin, calcium chloride, and Kayexalate/sorbitol.
- *Hypokalemia:* This is associated with wide complex QRS. Other ECG characteristics may include flattened T waves, prominent U waves, prolonged QT interval, and wide complex tachycardia. Historical evidence may include abnormal loss of potassium and/or diuretic use. Treatment options include rapid but controlled infusion of potassium and adding magnesium during cardiac arrest.
- *Hypothermia:* This would rarely be encountered with patients in the electrophysiology lab. The patient's history would include exposure to cold with associated decrease in central body temperature.

T's:

- *Toxins (tablets or drug overdose):* There are highly variable effects on the ECG due to the wide variety of possible medications, but the predominant effect would be the prolongation of the QT interval. A history and physical exam may include bradycardia and changes in the neurologic exam. When dealing with patients outside of the EP lab, include drug screens, lavage, activated charcoal, lactose per protocol, and specific antidotes depending on the cause. Lab treatment may include naloxone or other reversing agent.
- *Tamponade:* This is often associated with narrow complex QRS and rapid rates. No pulse may be felt with CPR and visible vein distension revealed on examination. The causes in the EP lab include device lead placement, cardiac catheter placement, transseptal sheath placement, or complications associated with ablation. The treatment is both pericardiocentesis and pericardial window.
- *Tension Pneumothorax:* In tension pneumothorax, the ECG can show narrow complex QRS with associated hypoxia. No pulse is felt during CPR. Physical exam reveals neck vein distension, tracheal deviation, unequal breath sounds, and is associated with difficulty to ventilate. The diagnosis can be confirmed by viewing the chest with use of fluoroscopy. Treatment options include needle decompression or placement of a chest tube. During procedures, it may be associated with placement of an internal

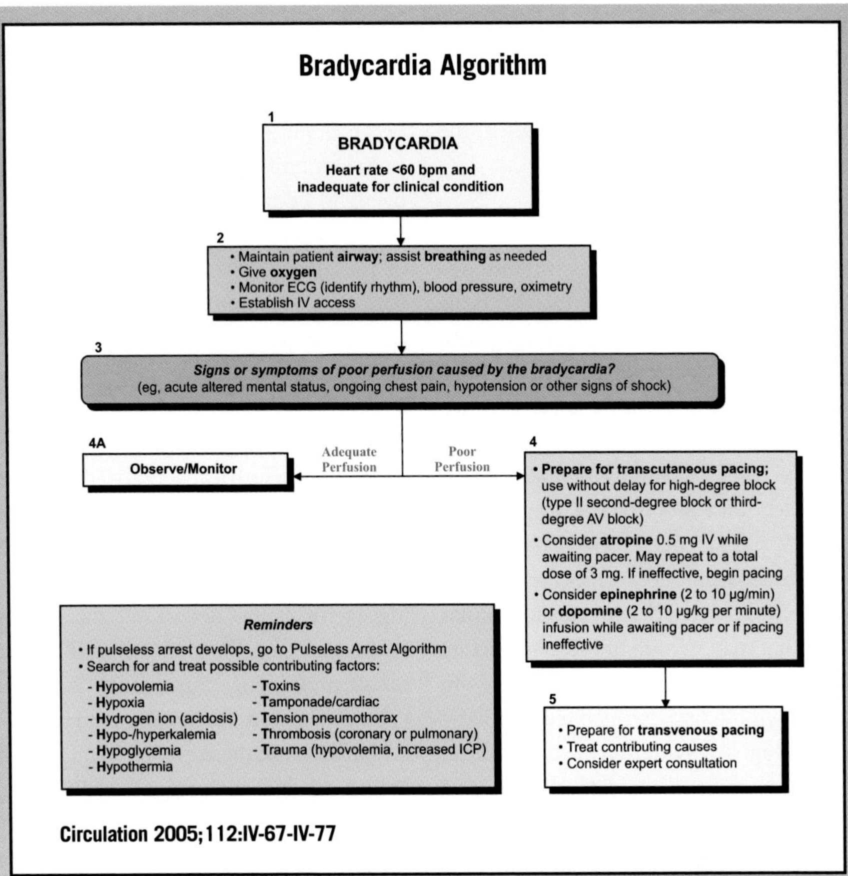

Bradycardia Algorithm
1
BRADYCARDIA
Heart rate <60 bpm and inadequate for clinical condition
2
• Maintain patient airway; assist breathing as needed
• Give oxygen
• Monitor ECG (identify rhythm), blood pressure, oximetry
• Establish IV access
3
Signs or symptoms of poor perfusion caused by the bradycardia?
(eg, acute altered mental status, ongoing chest pain, hypotension or other signs of shock)
4A
Observe/Monitor
Adequate Perfusion
Poor Perfusion
4
• Prepare for transcutaneous pacing; use without delay for high-degree block (type II second-degree block or third-degree AV block)
• Consider atropine 0.5 mg IV while awaiting pacer. May repeat to a total dose of 3 mg. If ineffective, begin pacing
• Consider epinephrine (2 to 10 μg/min) or dopomine (2 to 10 μg/kg per minute) infusion while awaiting pacer or if pacing ineffective
Reminders
• If pulseless arrest develops, go to Pulseless Arrest Algorithm
• Search for and treat possible contributing factors:
- Hypovolemia
- Hypoxia
- Hydrogen ion (acidosis)
- Hypo-/hyperkalemia
- Hypoglycemia
- Hypothermia
- Toxins
- Tamponade/cardiac
- Tension pneumothorax
- Thrombosis (coronary or pulmonary)
- Trauma (hypovolemia, increased ICP)
5
• Prepare for transvenous pacing
• Treat contributing causes
• Consider expert consultation
Circulation 2005;112:IV-67-IV-77

Figure 5.2: Bradycardia Algorithm (reprinted with permission from: ECC Committee, Subcommittees and Task Forces of the American Heart Association. 2005 American Heart Association Guidelines for Cardiopulmonary Resuscitation and Emergency Cardiovascular Care. *Circulation* 2005 Dec 13;112[Suppl I]:IV-67-IV-77).

jugular line or with subclavian access during lead placement.

- *Thrombosis of the Heart (acute myocardial infarction or heart attack)*: Clues from the ECG include multiple abnormalities with the 12-lead electrocardiogram: Q waves, ST segment changes, and T wave changes with inversions. Our recommendations include dealing with acute clinical changes and consulting the cardiac cath lab team to perform emergent cardiac catheterization with potential intervention.
- *Thrombosis of the Lungs (pulmonary embolism)*: ECG will show rapid rates with narrow QRS complexes. No palpable pulse is a usual finding during CPR. Physical examination reveals visible neck vein distension on examination. Intervention may include embolectomy or fibrinolytics.
- *Trauma*: Due to trauma, the ECG clues are highly variable. With increased intracranial pressure, bradycardia will be present. Hypovolemia associated

with trauma may lead to tachycardia. Recommendations with trauma include reviewing all H's and T's with treatment directed at reversing the underlying etiology.

Treatment of Bradycardia

Bradycardia is defined as any rhythm disorder with a heart rate of less than 60 beats per minute. This can be a normal finding with well-conditioned athletes at rest. The rhythms associated with bradycardia include sinus bradycardia, first-degree AV block, second-degree AV block (Mobitz type I, also called Wenckebach, and Mobitz type II), or third-degree AV block. Third-degree and Mobitz type II second-degree heart block are the most likely blocks associated with cardiovascular collapse that may require immediate pacing. Staff needs to assess the patient if there are signs and symptoms associated with the slow heart rate. Signs of symptomatic bradycardia may include chest discomfort, shortness of breath, decreased level of consciousness, weakness, fatigue, lightheadedness, dizziness, and presyncope or syncope. Treatment options for symptomatic bradycardia include medication or interventional treatment. Medications include atropine 0.5 mg IV, and 0.5 mg may be repeated to a total dose of 3.0 mg. Epinephrine or dopamine drips may be used while preparing for transvenous pacing. See figure 5.2 for more information.

Treatment of Tachycardia

The treatment of symptomatic tachycardia is a complex algorithm (figure 5.3). The ABC's of ACLS apply to the treatment strategy: provide oxygen, monitor ECG, and identify and treat reversible causes (H's and T's). The staff needs to establish if the patient is stable or unstable. If the patient is unstable, synchronized cardioversion needs to be performed if it is determined that the tachycardia is not sinus tachycardia. If the patient becomes pulseless, the staff needs to use the pulseless arrest algorithm. The tachycardia needs to be interpreted to determine if the rhythm is narrow or wide as well as regular or irregular. Medication treatment is highly variable based on if the QRS complex is narrow or wide, regular or irregular, and if tachycardia is ventricular or supraventricular.

Treatment of Pulseless Electrical Activity

Pulseless electrical activity (PEA) is associated with adverse outcomes. Rapid assessment with an aggressive treatment strategy with hopes of reversing a H or T contributing factor helps determine the outcome. When assessing the situation and searching for an underlying cause, many issues need to be considered. Reviewing the H's and T's is helpful, since these are the frequent causes of PEA. Careful analysis of the ECG can give clues to the underlying etiology. Quickly assess and treat hypovolemia, since this is easily treated. Look for potential adverse effects related to the procedure being performed (pneumothorax, tamponade, hypoxia, etc.). Positive outcomes are related to early detection and aggressive treatment of the underlying cause.

Effective Team Dynamics During Resuscitation

There are many tasks performed during resuscitation. Successful outcomes are directly affected by the medical expertise, knowledge of ACLS, and effective team communication during the acute event. The staff needs to be trained and educated in order to understand their role during resuscitation and to

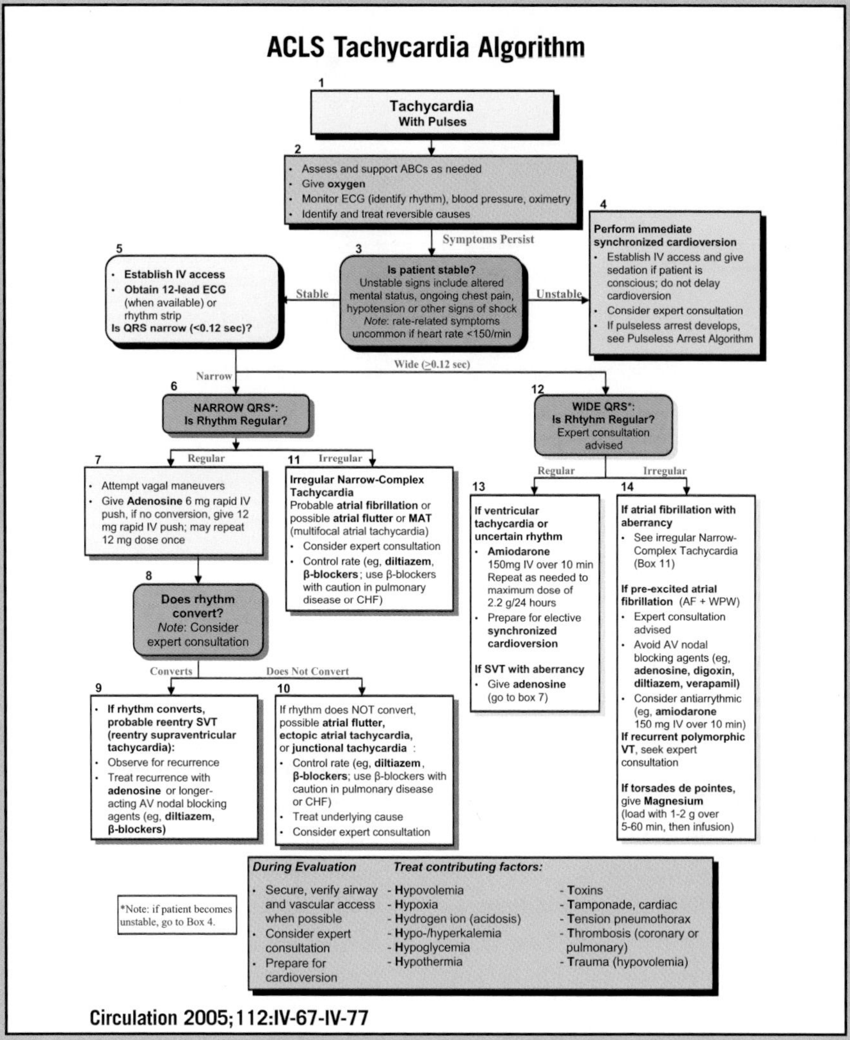

Figure 5.3: ACLS Tachycardia Algorithm (reprinted with permission from: ECC Committee, Subcommittees and Task Forces of the American Heart Association. 2005 American Heart Association Guidelines for Cardiopulmonary Resuscitation and Emergency Cardiovascular Care. *Circulation* 2005 Dec 13;112[Suppl I]:IV-67-IV-77).

know the role of all participants. The staff also needs to understand what they are authorized to perform that is within the scope of their practice.

There are eight elements of effective resuscitation team dynamics according to the ACLS guidelines:

1) *Closed-loop communication:* The team leader gives a message, order, or assignment to a team member. The team leader confirms that the message was received and understood. Then the team leader listens for confirmation from the team member who was delegated that task.

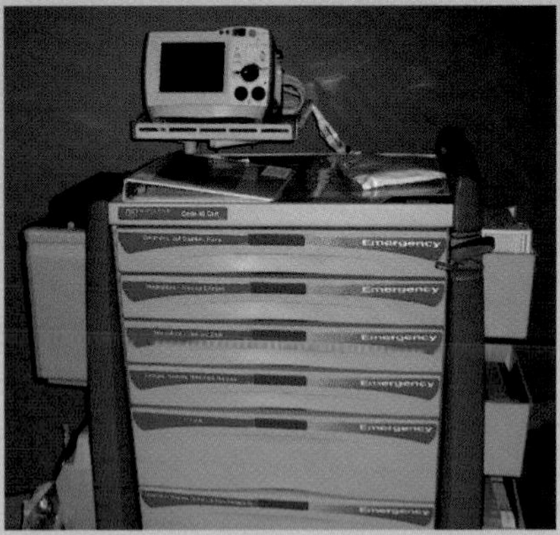

Figure 5.4: An example of a crash cart.

2) *Clear message:* Concise communication spoken with distinctive speech in a controlled voice in a calm manner.
3) *Clear roles and responsibilities:* Every team member needs to understand their role and responsibilities. The team leader should clearly delegate tasks, and team members should communicate when and if they can handle additional responsibilities.
4) *Knowing one's limitations:* Everyone should know their own limitations as well as those of the team. This helps evaluate the need to call for backup assistance if required.
5) *Knowledge sharing:* Sharing information is a critical component of effective team performance. Team members should inform the team leader of any changes in the patient's status to assure that decisions are made with all available information.
6) *Constructive intervention:* The team leader or team member should intervene if an action that is going to occur may be inappropriate at that time. Constructive input needs to be provided tactfully to avoid confrontation.

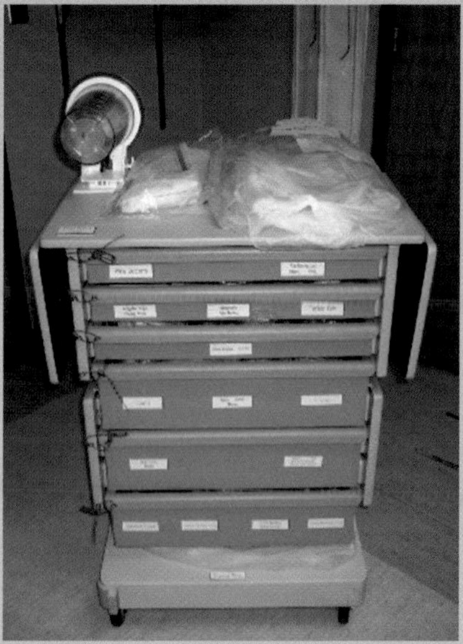

Figure 5.5: An example of a thoracotomy (chest opening) cart.

7) *Reevaluation and summarization:* The team leader needs to monitor and reevaluate the patient's status, review the interventions that have been performed, and assess the impact of the interventions. This information needs to be summarized out loud in order to update the team.
8) *Mutual respect:* The best teams are composed of members who share a mutual respect for one another and work in a collegial manner.

Emergency Equipment/Supplies for the EP Lab

The EP staff needs to be prepared for a wide variety of emergency situations that can occur in the EP lab setting. These supplies and equipment need to be checked daily to assure for availability, functionality, and sterility.

Along with the necessary equipment associated with performing procedures

Table 5.2: Information on ACLS Medications

EP Laboratory Emergency Drugs

Drug	Indication	Dosage/Directions
Classification: Antiarrhythmic Agents:		
Amiodarone	Recurrent VT/VF	• Maximum cumulative: 2.2 g over 24 hours • Start with IV bolus of 150 mg over 10 minutes • Infuse 360 mg IV over next 6 hours (1 mg/min) • Maintenance infusion 540 mg IV over next 18 hours (0.5 mg/min)
Lidocaine	VT or VF	• Based on no previous administration during event • Loading dose 1.0-1.5 mg/kg • Follow by 0.5-0.75 mg/kg every 5-10 minutes • Total doses up to total of 3 mg/kg
Magnesium Sulfate	Recurrent torsades de pointes associated with long QT intervals	• Loading dose of 1-2 g IV/IO diluted in 10 ml D5W • Infuse over 5-20 minutes • Indicated is known or suspected low serum magnesium
Pulseless Electrical Activity (PEA)/Asystole:		
Epinephrine	PEA/Asystole	• 1 mg IV/IO • Repeat every 3-5 minutes
Vasopressin	PEA/Asystole	• 40 U IV/IO • Can substitute vasopressor for first or second dose of epinephrine
Atropine	Slow PEA/ Asystole	• 1 mg IV/IO • Repeat every 3-5 minutes up to 3 doses
Symptomatic Bradycardia:		
Atropine	Symptomatic Bradycardia	• 0.5 mg IV and may repeat to total dose of 3 mg • Prepare for transcutaneous pacing (TCP)
Epinephrine	Symptomatic Bradycardia	• 2-10 mcq/min • Use if atropine ineffective • Prepare and start TCP
Dopamine	Symptomatic Bradycardia	• 2-10 mcq/kg per minute • Use if atropine ineffective • Prepare and start TCP
Narrow QRS Tachycardia:		
Adenosine	Narrow regular tachycardia	• 6 mg IV push • 12 mg IV push if SVT does not convert in 1-2 minutes • Repeat 12 mg IV push if SVT does not convert in 1-2 minutes • Give in large vein over 1 second followed by 20 ml saline

(fluoroscopy, recording system, stimulator, 3-D mapping system, intracardiac ultrasound, etc.) and the standard emergency crash cart (figure 5.4), other items are necessary to operate a safe laboratory practice. Biphasic defibrillators have become a standard in the lab in favor of monophasic systems due to superior conversion success rates. These systems need to be checked daily in order to assure proper functionality. These daily checks need to be documented with the records saved as part of quality assurance. Laboratories should also have access to rapid laboratory testing devices (such as Abbott Laboratories's i-STAT, a hand-held portable system that performs a comprehensive panel of critical laboratory tests at the patient's point-of-care) in order to properly monitor ABGs, electrolytes, Hgb/Hct, and blood sugars during the procedure and if emergencies develop. These systems also require regular quality assurance checks to assure accuracy.

Surgical back-up equipment also needs to be considered for the laboratory setting. These specialty carts/trays include pericardiocentesis trays with vacuum collection bottles, chest tube trays with thoraceal, tracheotomy trays, and a cardiac surgery thoracotomy (chest opening) cart (figure 5.5). During emergencies, delays in appropriate care can mean the difference between life and death, so it is imperative to have the appropriate equipment readily available and in proper working order.

Table 5.2 shows useful information related to commonly used ACLS medications. This table includes the indications, dosages, frequency of delivery, and side effects. The table should serve as a useful review for those who are certifying or recertifying in ACLS. Please check the current ACLS manual for any updates related to these medications.

Chapter 6

The Electrophysiology Laboratory

The electrophysiology laboratory is a unique place for the diagnosis and treatment of cardiac arrhythmias. In general, it is an invasive laboratory very similar to the cardiac catheterization laboratory. The laboratory should be electrically isolated (free of outside electrical noise), since in addition to recording standard body surface electrocardiograms, high-fidelity intracardiac electrograms (recordings from inside the myocardium) are recorded.

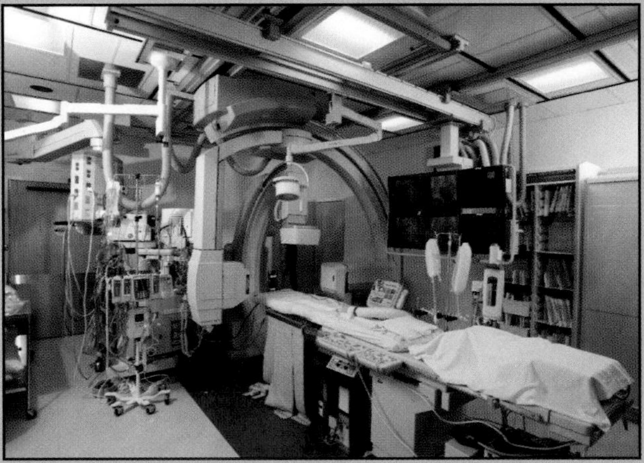

Figure 6.1: A typical electrophysiology laboratory (reprinted with permission from *EP Lab Digest* 2009;2:12, courtesy of Duke Medical Center).

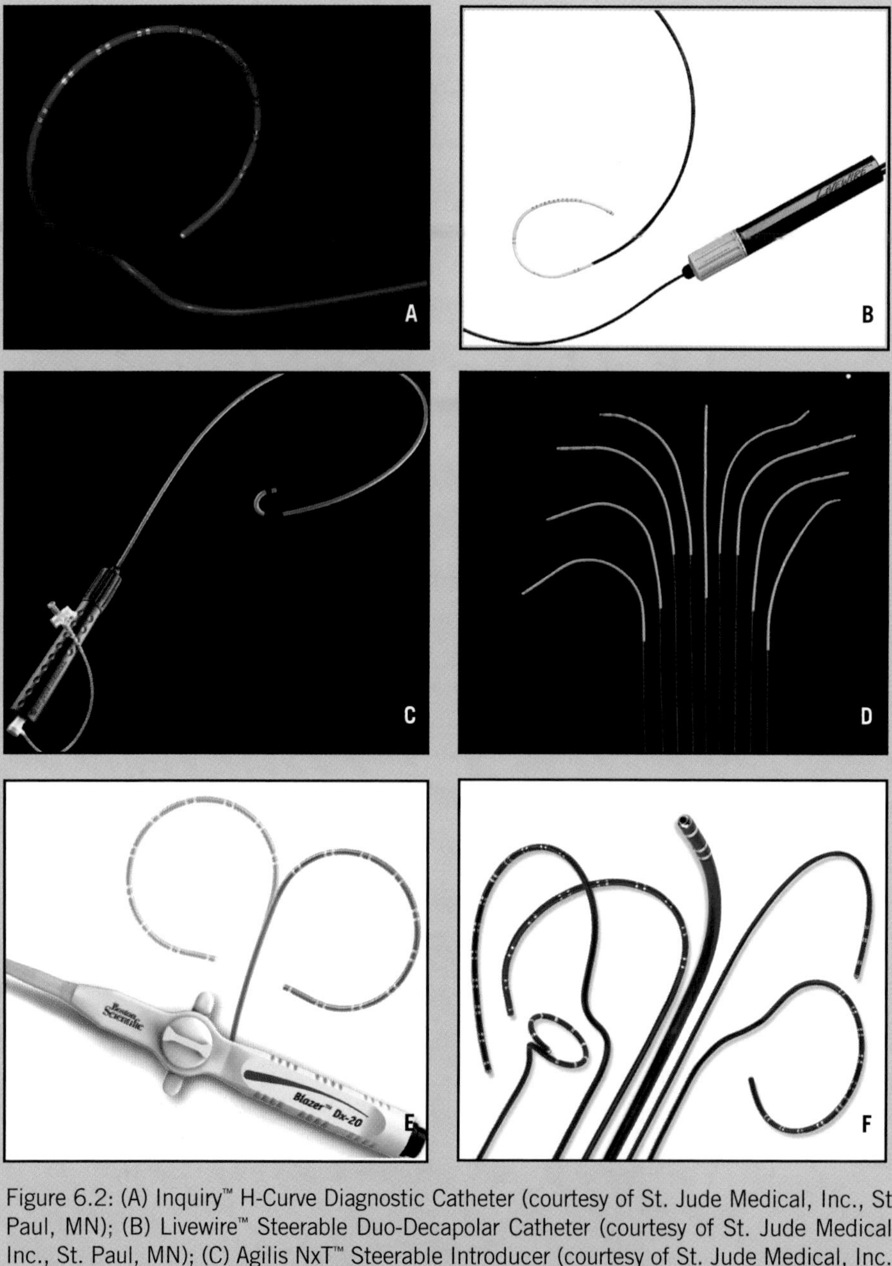

Figure 6.2: (A) Inquiry™ H-Curve Diagnostic Catheter (courtesy of St. Jude Medical, Inc., St. Paul, MN); (B) Livewire™ Steerable Duo-Decapolar Catheter (courtesy of St. Jude Medical, Inc., St. Paul, MN); (C) Agilis NxT™ Steerable Introducer (courtesy of St. Jude Medical, Inc., St. Paul, MN); (D) Fixed-curve diagnostics (courtesy of St. Jude Medical, Inc., St. Paul, MN); (E) Blazer™ Dx-20 bidirectional steerable diagnostic catheter (courtesy of Boston Scientific, Natick, MA); (F) IBI Catheters (courtesy of Boston Scientific, Natick, MA).

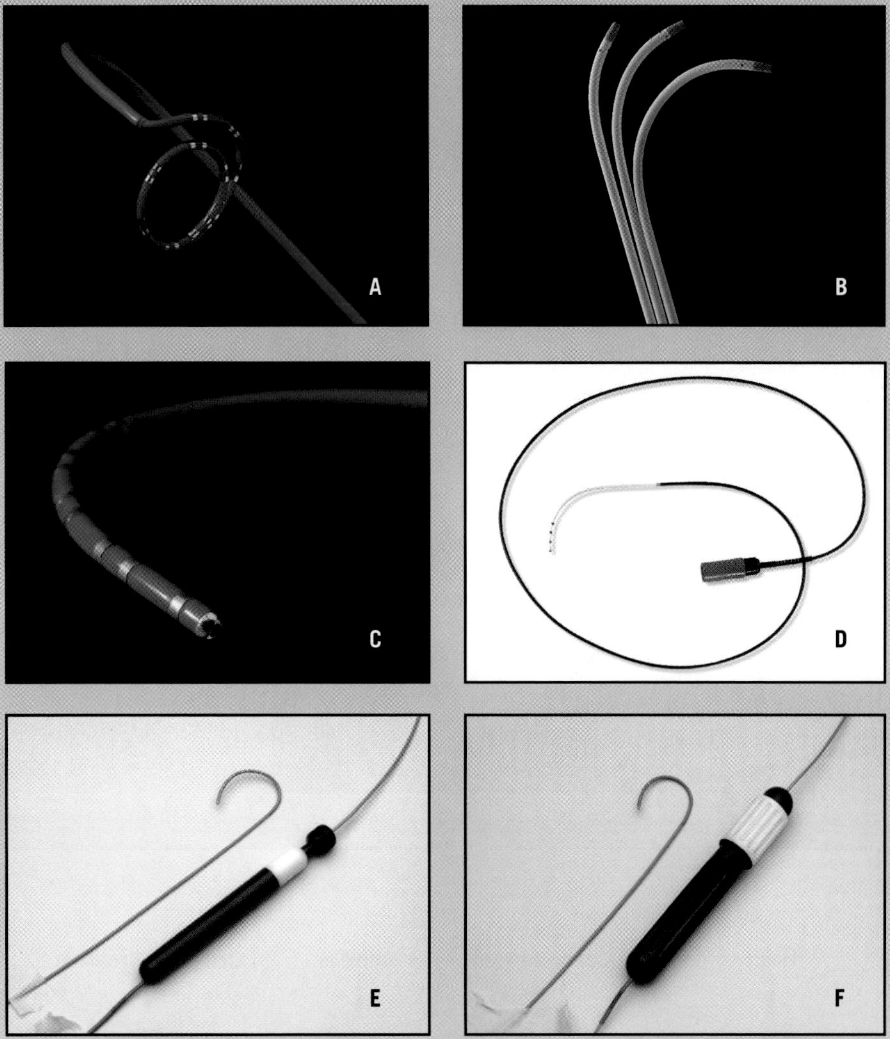

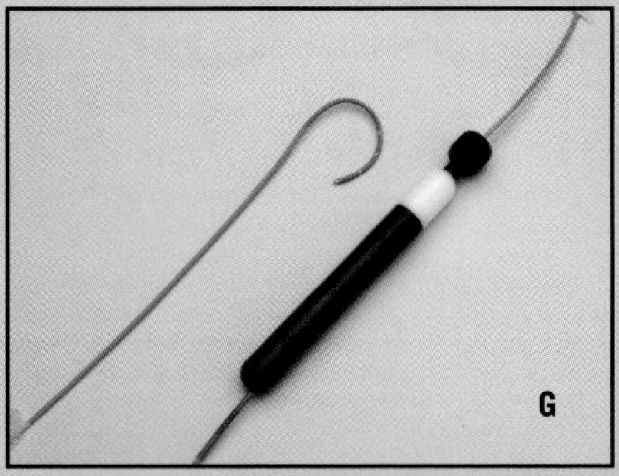

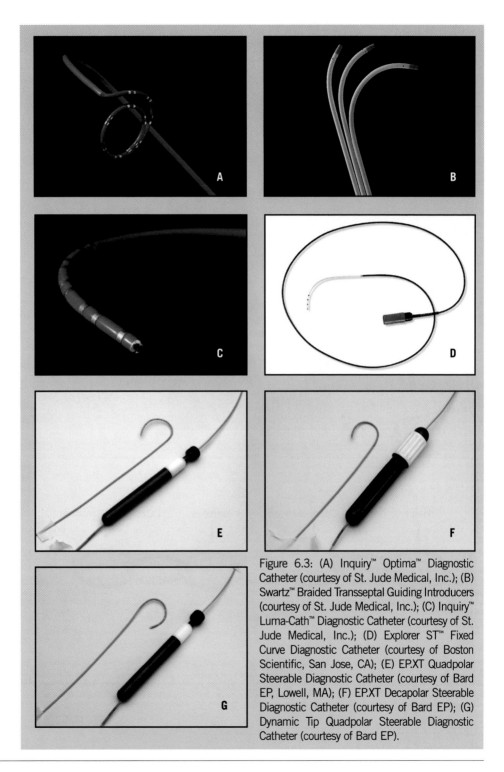

Figure 6.3: (A) Inquiry™ Optima™ Diagnostic Catheter (courtesy of St. Jude Medical, Inc.); (B) Swartz™ Braided Transseptal Guiding Introducers (courtesy of St. Jude Medical, Inc.); (C) Inquiry™ Luma-Cath™ Diagnostic Catheter (courtesy of St. Jude Medical, Inc.); (D) Explorer ST™ Fixed Curve Diagnostic Catheter (courtesy of Boston Scientific, San Jose, CA); (E) EP.XT Quadpolar Steerable Diagnostic Catheter (courtesy of Bard EP, Lowell, MA); (F) EP.XT Decapolar Steerable Diagnostic Catheter (courtesy of Bard EP); (G) Dynamic Tip Quadpolar Steerable Diagnostic Catheter (courtesy of Bard EP).

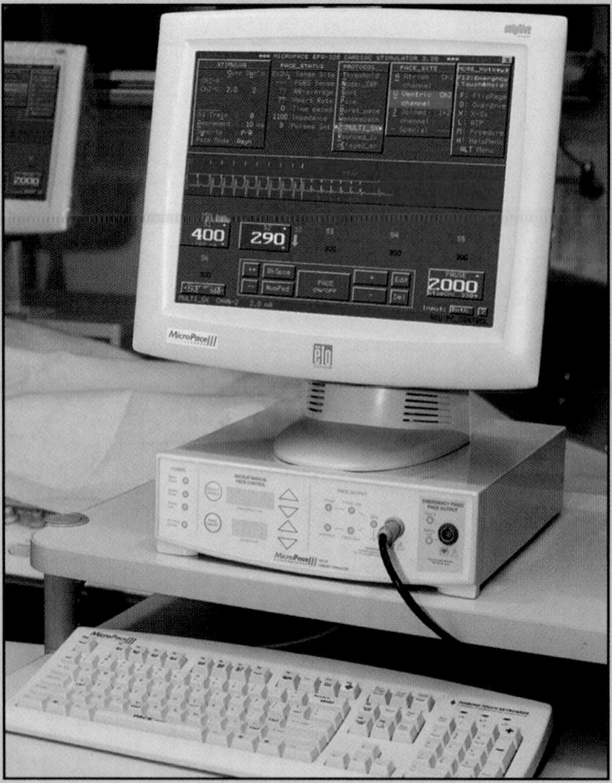

Figure 6.4: The stimulator, a computer used to deliver electrical impulses in order to pace the heart, deliver stimuli, and perform programmed electrical stimulation. Whether computer-based or a manual system, pacing outputs, rates, and premature impulses can be adjusted during electrophysiology studies. This photo shows the MicroPace Stimulator (Bard EP, Lowell, MA) with touch screen that can be used alone or in conjunction with the EP Recording System (Bard LabSystem PRO EP Recording System). (Photo courtesy of Bard EP, Lowell, MA.)

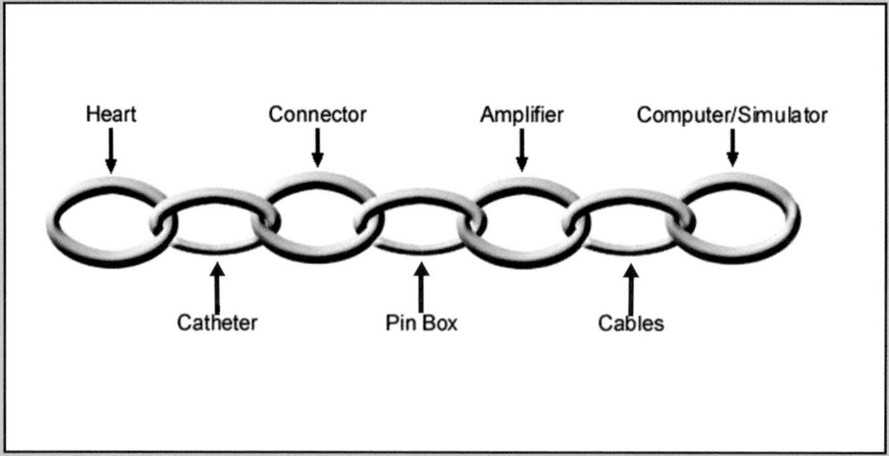

Figure 6.5: The vital equipment used in a typical electrophysiological procedure and the order in which the equipment is connected. This forms the "links in the chain" necessary for pacing and electrical signal analysis. Any breaks in the links can cause a problem in the lab.

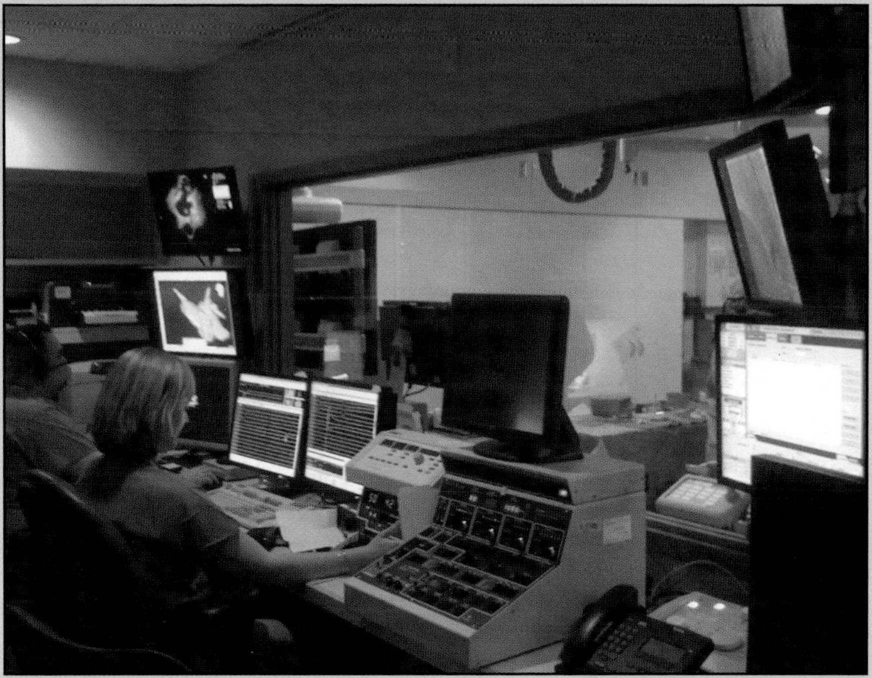

Figure 6.6: The typical control room and computers used to aid the doctor and staff. (Courtesy of Laurence Epstein, M.D., Brigham and Women's Hospital, Boston, MA).

The lab contains a fluoroscopy table that in some cases may be able to tilt the head upward as well as downward (as in the Trendelenburg position, in which the feet are raised above the head to help pool venous blood back into the central circulation). The tilting motion may be helpful in gaining access to the blood vessels in order to insert catheter and/or introducer sheaths. It is also helpful if the patient has low blood pressure. In some laboratories, the table can tilt upward at least 60 degrees to facilitate head-up tilt-table testing (the procedure to diagnose vasovagal syncope or neurocardiogenic syncope). This table should be able to tilt rapidly up and down, and it should be stable enough to accommodate the weight of the patient.

In the electrophysiology laboratory, the electrode catheters are positioned percutaneously through the femoral vein and/or artery into the heart. The catheters record electrical activity from their locations within the heart. They are connected to a pin box and an amplifier that attaches to a computerized recording system where real-time and digital analysis can be performed. Figures 6.2 and 6.3 show an array of diagnostic catheters that can be used during an electrophysiology study.

Also in the electrophysiology lab is a stimulator (figure 6.4) that can interface with the computerized system to provide pacing capabilities. The signals are routinely filtered at 30 hertz (Hz) to 500 Hz; a notch

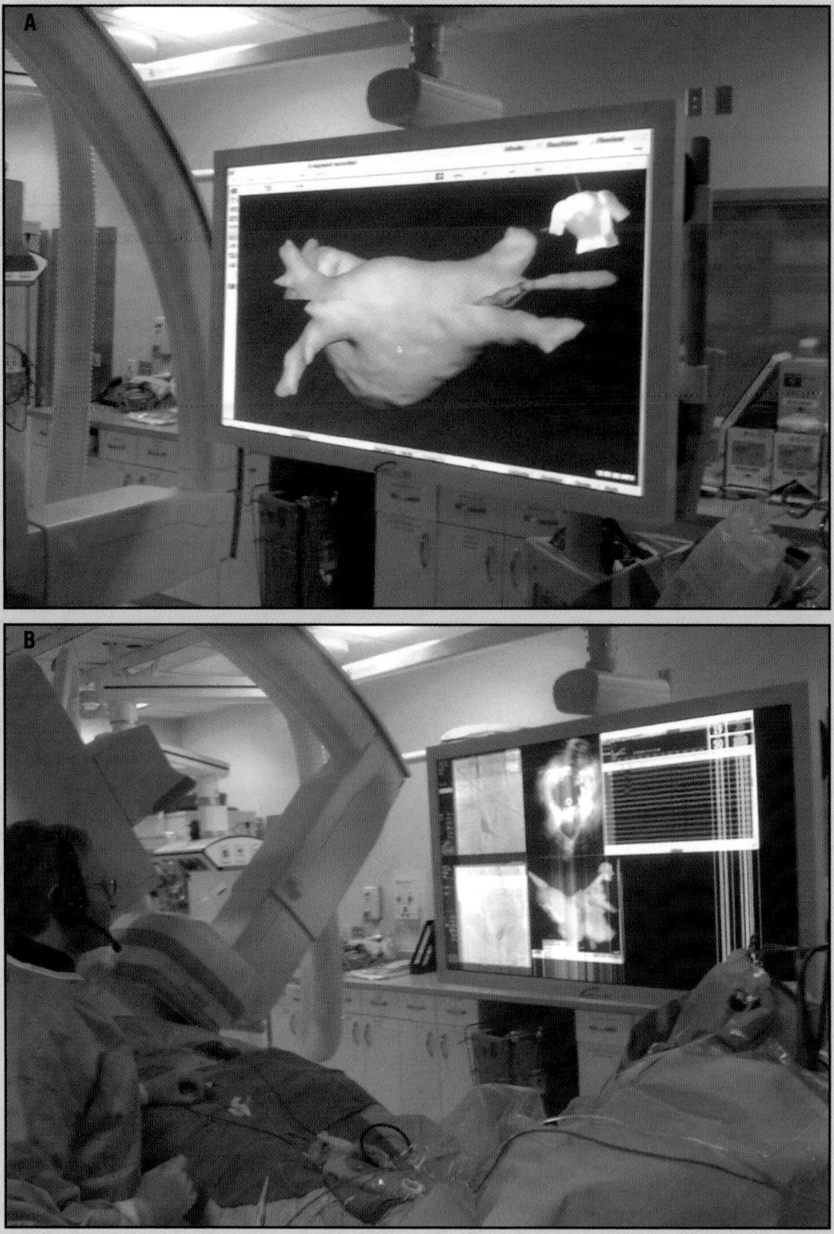

Figure 6.7: (A) This shows a large flat-panel monitor (Cardio-View™, Carrot Medical, Newton, MA) displaying an image of the left atrium and pulmonary veins. (B) This single monitor can be broken into a myriad of smaller images simultaneously demonstrating surface and intracardiac electrograms, fluoroscopy images, intracardiac echo images, and non-fluoroscopic three-dimensional reconstructed images (courtesy of Laurence Epstein, M.D., Brigham and Women's Hospital, Boston, MA).

filter can eliminate the 60 Hz of noise from other electrical equipment.

Figure 6.5 shows the "links in the chain" of an electrophysiology laboratory from patient to computer stimulator. Any breaks in a link in the chain can prevent pacing and/or appropriate intracardiac or surface electrogram analysis.

The laboratory may be one encompassing room or segregated into a control room and procedural room (figure 6.6). The latter set-up is preferable to minimize the fluoroscopy exposure to the operators when they are using the stimulating and recording equipment. Figure 6.7 shows a large, single flat-panel monitor that could integrate simultaneously a number of imaging modalities. The electrophysiology laboratory requires at least two external defibrillators (figures 6.8-6.10), one used as a backup in case the primary one fails. The defibrillator's main purpose is to be able to defibrillate a patient should a tachyarrhythmia occur; it also can be used to monitor the patient's heart rate, blood pressure, and possibly other vital signs during the electrophysiology procedure. Many defibrillators have external pacing capabilities through large external skin patches.

In addition, pulse oximetry with audible tones that change with desaturation are also useful in monitoring patients with impaired cardiac function. End tidal C02 monitoring may also be useful in patients with obstructive sleep apnea and other respiratory diseases. The latter will likely be the standard of care for all monitored deep sedation cases.

A standard automatic external defibrillator (AED) is often used in public forums to treat ventricular tachycardia and ventricular fibrillation. The AED is a simplified version of the defibrillator used in the EP lab and is geared more for use by the general public. Public not-for-profit organizations such as the Sudden Cardiac Arrest Association are committed to the treatment of cardiac arrest and public awareness. The more AEDs that are out in the community (*e.g.*, churches, synagogues, schools, stadiums, libraries, museums, etc.), the more likely patients will survive a witnessed cardiac arrest. AEDs may also be used in pacemaker clinics in order to easily treat spontaneous or induced ventricular arrhythmias. Please note that AEDs are too limited for general inclusion in standard electrophysiology laboratories per se. This is because they do not visualize the electrocardiogram during monitoring, and have limited defibrillation (and no pacing) capabilities.

Tilt-table testing can be performed in an electrophysiology laboratory with the appropriate table. Most institutions and offices, however, have a separate room with a tilting table that can provide such testing. This separate room should also be equipped with monitoring equipment similar to that in the electrophysiology laboratory, including a peripheral automated blood pressure monitor, oximeter, and a defibrillator with external pacing capabilities. Intravenous delivery pumps for medication such as isoproterenol and for normal saline should be available as well.

The laboratory room and environment should be clean and professional and as free from noise and talking as possible in order to be conducive to patient care. Ideally it should be off a corridor or area related to a recovery room. In addition, a

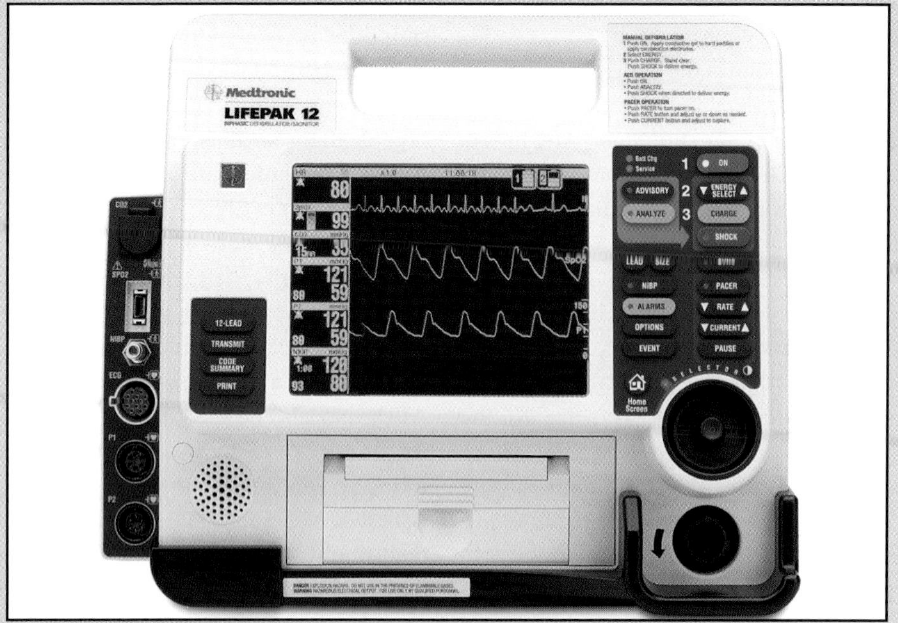

Figure 6.8: The LIFEPAK® 12 defibrillator/monitor (courtesy of Physio-Control, Inc., Redmond, WA).

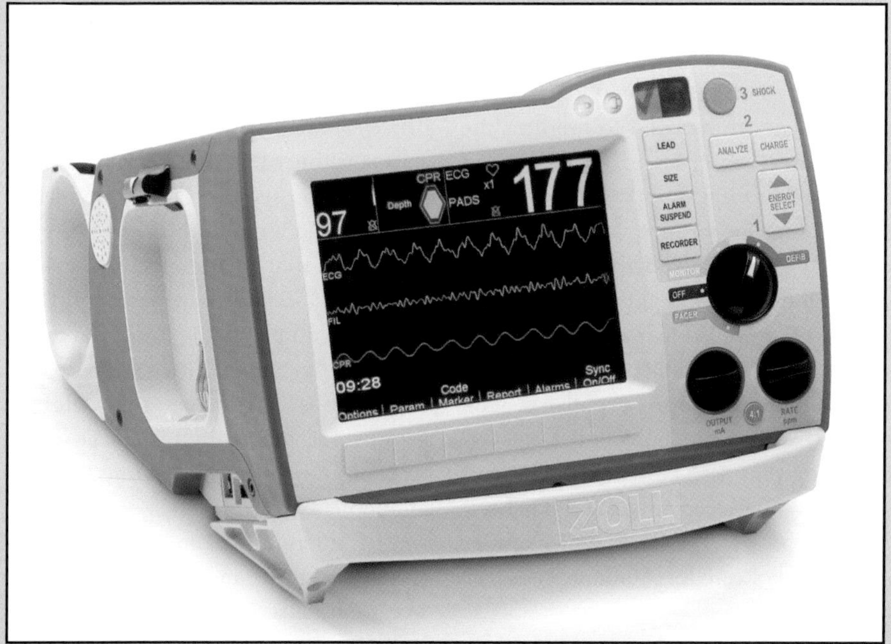

Figure 6.9: The R Series® ALS defibrillator with See-Thru CPR® (courtesy of Zoll Medical Corporation, Chelmsford, MA).

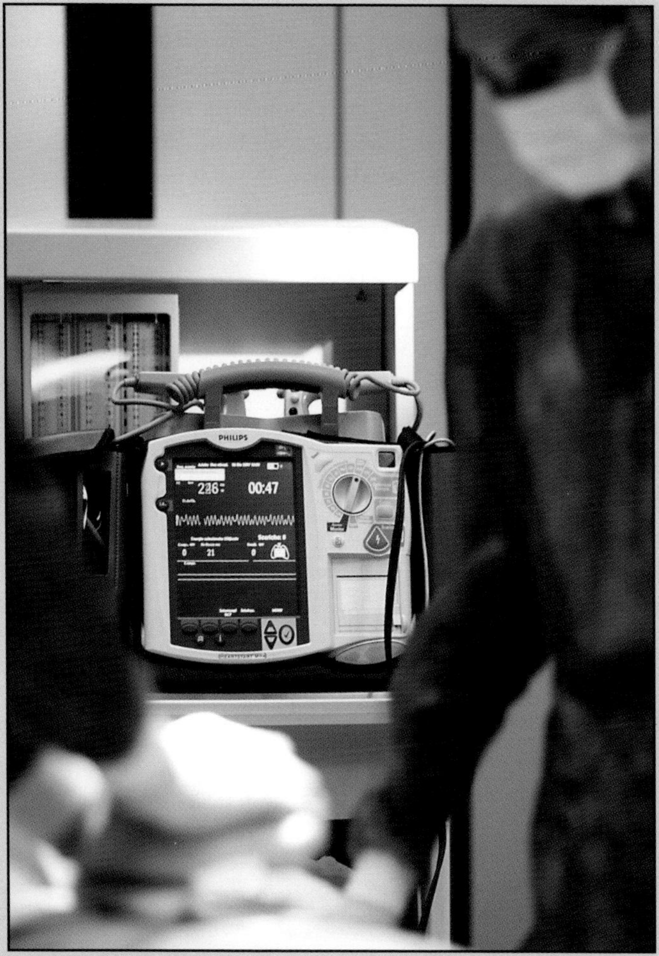

Figure 6.10: The Philips HeartStart MRx monitor/defibrillator (courtesy of Philips Healthcare, Andover, MA).

scrub sink should be outside the main procedure room.

For pacemaker or defibrillator implantation to be performed, the laboratories need to be terminally cleaned and have adequate air circulation and ventilation. These laboratories do not need to be of an operating-room standard, but they should be as close to that as possible. Several studies have documented the safety of implantation of permanent pacemakers and defibrillators in cardiac catheterization laboratories. The infection rate in these rooms is no higher than in the operating-room environment; however, cleanliness and sterility remain essential to implant procedures.

All the rooms described need to have enough circulation space to provide adequate delivery of oxygen, intubation if necessary, and cardiopulmonary resuscitation.

All electrophysiology procedure rooms must have immediate accessibility to a crash cart with standard emergency medical equipment and intubation tools. In addition, the electrophysiology laboratory should have a pericardiocentesis tray immediately available in case of emergent cardiac tamponade (in which blood accumulates in the pericardial sac surrounding the heart and impedes the blood flow out of the heart resulting from myocardial perforation).

Chapter 7

Radiation Protection

Radiation protection in electrophysiology is essential to all patients and personnel in order to minimize the cumulative effects to the bone marrow and other radiation-sensitive tissue as well as the possible risk of cancer. The electrophysiology laboratory (including all associated operating rooms) should strive for the ALARA principle, which stands for radiation exposure should be "As Low as Reasonably Achievable."

In order to minimize radiation exposure, there are three factors that need to be considered: 1) time, 2) distance, and 3) shielding. The amount of radiation exposure is directly related to the exposure time of the procedure. In particular, the current needed to generate x-rays, mAs (milliampere-seconds), should be maintained as low as possible. The image intensifier to object (patient) distance must be kept to a minimum at all times to reduce exposure from scattered radiation to both the operator and assisting personnel. The further the image intensifier is from the patient, the greater the radiation required to produce a diagnostic image with subsequent increase of scatter and radiation exposure to the staff. All non-essential personnel should be at least six feet from the source of the scattered radiation, the patient, during fluoroscopy. In addition, the duration of fluoroscopy exposure for long and complex electrophysiology procedures (*e.g.*, catheter ablations and biventricular implants) should be less than 60 minutes in order to minimize the potential for a radiation burn to the patient's skin.

Radiation protective shielding is barrier protection, which limits the effects of ionizing radiation by limiting its penetration.

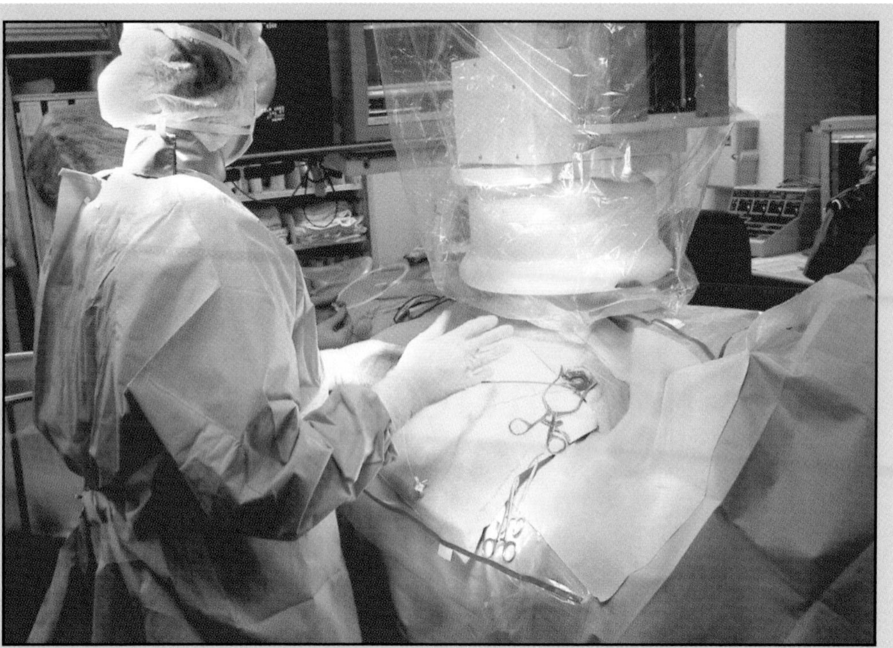

Figure 7.1: RADPAD® EP shield used during a biventricular pacing procedure (courtesy of Worldwide Innovations & Technologies, Inc., Overland Park, KS).

This type of shielding can occur in several forms. First, pull-down shields should be utilized. These are leaded acrylic shields that hang from a boom from the ceiling and can be interposed between the patient, the scattered radiation source, and the operator. Second, radiation protective drapes, which hang down from the table sides to the floor, can help limit the radiation exposure to the operator. Third, lead aprons including thyroid shields should be worn by all staff present in the laboratory. Fourth, radiation protective drapes positioned on the patient, specifically designed to minimize scatter, can help further reduce radiation exposure to the electrophysiology staff and operators. In particular, a shield that has been utilized in our laboratory (RADPAD®, Worldwide Innovations & Technologies, Inc., Overland Park, Kansas) has helped to reduce radiation exposures to the operator by up to 50 percent. Figure 7.1 shows a RADPAD® EP shield used during biventricular pacing procedures. Specific drapes have also been designed for a variety of electrophysiology procedures (RADPAD® Prometheus, Worldwide Innovations & Technologies, Inc.); figure 7.2 shows such a drape designed for electrophysiologists. Fifth, lead glasses and gloves may also be helpful. The glasses should be worn by the operators in order to minimize the risk of cataracts (especially high-volume operators). Lead gloves may be useful for direct beam radiation exposure; however, this type of exposure should be avoided unless absolutely necessary.

RADPAD® Prometheus Left Side Pacemaker/ICD Drape (Cat.#4920)

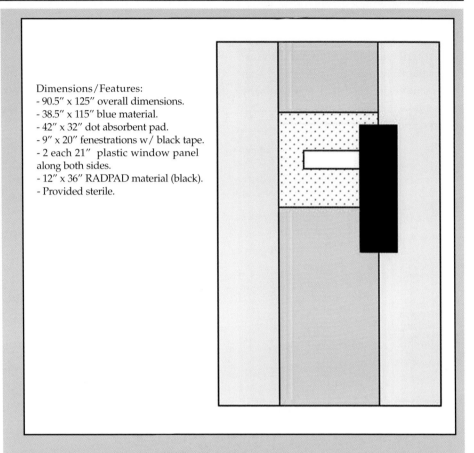

Dimensions/Features:
- 90.5″ x 125″ overall dimensions.
- 38.5″ x 115″ blue material.
- 42″ x 32″ dot absorbent pad.
- 9″ x 20″ fenestrations w/ black tape.
- 2 each 21″ plastic window panel along both sides.
- 12″ x 36″ RADPAD material (black).
- Provided sterile.

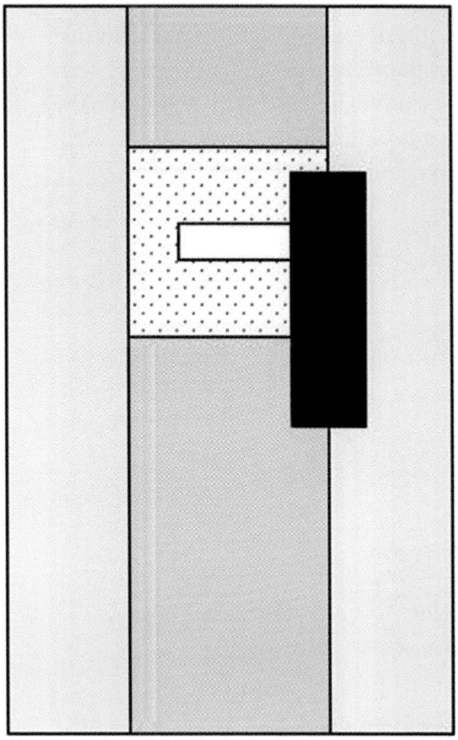

Figure 7.2: Shows a drape designed for electrophysiologists (RADPAD® Prometheus Left Side Pacemaker/ICD Drape (Cat. #4920), courtesy of Worldwide Innovations & Technologies, Inc., Overland Park, KS) (reprinted with permission from *EP Lab Digest* 2004;8:1,12).

Newer technology has incorporated robotics into catheter manipulation (see Chapter 31). This technology has permitted remote catheter manipulation by the electrophysiology operator (at a further distance from the x-ray equipment and even in a shielded control room). This approach has helped minimize direct radiation exposure to the operator, who now at times may be able to remove their lead apron shields while manipulating a catheter from a shielded control room.

All equipment must be properly maintained, inspected, and monitored by the Radiation Safety Department, which is overseen by the Radiation Safety Officer. Importantly, all electrophysiology staff should wear radiation monitoring devices, so exposures can be reviewed monthly and cumulatively on a yearly basis in accordance with the radiation safety program. Annual radiation exposures for all electrophysiology staff must be less than 5 rem per year. Pregnant staff levels should be less than one-tenth the allowable annual exposure of a typical staff member (less than 0.5 rem).

Overall, an effective radiation safety program at a hospital will help minimize the exposure of radiation to all staff members, operators, and patients. Working together with the Director of the Electrophysiology Laboratory, the Radiation Safety Officer can help to optimize the clinical outcomes of the Electrophysiology Program.

Part 1: Quiz

Test your knowledge of Part 1:

Question 1. Match the individual to their contribution in electrophysiology or implantable devices:

A. Mirowski and Mower	1. Implantable defibrillator
B. Einthoven	2. Catheter ablation
C. Scheinman	3. Atrial fibrillation ablation
D. Haïssaguerre	4. Electrocardiogram

Question 2. An anatomical landmark for mapping in catheter ablation surrounded by the tendon of Todaro, the coronary sinus ostium, and the septal leaflet of the tricuspid valve is called:

A. Eustachian valve
B. The sinus node
C. The triangle of Koch
D. Bachman's bundle

Question 3. The cardiac action potential is a recording of:

A. The changes in cardiac output of the heart over time.
B. The changes of electrical potential over time recorded from inside a heart muscle cell.
C. The changes in electrical conduction recorded from the body surface.
D. The change in the contractility of the heart over time.

Question 4. Match the phases of the action potential represented as activity:

A. Depolarization	1. Phase 4
B. Repolarization	2. Phases 1 through 3
C. Resting	3. Phase 0

Question 5. Which of the following intervals is abnormal?

A. PR interval of 150 milliseconds
B. QRS duration of 100 milliseconds
C. QT interval of 600 milliseconds
D. Corrected QT interval of 430 milliseconds

Question 6. In order to perform programed electrical stimulation in a patient in the electrophysiology laboratory, it is important to have:

A. Positive pressure ventilation.
B. Uninterrupted links in the chain between the stimulator, cables, amplifier, pin box, connector, catheter, and heart.
C. A tilt table.
D. Temperature monitoring via the esophagus.

Question 7. The minimum standard of defibrillators necessary for an electrophysiology laboratory is:

A. One
B. Two
C. Three
D. Four

Question 8. The ALARA principle means that radiation exposure should be:

A. At Low Amplitude Receiving Analysis
B. At Longitudinal Atmospheric Radiation Altitudes
C. As Low as Reasonably Achievable
D. After Long Ablation Radiofrequency Attempts

Question 9. All equipment must be properly maintained, inspected, and monitored by:

A. The radiation safety officer
B. The police officer
C. The fire and safety department
D. Administration

Question 10. Which of the following is considered barrier protection, which limits radiation exposure to the operator?

A. Pull-down shields
B. Sterile gowns
C. Sterile gloves
D. The crash cart

Answer key:
1. (A: 1, B: 4, C: 2, D: 3)
2. C
3. B
4. (A: 3, B: 2, C: 1)
5. C
6. B
7. B
8. C
9. A
10. A

Part 2

THE ELECTROPHYSIOLOGY STUDY AND BASIC ARRHYTHMIAS

Chapter 8

Venous and Arterial Access

In the beginning of an electrophysiology study, it is important to gain venous and/or arterial access. This is essentially placing an intravenous catheter (an introducer sheath) into a vein and/or artery. For electrophysiology procedures, it is not uncommon to place three introducer sheaths into a single femoral vein.

First, the femoral artery and/or vein must be located so that the operator can access the circulation in order to perform an electrophysiology study. The operator can identify the appropriate location by palpating the groin area of the patient near the iliac crest and the ischial tuberosity, as well as the symphysis pubis.

The inguinal ligament extends from the iliac crest down to the symphysis pubis. About two-thirds of the way medial between this location, one should be able to palpate the femoral artery, below the femoral ligament. There is a triangle in which the femoral nerve, artery, and vein are located from lateral to medial (figure 8.1). By using the mnemonic NAVel, you can remember that the nerve, the artery, and the vein are always facing the navel whether one proceeds from the right or left side. In other words, the nerve (N) is most lateral, followed by the artery (A), and then the vein (V) as the most medial of the structures.

Once the patient is prepped and draped in usual sterile manner, lidocaine or a similar injectable anesthetic is used as a local anesthetic before femoral venous access is attempted. The skin is anesthetized subcutaneously medial to the artery with a 22-gauge needle down to the femoral vein until blood return occurs, which

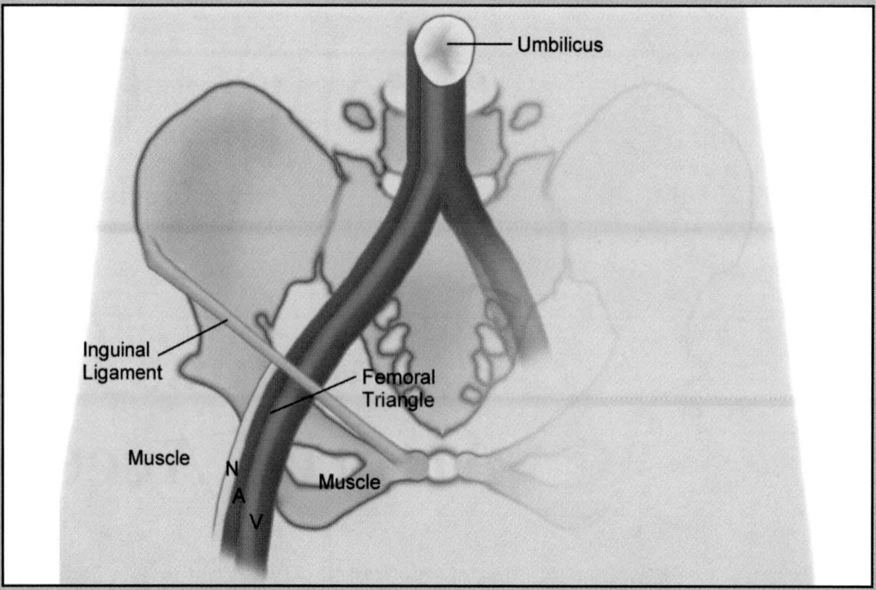

Figure 8.1: The anatomic positions of the femoral artery and vein. Note the use of the mnemonic NAVel helps identify structures in the femoral triangle.

demonstrates the exact location of the blood vessel.

The needle is disconnected from the syringe, and a large-bore introducer needle is placed parallel to the 22-gauge finder needle until venous access is achieved. If the artery is inadvertently hit, the needle is removed, and pressure is applied for three to five minutes until hemostasis occurs. If the vein is hit appropriately, the hub of the syringe is removed from the needle, and a soft J-tip guidewire is placed into the vessel. If any evidence of obstruction occurs, the guidewire is pulled back, and free blood flow from the needle is obtained via the use of a syringe. If necessary, this step is repeated until the guidewire freely flows into the circulation. Fluoroscopy or contrast dye may be needed to help define any obstruction.

Once the guidewire is safely in the blood vessel, the needle is removed, and another venopuncture is performed. The location of this second venopuncture is about one-quarter of an inch to one-eighth of an inch above or below the original insertion site to find the blood vessel along the same plane from which venous access was previously obtained. Again, once the wire is advanced appropriately into that vessel, the needle is pulled back, and the wire is left in place. Should a third wire be desired, the same sequence would be followed. Figure 8.2 shows the sequential steps necessary to insert introducer sheaths into the femoral vein.

It is important to note that sheaths are not placed into the blood vessel and along the guidewire until all the guidewires are in appropriate positions. If the patient has

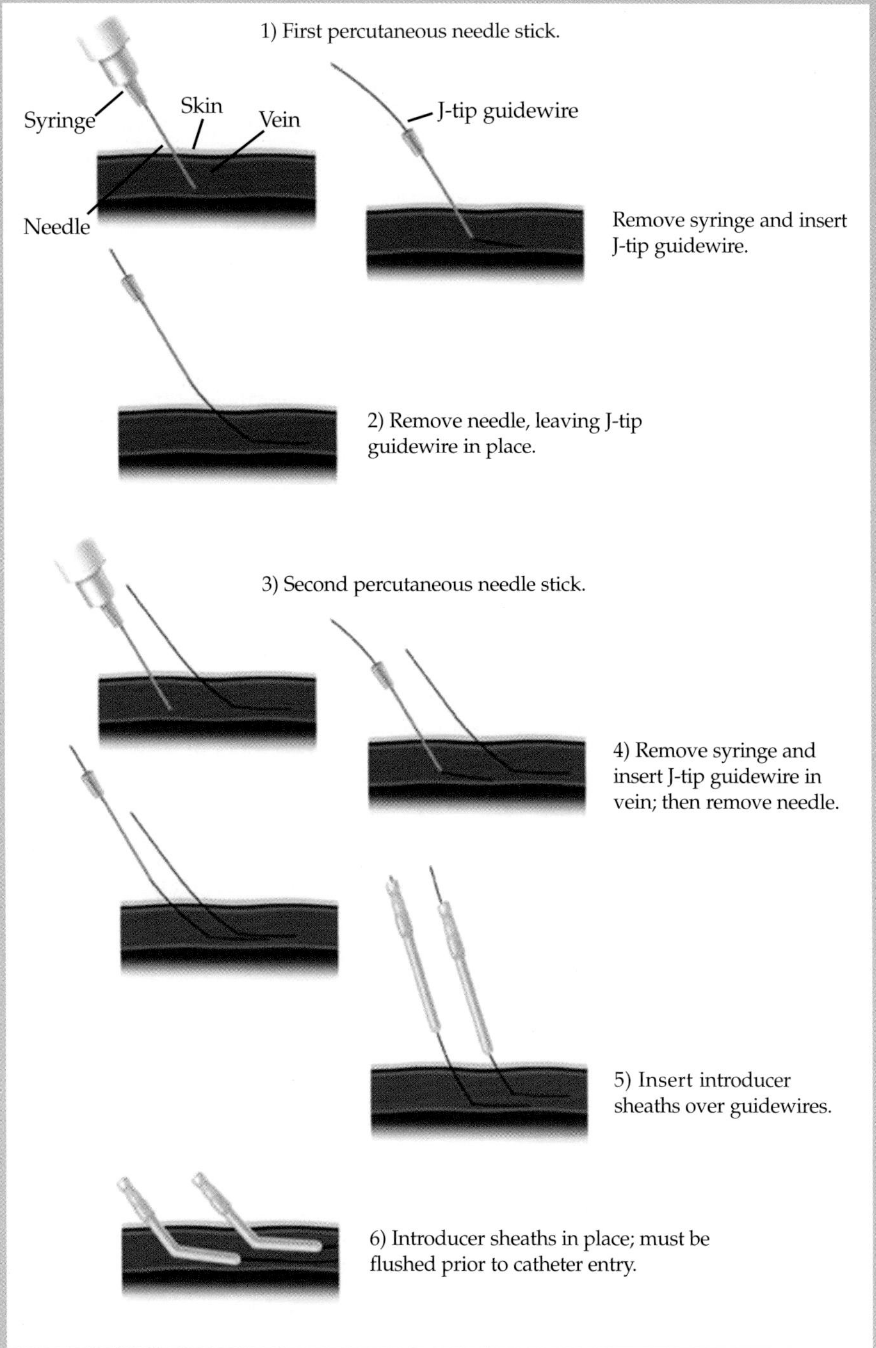
1) First percutaneous needle stick.
Syringe
Skin
Vein
Needle
J-tip guidewire
Remove syringe and insert J-tip guidewire.
2) Remove needle, leaving J-tip guidewire in place.
3) Second percutaneous needle stick.
4) Remove syringe and insert J-tip guidewire in vein; then remove needle.
5) Insert introducer sheaths over guidewires.
6) Introducer sheaths in place; must be flushed prior to catheter entry.

Figure 8.2: The sequential steps needed to access the femoral vein and introduce the proper catheters into the heart.

a sheath placed and then a wire is added, there is a risk of sticking a needle in the sheath and shearing it, which in turn could cause a foreign body to become dislodged. The author has observed this phenomenon, and the sheath required retrieval from the circulation.

Femoral arterial access is performed in a similar manner, except palpation is directly over the blood vessel, so that the pulsations of the femoral artery can be felt. Subcutaneous anesthetic is administered over the femoral artery. A finder needle is often unnecessary for this procedure because of the ease of arterial palpation. By taking the introducer needle with a syringe and directly hitting the femoral artery, one can observe unimpeded blood flow; when it is then disconnected from the hub of the syringe, a free flow of pulsatile arterial blood clearly identifies direct access into the femoral artery.

A soft J-tip guidewire is placed through the syringe needle; the needle is then removed. The introducer sheath is subsequently placed over this, and finally the dilator and the guidewire are withdrawn. The side port is then flushed, ensuring that no bubbles enter the arterial circulation.

It is important to note that if the catheter inserted into the introducer sheath with a side port is the same size as the introducer sheath itself, it will be very difficult to draw blood back from the introducer and to administer intravenous fluids. Therefore, the introducer sheath used for this purpose should be one French size larger than the catheter inserted. For example, if a 6 French introducer sheath is used and intravenous fluids need to be administered and blood needs to be withdrawn, a 5 French catheter should be used for the study.

Specifically-designed long preformed sheaths and needles have been developed for atrial transseptal procedures. These sheaths are placed from the femoral vein up into the superior vena cava and withdrawn back to the fossa ovalis. A transseptal needle is carefully advanced from the right to left atrium with advancement of the sheath over the needle to permit direct left-sided catheter access. Additional complications include aortic and myocardial perforation (cardiac tamponade), air embolism and thromboembolism (the latter two resulting in neurologic sequelae, *i.e.*, transient or permanent cerebrovascular injury). Attention to detail, including hemodynamic monitoring, anticoagulation, and sheath flushing throughout the procedure, is essential. The pericardiocentesis tray may be useful for emergent treatment of cardiac tamponade.

Potential complications from vascular access include bleeding, infection, clot formation (hematoma), deep venous thrombosis and possible pulmonary embolus, pseudoaneurysm, retroperitoneal bleed, and an arteriovenous fistula. Appropriate hemostasis must be obtained post procedure with particular attention to changes in groin swelling, pain, and peripheral pulses. If a problem is suspected, a Doppler study/ultrasound and/or computer-axis tomography may be useful, and if a complication is confirmed, vascular surgical assistance may be necessary.

Chapter 9

Assessment of Conduction and Refractoriness

One of the critical components of an electrophysiology study is the evaluation of conduction. Concepts presented in this chapter are in the order in which they are usually evaluated during a routine electrophysiology study. The first concept, conduction, can be assessed by pacing a proximal structure and assessing the delivery of the electrical impulse to a more distal structure. For example, atrioventricular conduction is assessed by pacing the atrium and examining the particular heart rate in which conduction block occurs, preventing ventricular depolarization. In addition, the site of the conduction block can also be assessed. The second concept relates to the response of cardiac tissue to premature extrastimuli: this is called refractoriness. In order to assess refractoriness of a particular myocardial structure (atrium, AV node, His bundle, or ventricle), programmed electrical stimulation is performed. In this manner, stimulation of a site of myocardium (atrium or ventricle) is performed in which 8–10 paced beats at a fixed heart rate are delivered. A premature stimulus after the constant drive train is then delivered at progressively shorter intervals.

First, it is important to place the intracardiac pacing catheters (standard four-poled catheters called quadripolar catheters) in the correct positions in the heart. A catheter is typically placed via introducer sheaths through the right femoral vein (or alternatively, the left femoral vein) and inserted so that one of the catheter's poles makes contact in the

Table 9.1: Normal Intracardiac Interval Measurements

Interval	Measurement	Normal Range (msec)
Intracardiac ECG		
AH Interval	Earliest rapid atrial deflection to onset of His deflection on His electrogram	65 to 140
HV Interval	Earliest His deflection on His electrogram to earliest surface ECG ventricular activation	35 to 55

high right atrium. Other locations such as the right atrial appendage or the lateral right atrium may also be acceptable.

A second catheter is positioned across the tricuspid valve so that contact is made against the septum. A recording of the His bundle is obtained so that an atrial and ventricular electrogram can be seen. A sharp potential should be seen between the atrium and ventricular electrogram; this is typically the His bundle potential. (Figure 9.1 shows fluoroscopic images of two catheters placed in the heart. The catheter on the left when viewing the image is in the high right atrium. The second catheter is across the tricuspid valve

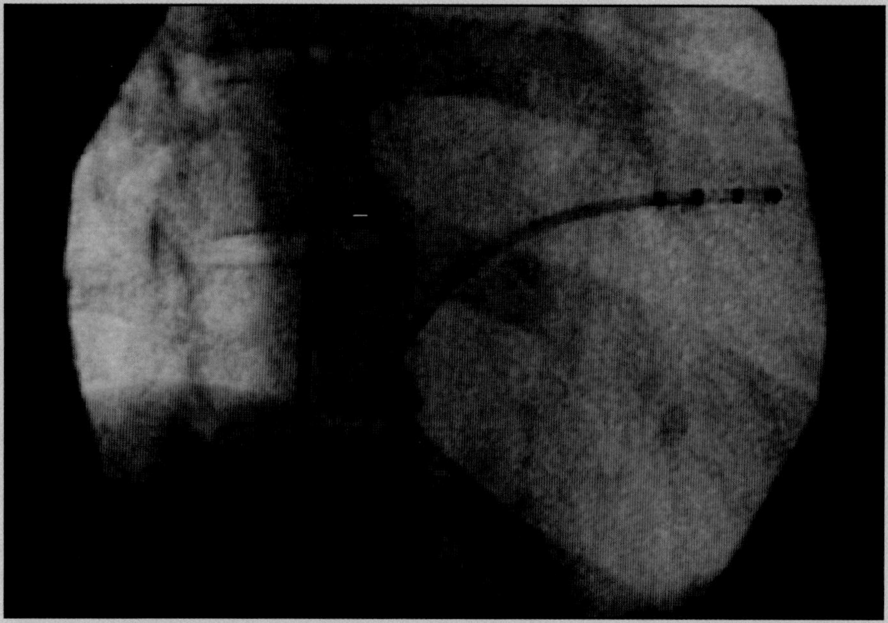

Figure 9.1: Fluoroscopic images of two catheters placed in the heart; one in the high right atrium and the other across the tricuspid valve to record the His bundle.

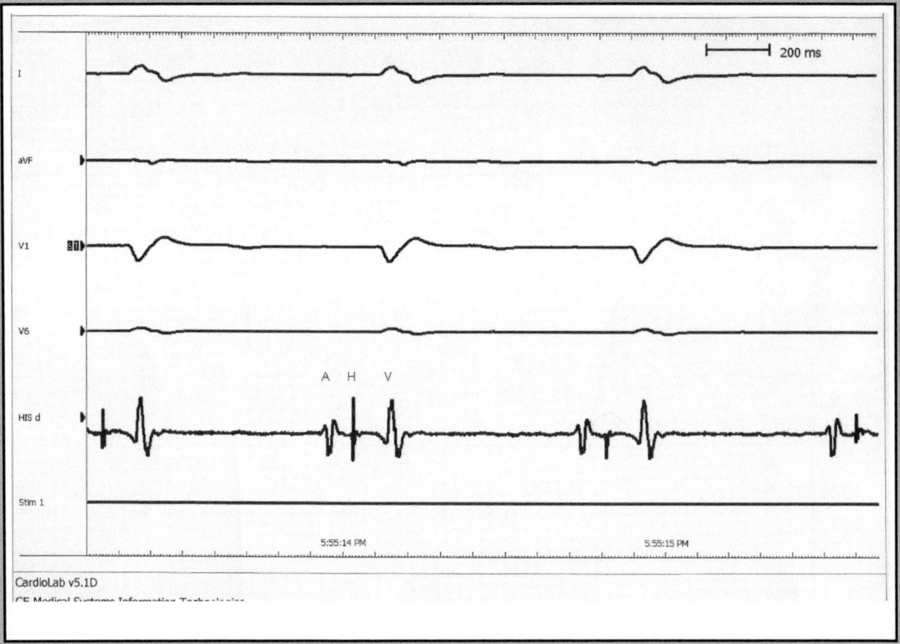

Figure 9.2: A traditional recording of the His bundle (H). The atrial and ventricular electrograms are indicated by A and V, respectively.

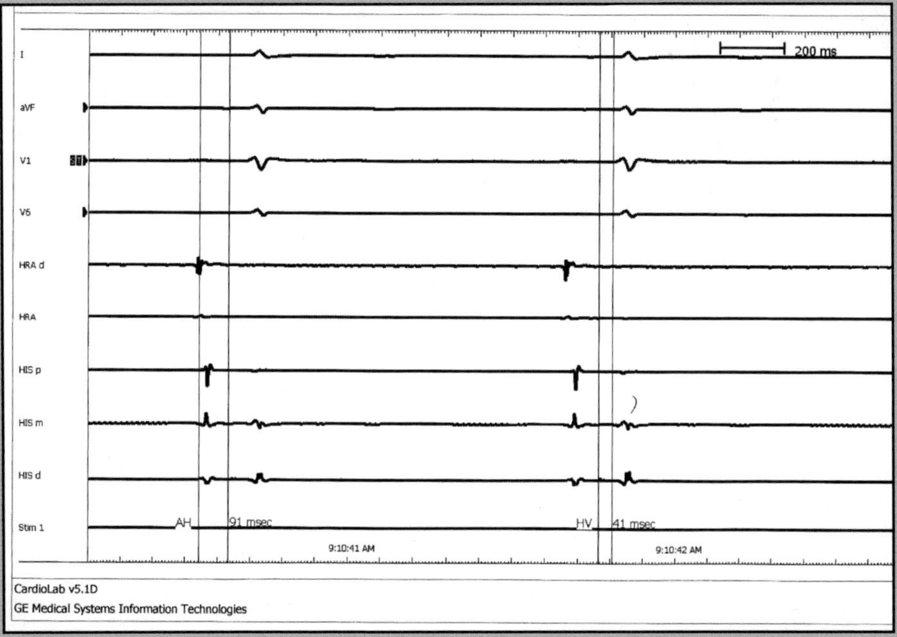

Figure 9.3: A measurement of the AH interval (a measure of AV nodal conduction) and the HV interval.

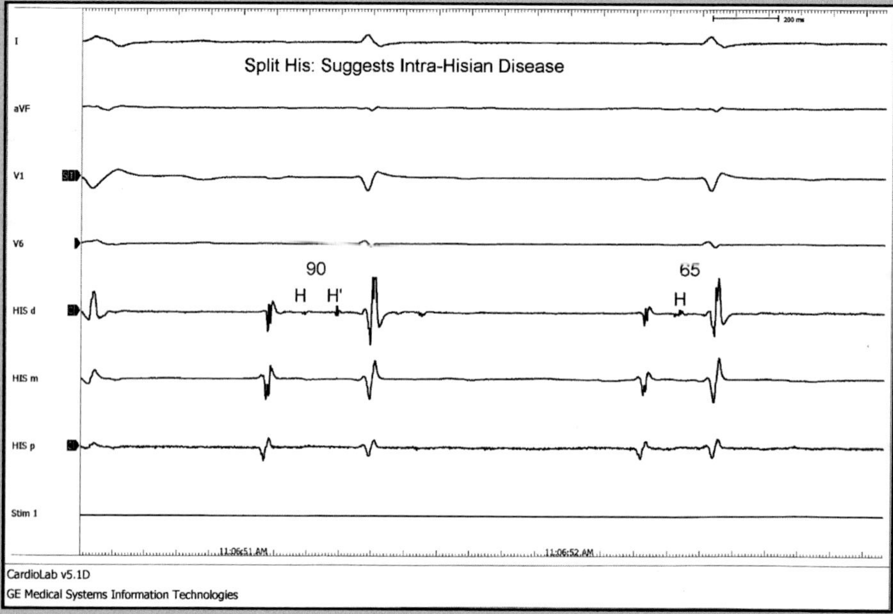

Figure 9.4: Demonstrates delay within the His bundle. The normal His bundle electrogram is not more than 25 msec in duration. This figure demonstrates marked intrahisian disease with a split His bundle electrogram having a proximal component (H) and a distal component (H') with significant intrahisian delay of 90 msec.

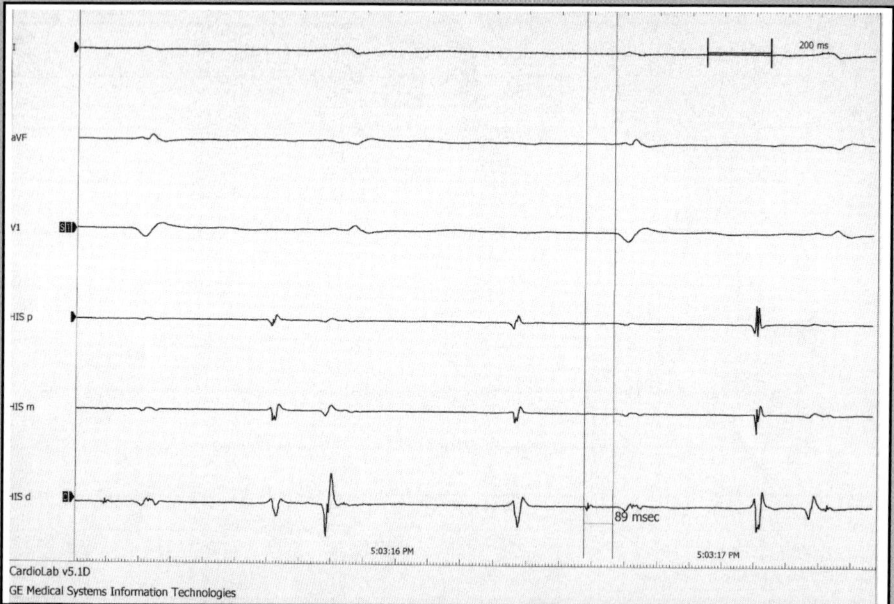

Figure 9.5: Shows an HV interval of 89 msec consistent with severe His-Purkinje disease.

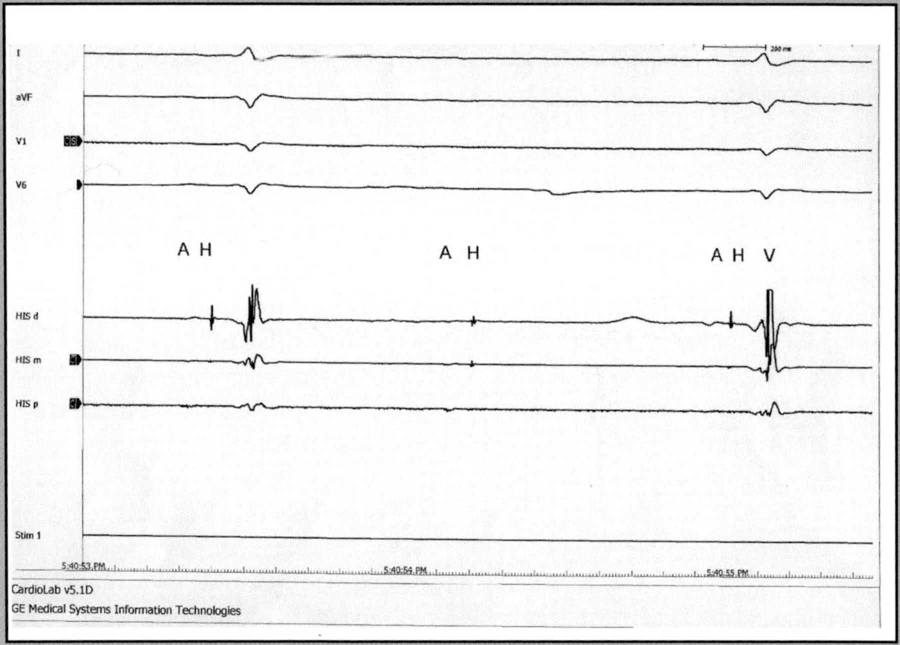

Figure 9.6: Shows Mobitz type 2 second-degree AV block with evidence of infrahisian conduction block.

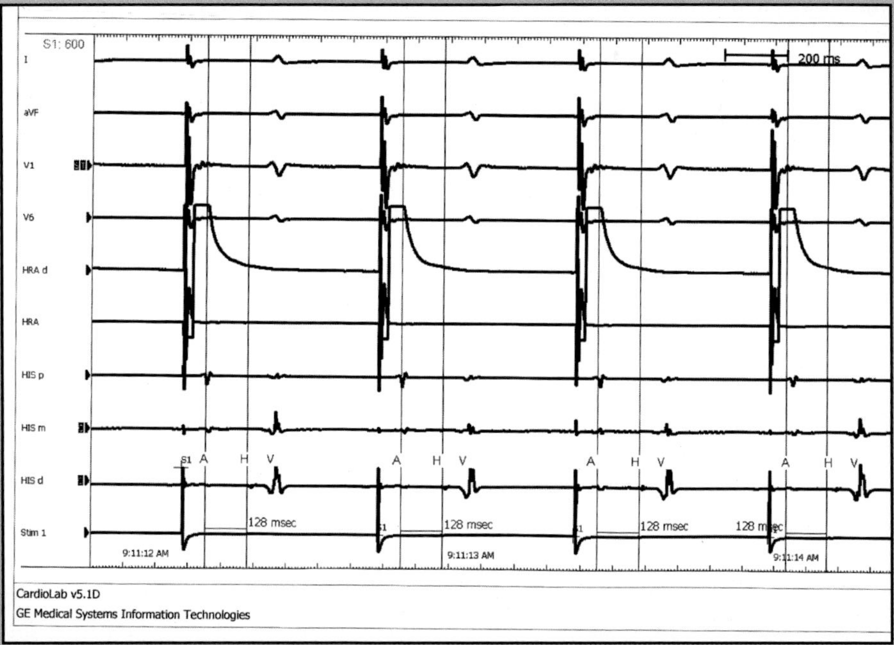

Figure 9.7: An AH interval of 128 msec during atrial pacing.

against the septum in a position to record a His bundle electrogram.)

Figure 9.2 shows the traditional recording of the His bundle. One can see the atrial recording (electrogram), which is indicated by an A. The His bundle recording is indicated by H, and the ventricular recording is indicated by V.

Conduction

Baseline Intracardiac Intervals

Figure 9.3 shows the measurement of the AH interval. The measurement is recorded in the His bundle recording and is taken from the earliest activation of the atrial signal to the earliest activation of the His bundle electrogram. A normal AH interval (a measure of the conduction time through the AV node) is 65 msec to 140 msec; figure 9.3 shows a normal AH interval of 91 msec. Table 9.1 shows the normal intracardiac measurements.

The HV interval is measured from the earliest activation in the His bundle recording to the earliest ventricular activation in any lead. A normal HV interval is between 35 and 55 msec. The HV interval of 41 msec in figure 9.3 is normal.

If the HV interval were less than 35 msec in adults (it can be < 35 mm in children), it would suggest the presence of an accessory pathway in which the accessory pathway preexcites the ventricle by bypassing the AV node. The presence of a bypass tract (preexcitation) associated with supraventricular tachycardia is called the Wolff-Parkinson-White (WPW) syndrome. The ECG typically shows a short PR interval (less than 120 msec) with slurring of the initial portion of the QRS (delta wave). (See Chapter 20 for more information on accessory pathways.)

HV prolongation occurs in the presence of His-Purkinje disease. The disease could be within the His bundle (intrahisian disease), signified by a markedly prolonged His bundle signal (more than 25 msec; figure 9.4). If the HV interval is greater than 70 msec, it is consistent with severe His-Purkinje disease (figure 9.5). Figure 9.6 shows an example of Mobitz type 2 second-degree AV block with evidence of infrahisian conduction block (block occurring below the His bundle).

Response to Atrial Pacing: Sinus Node, AV Node, and His-Purkinje Function Assessment

After the baseline intervals are measured, the atrium is paced at 100 beats per minute. In clinical electrophysiology, operators use the time period between each beat and refer to this as cycle length (often recorded in msec). One hundred beats per minute is equivalent to a 600-msec cycle length. A simple formula can convert cycle length to heart rate and vice versa:

Cycle length (msec) =
60,000 ÷ heart rate (beats per minute)

Heart rate (beats per minute) =
60,000 ÷ cycle length (msec)

In figure 9.7, the patient's right atrium is paced at 600-msec cycle length (100 beats per minute). The AH interval is 128 msec during the atrial pacing.

Sinus Node and AV Node Function

After 30 seconds of atrial pacing, the sinus node has a recovery period. Normal sinus node recovery time (SNRT) is less than or equal to 1,500 msec, as seen in figure 9.8.

In figure 9.9, the atrium is paced at 500 msec (120 beats per minute), and the AH interval continues to prolong to 160 msec. This is an example of the decremental (or delaying) properties of the AV node.

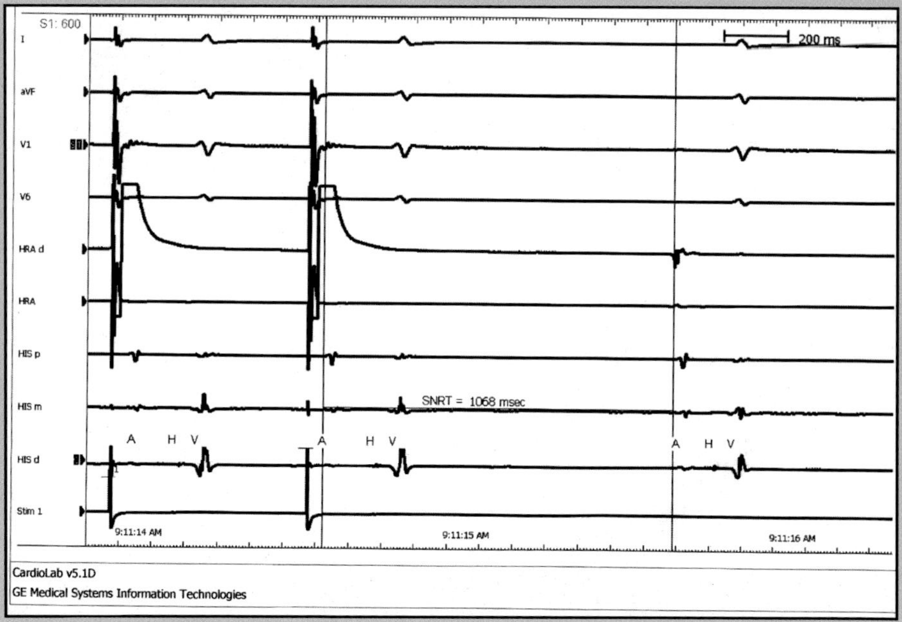

Figure 9.8: A normal sinus node recovery time is less than or equal to 1,500 msec.

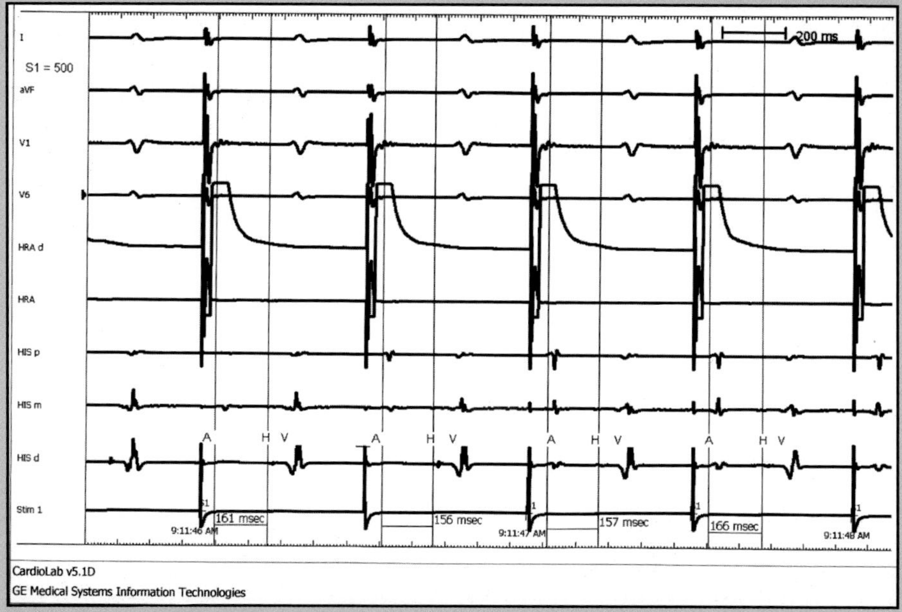

Figure 9.9: An example of the decremental (or delaying) properties of the AV node—the faster the atrium is paced, the longer the AH interval, until AV nodal blockade occurs (see figure 9.11).

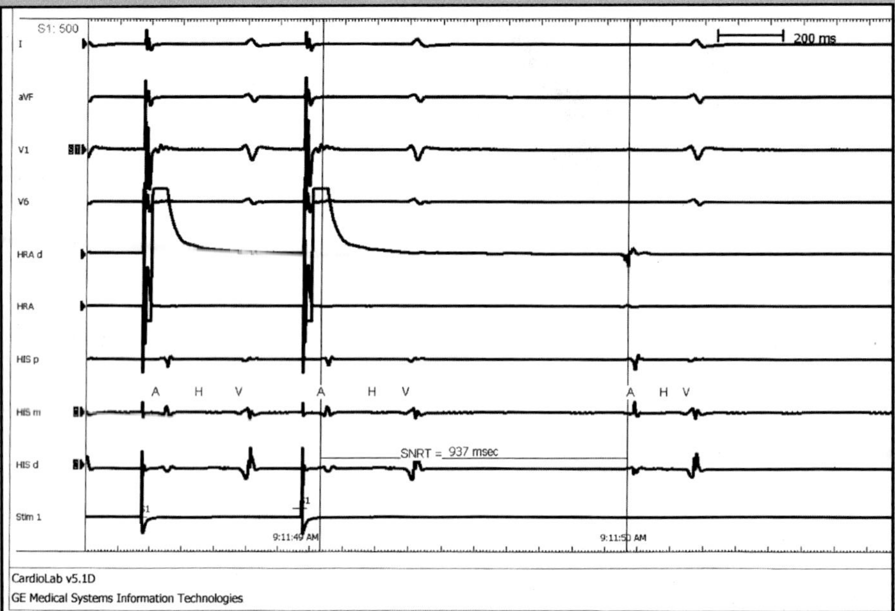

Figure 9.10: Upon the stopping of pacing, there is a sinus node recovery time of 937 msec.

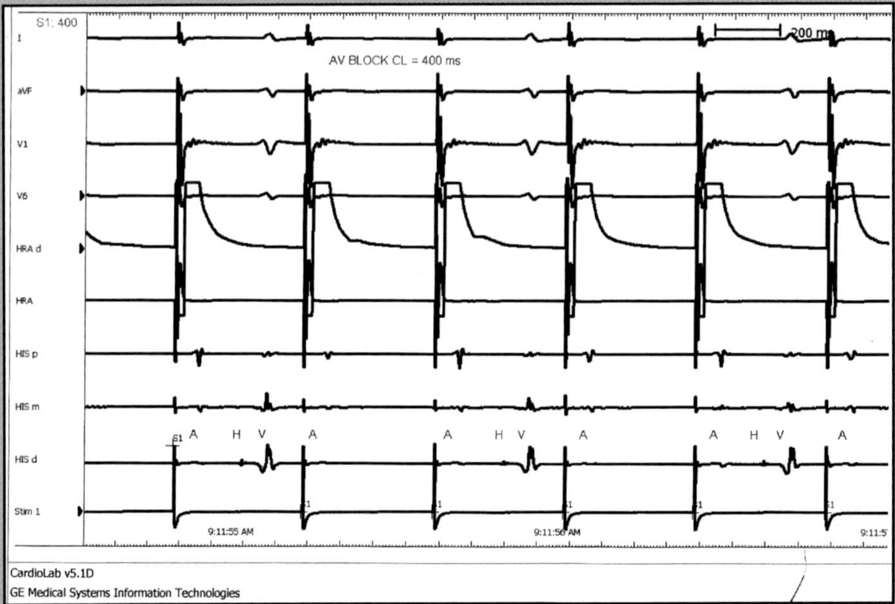

Figure 9.11: Atrial pacing at 400-msec cycle length (150 beats per minute). After the first stimulus is an atrial paced beat, followed by normal AV nodal conduction. The second atrial paced complex demonstrates block in the AV node at an AV block cycle length of 400 msec.

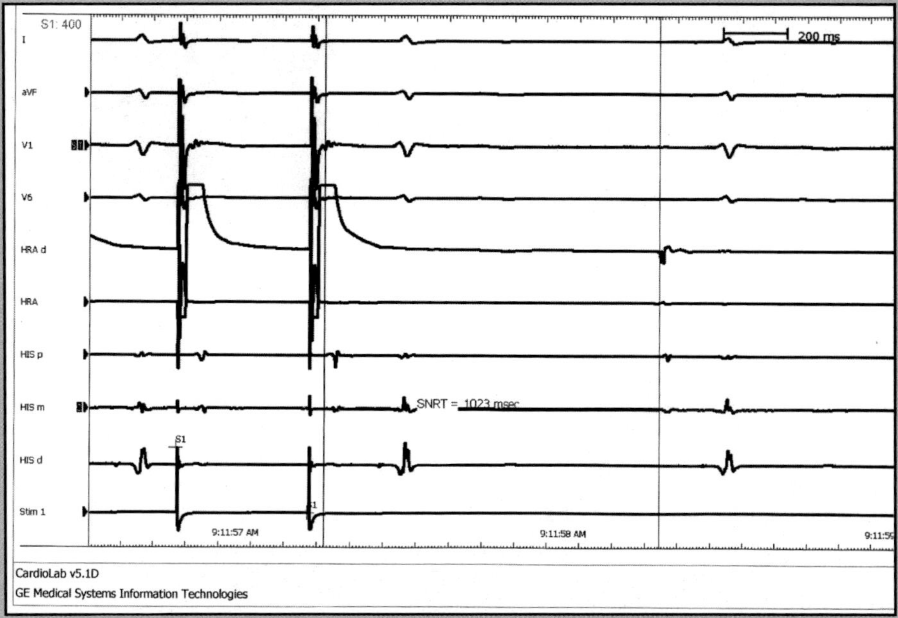

Figure 9.12: A sinus node recovery time at 400 msec of 1,023 msec. This is consistent with a normal sinus node recovery time.

In figure 9.10, upon stopping pacing, a SNRT of 937 msec is observed. Usually SNRT will increase but then decrease with more rapid paced rates due to entrance block into the sinus node.

In figure 9.11, atrial pacing at 400-msec cycle length (150 beats per minute) is observed. After the first stimulus there is an atrial paced beat followed by normal AV nodal conduction. The second paced complex, however, demonstrates no conduction to the His bundle and/or the ventricle. Conduction is blocked above the His bundle (in the AV node) with an AV block cycle length of 400 msec. This is normal AV nodal function. If the AV node conduction were diseased or affected by medications such as beta blockers and/or calcium channel blockers, conduction block might occur at cycle lengths in the 500 to 600 msec plus range. In addition, there can be enhanced AV nodal conduction in which conduction block does not occur until a cycle length of 300 msec. In this situation, there is a very little decremental conduction in the AV node.

Figure 9.12 shows the SNRT at a drive cycle length of 400 msec of 1,023 msec. This is consistent with a normal sinus node recovery time. In the electrophysiology report, only the maximum SNRT (*e.g.*, 1,068 msec), which was obtained during atrial pacing at 600 msec, is recorded. The SNRT then should be corrected for the baseline sinus cycle length that immediately preceded the pacing. The formula for determining corrected sinus node recovery time (CSNRT) is:

CSNRT = baseline sinus cycle length (SCL) - SNRT

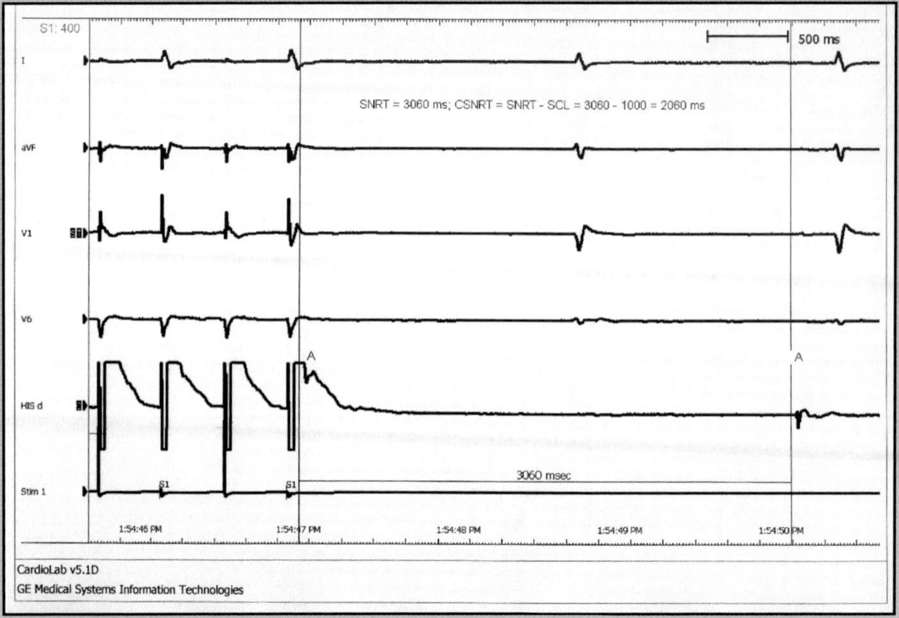

Figure 9.13: Shows severe sinus node dysfunction with a prolonged SNRT of 3,060 msec (CSNRT = 2.060 msec).

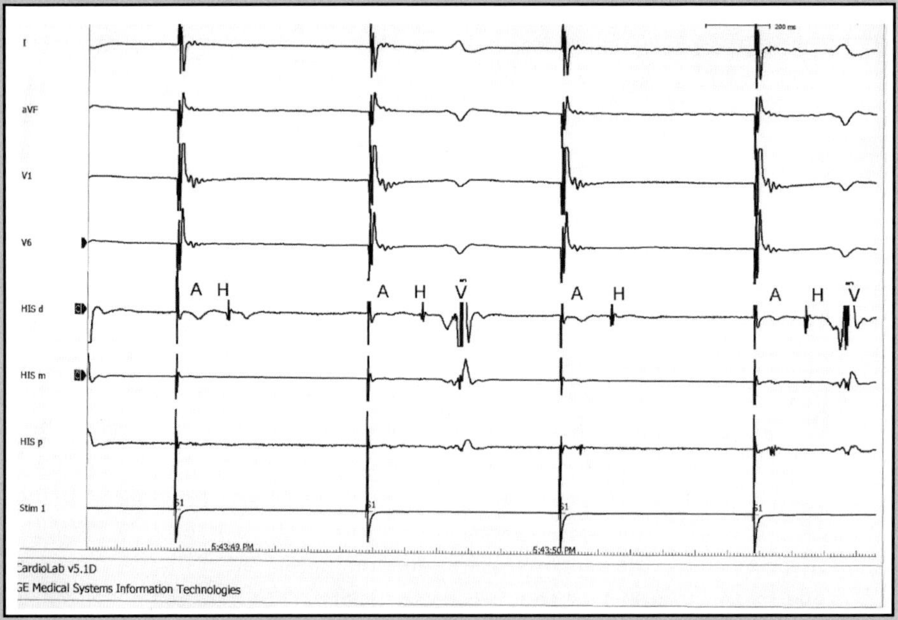

Figure 9.14: Shows infrahisian block occurring during atrial pacing a cycle length of 600 msec indicative of severe His-Purkinje disease.

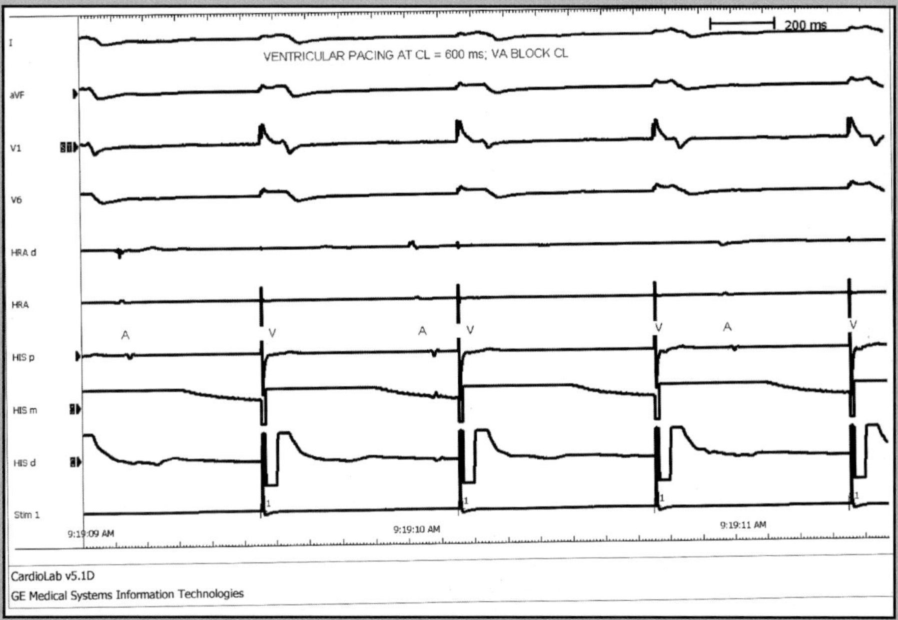

Figure 9.15: No retrograde conduction is seen while the right ventricle is paced at 600-msec cycle length.

A normal CSNRT should be less than or equal to 550 msec. In this case, the baseline sinus cycle length was approximately 1,000 msec. By subtracting the sinus cycle length from the sinus node recovery time, one derives a corrected sinus node recovery time of 68 msec, which is within normal limits. Figure 9.13 shows a prolonged SNRT of 3,060 msec consistent with significant sinus node dysfunction.

His-Purkinje Function

Finally, during atrial pacing, conduction block can occur below the His bundle. This is called infrahisian block, and is abnormal at atrial paced rates less than 150 beats/minute (or > 400 msec cycle length). In addition, infrahisian block occurring at higher atrial paced rates may be pathological, especially if the block occurs in the His-Purkinje system after consecutively conducted beats. Figure 9.14 shows infrahisian block occurring at an atrial paced cycle length of 600 msec.

Response to Ventricular Pacing

In addition, conduction from the ventricle to the atrium (retrograde conduction) can be assessed by pacing the ventricle and recording from the atrium. Figure 9.15 shows no ventricular retrograde conduction at a ventricular-paced cycle length of 600 msec.

It is important to assess conduction in both the anterograde (from the atrium to the ventricle) and the pattern of retrograde atrial activation. Retrograde conduction may be important in determining whether the patient is prone to pacemaker syndrome (feeling the effects of retrograde conduction) or pacemaker-mediated tachycardia (the pacemaker senses the retrograde

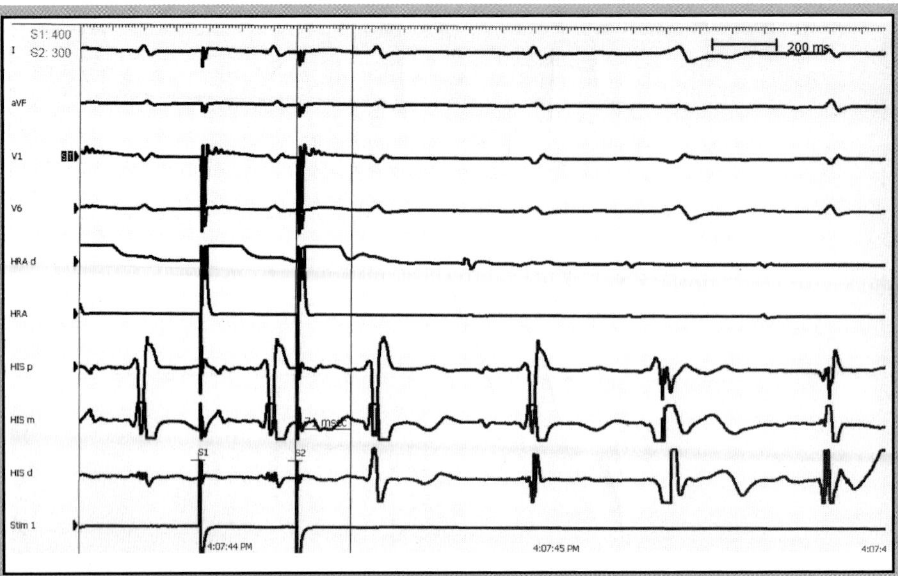

Figure 9.16: Shows programmed atrial stimulation in which pacing is performed at 150 beats per minute (cycle length of 400 msec).

atrial activity and conducts at the upper rate limit of the device). This is a routine part of the conduction portion of the electrophysiology study.

For more information on electrophysiology study indications, please refer to table 14.1 in Chapter 14.

Refractoriness

After assessing conduction, programmed electrical stimulation is performed by pacing a given chamber of the heart and introducing progressively premature extrastimuli. When looking at intracardiac electrograms, a stimulus channel often exists in which the electrical stimulus generated by the stimulator may be seen. S1 indicates a constant pacing drive train of these stimuli. S2 is the delivery of the first extrastimulus (often early or premature). The atrial or ventricular electrogram component following S1 may be indicated as A1 or V1, respectively, and the corresponding atrial or ventricular electrogram component following S2 may be indicated as A2 or V2. It is conceivable that a stimulus is delivered without a corresponding atrial or ventricular electrogram, either due to loss of capture or the delivery of the stimulus within the refractory period of the tissue as defined below. For more details, please see Chapter 14: Programmed Electrical Stimulation. Figure 9.16 shows programmed atrial stimulation in which pacing is performed at 150 beats per minute (cycle length of 400 msec). A premature atrial complex is delivered at a coupling (the distance from the last paced stimulus to the premature stimulus) cycle length of 300 msec. The AH interval is approximately 171 msec. Figure 9.17 shows progressive shortening of the premature complex (A1A2 of 280 msec). The AH interval is prolonged to 178 msec, exhibiting the decremental properties (delay) of the AV node. Figure 9.18 shows an even further shortening of the atrial

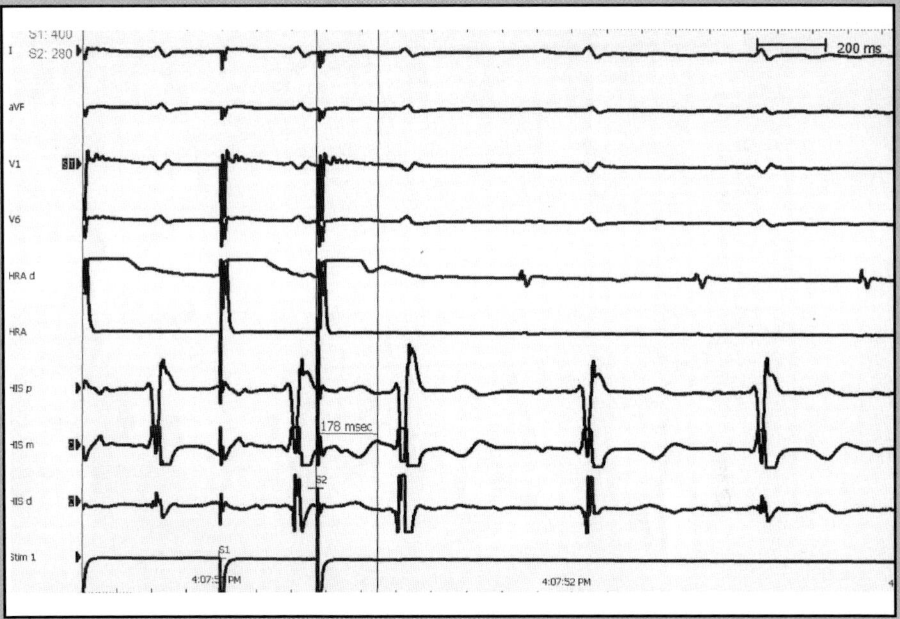

Figure 9.17: Shows progressive shortening of the premature complex (A1A2 of 280 msec). The AH interval is prolonged to 178 msec, exhibiting the decremental property (delay) of the AV node.

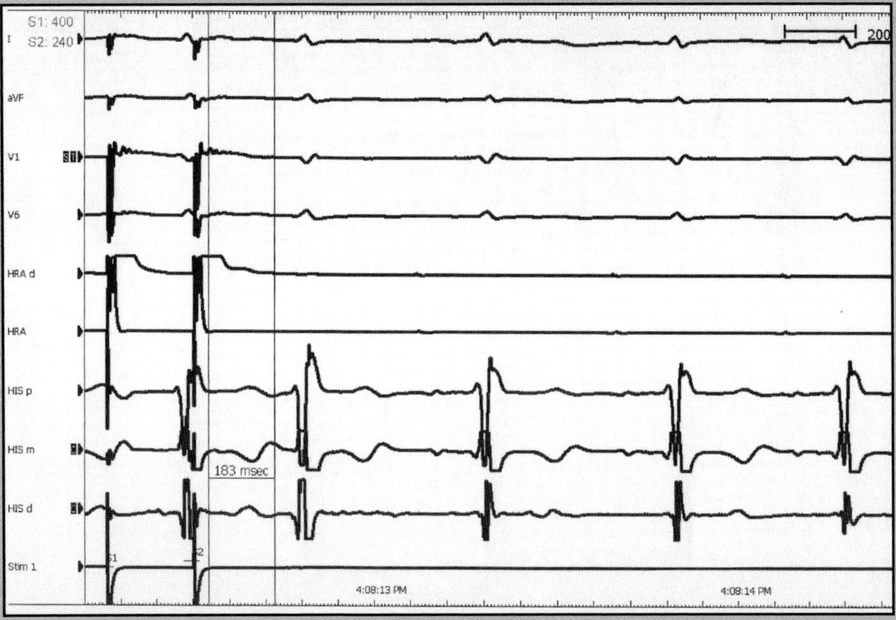

Figure 9.18: Shows an even further shortening of the atrial extrastimuli (A1A2 of 240 msec). The AH interval continues to prolong to 183 msec.

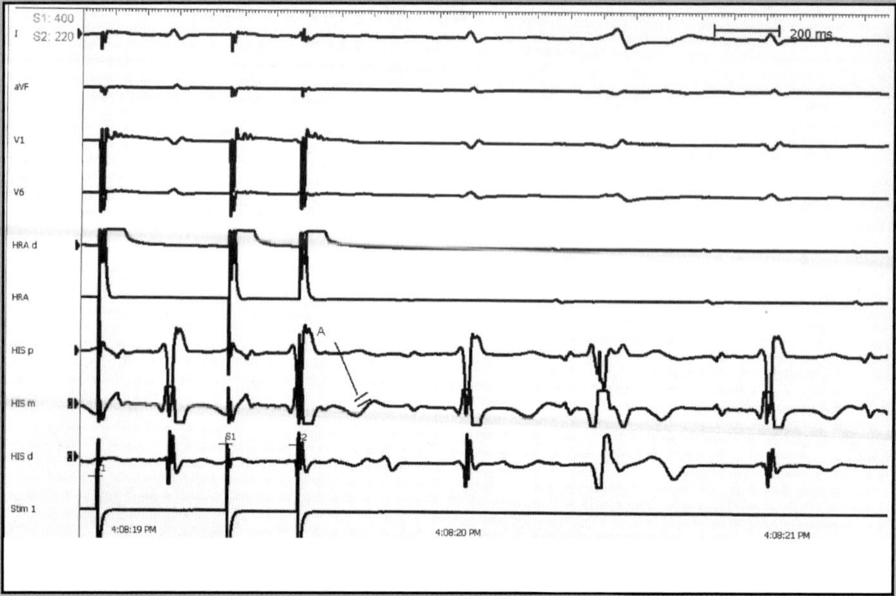

Figure 9.19: Demonstrates that at an even shorter premature coupling interval of 220 msec (A1A2 = 220 msec), there is no conduction to the His bundle of the atrial extrastimuli. This blocked premature beat demonstrates the AV node effective refractory period.

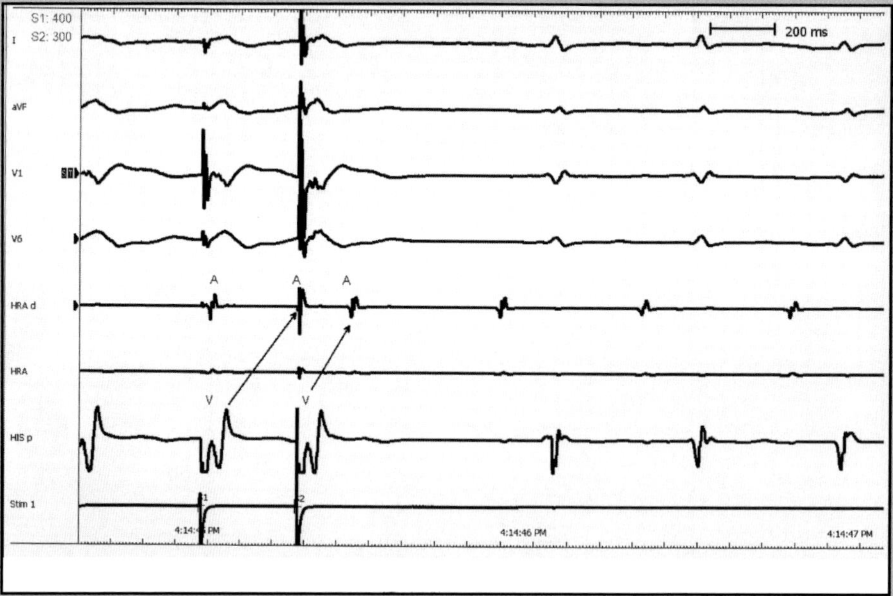

Figure 9.20: Ventricular programmed stimulation is performed in which pacing from the ventricle occurs at a cycle length of 400 msec.

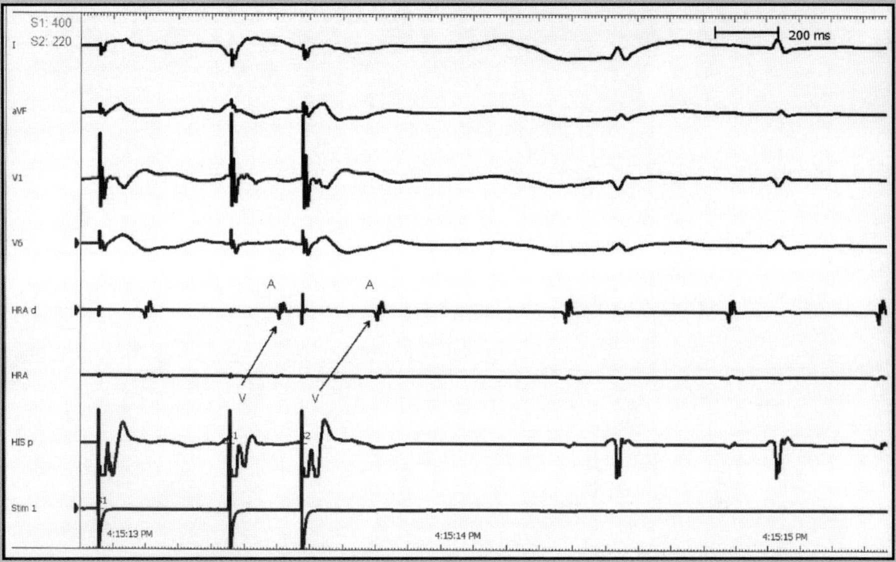

Figure 9.21: Demonstrates an increasing delay in the retrograde conduction as a result of a further shortening of ventricular premature complex coupling interval to the drive cycle length (V1V2 = 220 msec).

extrastimuli (A1A2 of 240 msec). The AH interval continues to prolong to 183 msec. Figure 9.19 demonstrates that at an even shorter premature coupling interval of 220 msec (A1A2 = 220 msec), there is no conduction to the His bundle of the atrial extrastimuli. Importantly, this blocked premature beat demonstrates the AV node effective refractory period (AVNERP). The "effective refractory period" (ERP) is the largest coupling interval in which a premature beat fails to conduct. The ERP is measured proximal to the refractory structure. In this example, a premature atrial complex fails to propagate to the His bundle. At a drive cycle length of 400 msec, the AVNERP is equal to 220 msec. Any further shortening of the atrial premature stimulation resulted in failure to stimulate the atrial tissue. This represents the atrial effective refractory period (AERP). Similarly, ventricular extrastimuli can be delivered in the same manner in order to assess the ventriculoatrial refractory period.

In figure 9.20, ventricular programmed stimulation is performed in which pacing from the ventricle occurs at a cycle length of 400 msec. The ventricular premature beat (V1V2 = 300 msec) is conducted to the atrial tissue, resulting in an atrial electrogram. In figure 9.21, there is an increasing delay in the retrograde conduction due to further shortening of ventricular premature complex coupling interval to the drive cycle length (V1V2 = 220 msec). Finally, in figure 9.22, ventricular extrastimuli delivered 180 msec from the ventricular drive cycle length (V1V2 = 180 msec) but failed to stimulate the ventricular tissue. This is representative of the ventricular effective refractory period (VERP). If the ventricle was captured via the extrastimuli but failed to conduct to the atrium, the ventriculoatrial effective refractory period (VAERP) would be

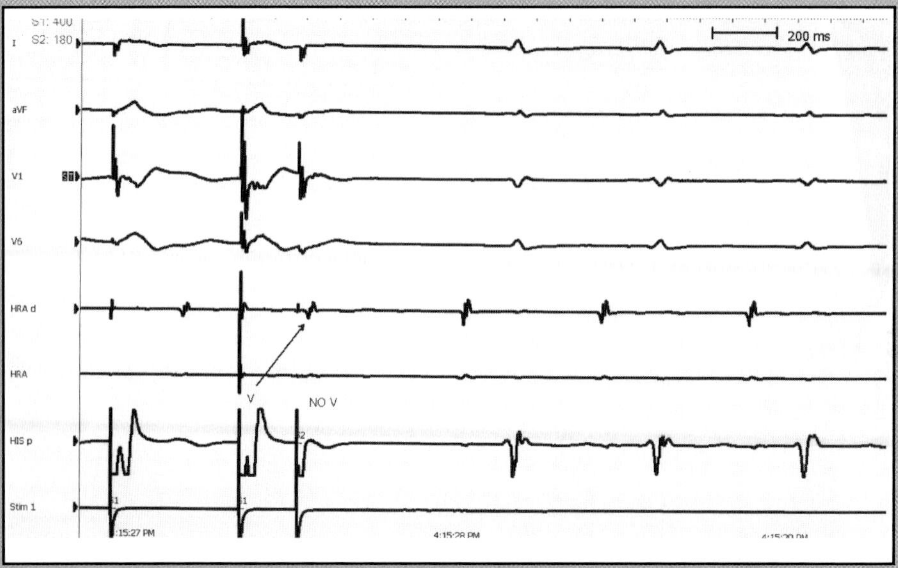

Figure 9.22: Ventricular extrastimuli delivered 180 msec from the ventricular drive cycle length (V1V2 = 180 msec), but failed to stimulate the ventricular tissue.

identified. Antiarrhythmic drugs as well as other medications have an effect on the ERPs of certain tissues. In particular, catecholamines (like isoproterenol) shorten the effective refractory period of the atrium, AV node, and the ventricle. Drugs such as amiodarone (see Chapter 11) increase the atrial, AV node, and ventricular effective refractory periods. Other less common refractory periods can also be determined. The relative refractory period is the longest coupling interval for which a premature extrastimuli exhibits delayed conduction through a given tissue. The functional refractory period measures the output from a given tissue and is defined by the shortest conducted interval between two delivered impulses (S1S2). For practical purposes, the ERP is used and measured almost exclusively in most electrophysiology laboratories.

Chapter 10

Mechanisms of Arrhythmias

Arrhythmias can be mechanistically separated into those due to abnormal impulse generation and those due to abnormal impulse conduction (table 10.1). The mechanisms of arrhythmias may be broken down into three categories: reentry, automaticity, and triggered arrhythmias.

Reentry

The reentry mechanism of arrhythmias has been well defined by Mines, who hypothesized that bidirectional conduction with unidirectional block leads to reentry. Figure 10.1 shows an example of reentry. This is very common in patients who have ventricular tachycardia with a scar in which there is slow conduction in one area, allowing for recovery with the ability for conduction to travel up another area, thus creating a circus movement tachycardia. Reentry is likely the mechanism responsible for the majority of clinically significant tachycardias.

For a reentrant tachycardia to exist, several conditions need to be met: 1) there must be a zone of tissue that conducts slowly; 2) unidirectional block must occur in part of the tissue involved in the reentrant circuit; and 3) the conduction velocity must be slow enough to allow the blocked tissue to recover.

Automaticity

In the second arrhythmia mechanism, automaticity, myocardial tissue may fire on its own periodically much like a pacemaker.

Table 10.1: Mechanisms of Arrhythmias

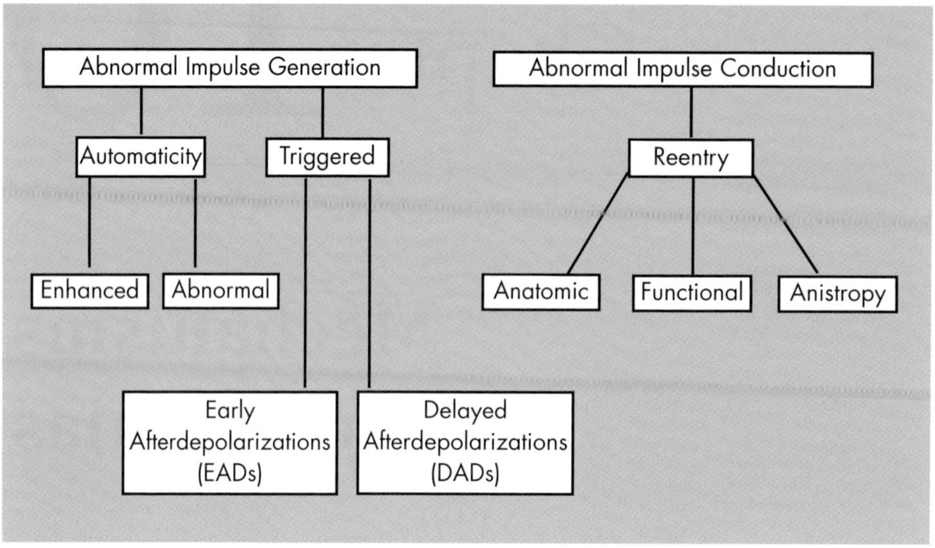

Automaticity refers to the ability of cardiac cells to spontaneously and repetitively depolarize in the absence of external stimulation. Conduction is the propagation of the depolarization across cells or tissue. When impairment of conduction is of clinical significance, it usually results in a bradycardia.

Normal automaticity is dictated by the rate of phase 4 depolarization. In abnormal automaticity, the rate of phase 4 depolarization may be slowed or the threshold potential increased—that is, the level that triggers the rapid phase 0 depolarization may be elevated. This would result in a bradycardia. Conversely, a tachycardia would result if the rate of phase 4 depolarization was increased or the threshold potential decreased. Arrhythmias caused by abnormal automaticity usually show gradual acceleration and deceleration ("warm-up and cool-down phenomena") (figure 10.2).

Triggered

The third method, a triggered arrhythmia, often occurs as a result of afterdepolarizations (figure 10.3). Little humps that occur after the action potential, that occur as a result of changes in membrane voltage, can trigger an arrhythmia. Early afterdepolarizations (EADs) occur during phase 2 or 3 of the action potential and may be related to the reopening of the L-type calcium channel. EADs may occur in long QT syndrome and may be induced by cesium.

Delayed afterdepolarizations (DADs) occur in phase 4 of the action potential and are most likely caused by changes in the transient inward current. Digitalis toxicity induced arrhythmias, accelerated idioventricular rhythm after myocardial infarction, and possibly even right ventricular outflow tract tachycardia may be caused by DADs. Treatments may be directed toward suppression of these afterdepolarizations

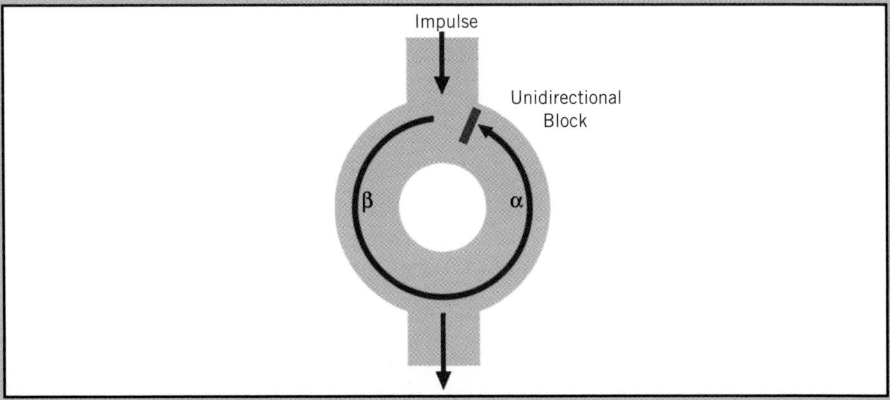

Figure 10.1: Demonstrates an example of reentry. An impulse finds 2 pathways (α and β); one is blocked (α = refractory), the other (β) permits conduction. The impulse can turn around and the original blocked pathway now can accept the impulse. A "circus movement" tachycardia results.

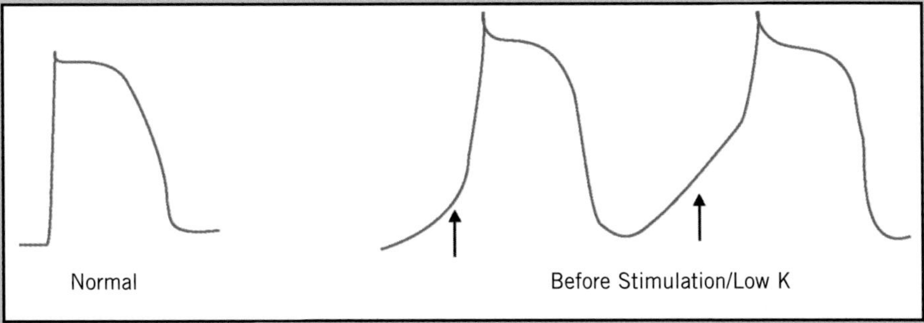

Figure 10.2: Shows automaticity which may enhance phase 4 depolarization (which might occur from catecholamines or hypokalemia).

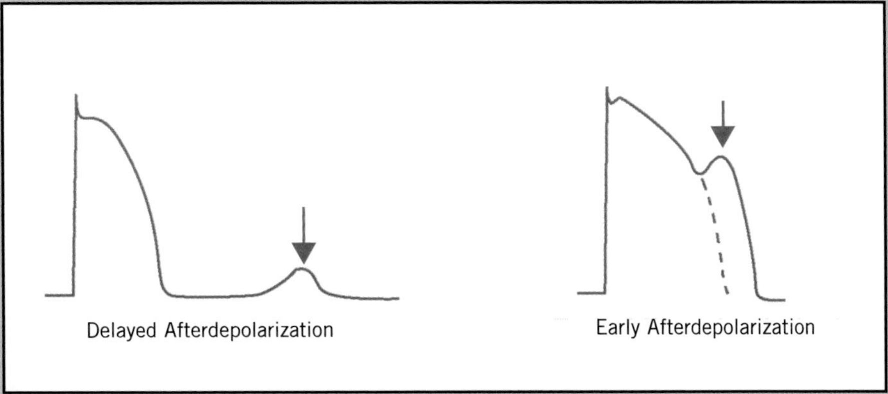

Figure 10.3: A triggered arrhythmia often occurs as a result of afterdepolarizations.

(either by treating drug toxicity, pharmacologic suppression of EADs or DADs, or ablating the inciting myocardial focus.

It is important to understand an arrhythmia's mechanism prior to treatment. First, if it is due to a reversible problem such as ischemia, drug toxicity, or an electrolyte abnormality, the treatment is to correct that abnormality. Second, reentrant arrhythmias can be treated by disrupting the reentrant circuit. For typical atrial flutter, creating a linear set of catheter ablation lesions which completely blocks the cavotricuspid isthmus (the region in which all flutter waves traverse) can achieve this goal. Similarly, catheter ablation of the critical slow zone for myocardial ventricular tachycardia in patients with coronary artery disease can result in a successful outcome. Third, focal tachycardias (*i.e.*, triggered or automatic) can be approached by catheter mapping and identification of the tachycardia's site of origin. Catheter ablation at that location can eliminate the tachycardia. In addition, linear block (around the orifice of the pulmonary veins) can prevent triggered potentials (arising from the pulmonary veins) from escaping and depolarizing the left atrium, which might provoke atrial fibrillation. Finally, drug therapy (pharmacotherapy) attempts to target critical mechanisms of action at the cellular level (see Chapter 11). Triggered arrhythmias, for example, may be suppressed by adenosine, calcium channel blockers or sodium channel blockers. An understanding of the mechanisms of both arrhythmias and the mechanism of action of medications is essential to optimal pharmacotherapy.

Chapter 11

Pharmacotherapy

The most widely used classification system for antiarrhythmic drugs is a modification of the system proposed by Vaughan Williams (table 11.1). It classifies drugs according to their effects on action potentials in individual cells. Class I drugs block sodium channels responsible for the fast response in atrial, ventricular, and Purkinje tissues, thus depressing conduction velocity. Class II drugs are beta-adrenergic receptor antagonists (or beta blockers). Class III drugs prolong cardiac repolarization, predominantly by blocking potassium channels during phases 2 and 3 of the action potential, thereby increasing tissue refractoriness. Class IV drugs block calcium channels (calcium channel blockers), depressing the slow response in sinus nodal and AV nodal cells, and perhaps in other cells as well.

This classification system is an oversimplification, however, and does not account for many other effects. Additionally, it does not account for the multiple effects a drug may have on cardiac cells. For example, sotalol has beta-blocking activity (Class II), but it also significantly prolongs the action potential duration (Class III). Another drug, amiodarone, has been shown to have Class I, II, III, and IV effects and perhaps others as well. Furthermore, many drugs undergo metabolism to electrophysiologically active metabolites, which may have electrophysiologic effects that differ from those of the parent compound.

Antiarrhythmic drugs are generally considered potential cardiac toxins and must be used with caution. Almost all antiarrhythmic

Table 11.1: Modified Vaughan Williams Classification of Antiarrhythmic Drugs

Class	Main Electrophysiologic Properties	Examples
Ia	Sodium-channel blockage Intermediate channel kinetics	Quinidine Procainamide
Ib	Sodium-channel blockade Rapid channel kinetics	Lidocaine Mexiletine Tocainide
Ic	Sodium-channel blockade Slow channel kinetics	Flecainide Propafenone Moricizine
II	Beta-adrenergic blockade	Propranolol Esmolol Acebutolol
III	Potassium-channel blockade Sodium-channel activation	Sotalol Amiodarone Ibutilide Dofetilide
IV	Calcium-channel blockade	Verapamil Diltiazem

drugs have the potential for producing proarrhythmia (figure 11.1). Proarrhythmia is the potentiation of life-threatening ventricular tachycardia and/or ventricular fibrillation (including torsades de pointes, a polymorphic ventricular tachycardia that twists upon an axis) and is often (but not necessarily) associated with QT prolongation.

The most commonly prescribed antiarrhythmic drugs are procainamide, lidocaine, mexiletine, flecainide, propafenone, sotalol, amiodarone, and dofetilide. These drugs are prescribed with the intent of effective control of cardiac arrhythmias.

Class Ia Antiarrhythmic Drugs

Class Ia drugs block the sodium channel and fast response, predominantly in atrial, ventricular, and Purkinje tissue. The maximum rate of rise of phase 0 of the action potential is depressed, slowing conduction velocity. The potency of channel blockade is moderate, and repolarization is prolonged. Class Ia antiarrhythmic drugs

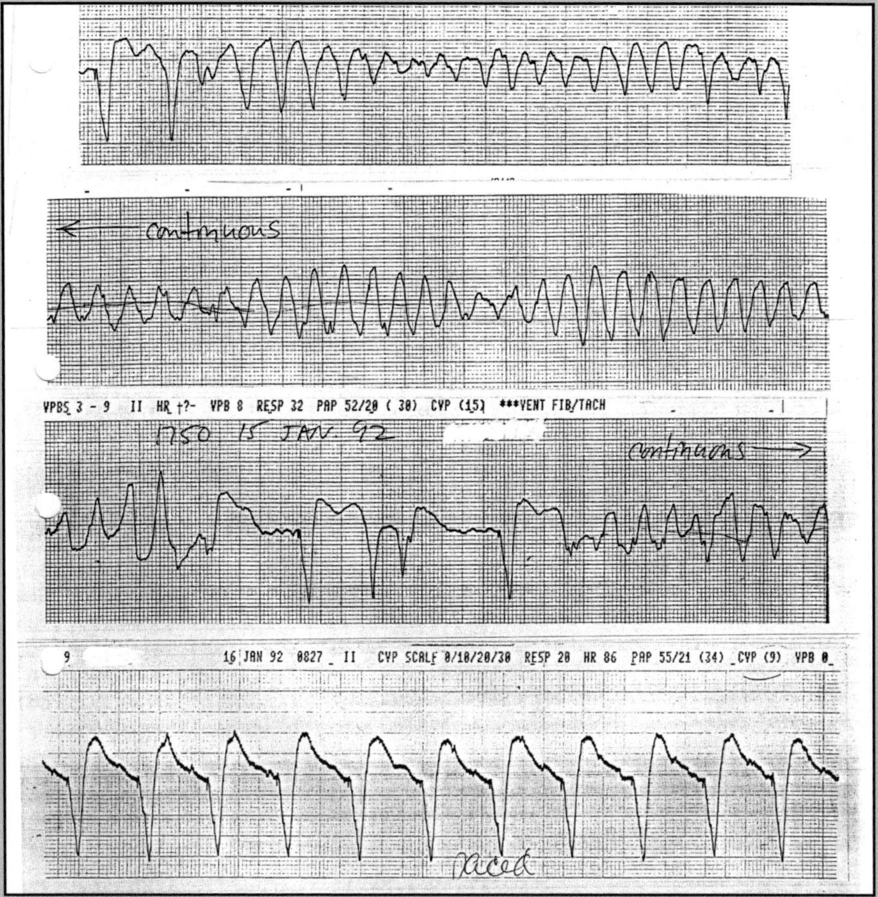

Figure 11.1: An example of amiodarone-induced torsade de pointes. When it occurs with amiodarone, it is almost always associated with hypokalemia. This condition is much more common with other antiarrhythmic drugs (in particular, Class Ia and other Class III drugs).

are effective for many atrial and ventricular tachyarrhythmias.

Procainamide is an antiarrhythmic medication derived from procaine hydrochloride (an anesthetic agent), but with less central nervous system (CNS) action. As a Class Ia medication, it decreases phase 0 of the action potential, decreases the amplitude of the action potential, and slows conduction velocity in atrial, ventricular, and Purkinje tissues. In addition, procainamide increases the effective refractory periods of atrial and ventricular cells. Sinus node automaticity is usually not affected. The metabolite of procainamide (N-acetyl procainamide, also called NAPA) has different electrophysiologic effects, predominantly Class III properties in which there is prolongation of the duration of the action potential (prolonging the QT and QRS intervals).

Procainamide can effectively suppress a variety of atrial, AV-nodal, and ventricular tachyarrhythmias; it can also benefit 20 to 30 percent of patients with sustained ventricular tachyarrhythmias. Procainamide is favored above other antiarrhythmic drugs in the acute medical treatment of wide-complex tachycardias of unknown etiology, including atrial fibrillation with ventricular preexcitation. It may also be infused during electrophysiologic testing to stress His-Purkinje conduction, to provoke a Brugada pattern on ECG (ST segment elevation in V1-3 in the setting of right bundle branch block), and occasionally to slow or suppress ventricular tachycardia. Failure to suppress inducibility of ventricular tachycardia by procainamide during electrophysiologic testing often predicts failure with other antiarrhythmic drugs.

The majority of procainamide's side effects are gastrointestinal, with nausea, vomiting, anorexia, or diarrhea occurring regularly. Dizziness, mental depression, and psychosis have been reported as well. Drug-induced fever, rash, and hepatitis may occur. A drug-induced lupus syndrome with arthralgias and arthritis has been reported in response to prolonged exposure to procainamide. Fortunately, unlike other Class Ia agents, procainamide does not significantly interfere with other drugs; prescribing amiodarone to a patient on procainamide is not recommended, however, since it increases procainamide levels, and the Class III effects of its metabolite, NAPA, plus amiodarone, may exacerbate QRS and QT prolongation and promote proarrhythmia. Increased NAPA levels can lead to torsades, especially in patients with poor renal function.

Class Ib Antiarrhythmic Drugs

Class Ib drugs also block sodium channels, but to a lesser degree than Class Ia drugs. Repolarization tends to be mildly shortened with the use of Class Ib drugs, and they often suppress premature ventricular contractions, but they are only occasionally effective as monotherapy for life-threatening ventricular tachyarrhythmias. Class Ib drugs are generally ineffective for atrial arrhythmias.

Lidocaine is an intravenous medication with local anesthetic and cardiac depressant characteristics that shortens the action potential duration and effective refractory period of Purkinje and ventricular tissues. At high concentrations, it depresses the rate of rise of phase 0 of the action potential and decreases conduction velocity in Purkinje fibers. In patients with severe His-Purkinje system disease, lidocaine may precipitate complete AV block. Lidocaine may occasionally depress both the sinus node and potential subsidiary escape pacemakers, causing asystolic pauses. The drug can be effective for the suppression of ventricular tachyarrhythmias, particularly in patients with myocardial ischemia. Prophylactic use of lidocaine after myocardial infarction, once quite common, has been abandoned.

The side effects of lidocaine most commonly involve the central nervous system. Early effects include dizziness and drowsiness, while prolonged use can produce hallucinations, confusion, and muscle tremor, which presage impending seizures, respiratory arrest, or cardiac arrest.

Mexiletine is an oral antiarrhythmic medication with electrophysiologic properties similar to those of lidocaine. Mexiletine decreases the rate of rise of phase 0 of the action potential and shortens the action potential's duration. The effective refractory period is decreased in Purkinje tissue but not in ventricular muscle. The slope of phase 4 diastolic depolarization is also decreased. In patients with normal His-Purkinje function, no significant changes are observed with the use of mexiletine, nor do any significant changes occur in the PR, QRS, or QT intervals.

Mexiletine may be used to suppress frequent and high-grade ventricular arrhythmias, including those that have failed to respond to Class Ia agents. Used alone, it is infrequently effective in suppressing life-threatening ventricular arrhythmias. In combination with Class Ia agents, however, efficacy increases, while toxicity decreases. It can also be used in concert with amiodarone or sotalol in patients with refractory ventricular tachycardia.

Side effects are common with mexiletine, occurring in up to 60 percent of patients in some series. The majority of side effects reported are related to the central nervous system and include dizziness, drowsiness, tremors, slurred speech, blurred vision, memory impairment, and mood swings. Seizures have rarely been reported; adverse cardiac effects such as worsening of congestive heart failure and proarrhythmic effects have also rarely been reported.

No specific adverse effects have been reported with the combination of mexiletine with other cardiotonic agents. Drugs interfering with hepatic enzymes do affect the metabolism of mexiletine, however.

Class Ic Antiarrhythmic Drugs

Class Ic drugs are potent sodium-channel blocking agents. They have little effect on repolarization. Class Ic drug effects are potentiated at increased heart rates due to its use-dependent effects. They are effective for a variety of atrial and ventricular tachyarrhythmias, and are highly effective in suppressing chronic ventricular ectopy.

Unfortunately, the marked slowing of conduction induced by these agents is an efficient mechanism to induce ventricular proarrhythmia. This effect is most marked in patients with significant structural heart disease, but may also occur in normal individuals, especially in the setting of rapid heart rates such as those induced by exercise.

Propafenone is an antiarrhythmic medication that has a weak beta-blocking activity. The drug is generally well tolerated. It is approved for the treatment of life-threatening ventricular arrhythmias and supraventricular arrhythmias in patients with structurally normal hearts. Propafenone is most useful in treating atrial fibrillation and/or atrial flutter in structurally normal hearts. It is rarely, if ever, used for ventricular tachycardia.

By blocking the fast inward sodium current in atrial, ventricular, and His-Purkinje tissue, propafenone decreases the rate of rise of phase 0 of the action potential. In addition, propafenone possesses weak beta-adrenergic and calcium-channel antagonist activities, and it suppresses delayed afterdepolarizations in ischemic Purkinje fibers. Electrocardiographic effects include prolongation of the PR and QRS intervals without significant change of the QT interval.

Like other Class Ic antiarrhythmic agents, propafenone is effective in suppressing frequent premature ventricular contractions, including complex forms. It should be used cautiously in patients with a history of myocardial infarction in view of the findings of the Cardiac Arrhythmia Suppression Trial (CAST), which showed an increased mortality in this population when treated with other Class Ic drugs (flecainide, encainide, and moricizine).

Side effects of propafenone include the worsening of ventricular arrhythmias (in approximately six percent). Gastrointestinal side effects and those related to the central nervous system are common, with dizziness, lightheadedness, nausea, vomiting, and a metallic taste the most common.

Flecainide is a potent antiarrhythmic, effective predominantly for treating supraventricular tachycardia. Although it is very effective at suppressing ventricular premature contraction in patients with a prior myocardial infarction, it is associated with a higher mortality than placebo in this population. A derivative of procainamide, flecainide exhibits potent sodium-channel blocking action, depression of phase 0 of the action potential, and slowing of conduction in a frequency- and dose-dependent manner throughout the heart. His-Purkinje tissue and ventricular muscle are affected the most, followed by atrial muscle, accessory pathways, and AV-nodal tissue. In most studies, the action potential duration is not significantly affected. Thus, flecainide is useful in suppressing both supraventricular and ventricular tachyarrhythmias and premature contractions. It is able to suppress chronic premature ventricular contractions by more than 75 percent and repetitive forms by more than 90 percent. Flecainide is effective at preventing supraventricular tachycardia, including atrial fibrillation and flutter, as well as accessory-pathway mediated tachycardias. It should not be used in patients with structural heart disease as a result of the CAST study.

The majority of side effects of flecainide are neurologic and cardiac, including blurred vision, headache, dizziness, paresthesia, tremors, skin rash, abdominal pain, diarrhea, and impotence, as well as worsening of arrhythmias, slowed conduction or heart block, and aggravation of congestive heart failure. Occasionally this medication in concert with a calcium-channel blocker, a beta-blocker, and/or digitalis may result in significant sinus node dysfunction. In addition, Class Ic agents may produce atrial flutter in the course of treating patients with atrial fibrillation.

Class II Antiarrhythmic Drugs

Class II drugs are beta-adrenergic blockers. Beta-blockers vary with respect to lipid solubility, membrane stabilizing effect, and relative specificity for the beta receptor, cardioselectivity, and partial agonist activity. Class II agents are useful for the treatment of many atrial and AV-nodal arrhythmias. They help with rate control of atrial fibrillation and flutter, as well as suppression of other types of supraventricular tachycardia by blocking the AV node. In addition, these medications can be helpful adjuncts in controlling ischemically-mediated arrhythmias (ventricular tachycardia/fibrillation).

Class III Antiarrhythmic Drugs

Class III drugs prolong the duration of action potential and increase refractoriness. The effect is often mediated by blockade of potassium channels during phase 2 or 3 of the action potential.

Amiodarone is an antianginal and antiarrhythmic drug. It increases the duration of ventricular and atrial muscle action by inhibiting sodium, potassium-activated myocardial adenosine triphosphatase. There is a resultant decrease in heart rate and vascular resistance.

Amiodarone has been shown to have Class I, II, III, and IV effects. It is a weak, noncompetitive inhibitor of alpha- and beta-adrenergic receptors. Its predominant action is to prolong the duration of the action potential and to increase refractoriness; it has only slight effects on the rate of rise of phase 0 of the action potential. Amiodarone slows the sinus rate and prolongs the PR, QRS, and QT intervals.

A large number of studies have documented the efficacy of amiodarone in suppressing supraventricular and ventricular arrhythmias, even when other agents were ineffective. Amiodarone is very effective in chronic maintenance of sinus rhythm in patients with atrial fibrillation, although it is not yet approved for that purpose.

Amiodarone affects almost every organ system. Corneal microdeposits are expected, abnormal thyroid function tests are common, and clinical hypothyroidism or hyperthyroidism becomes evident in two to four percent of patients. A blue-gray skin discoloration may occur as well as photosensitivity. Liver function abnormalities, neuropathy, myositis, and severe hepatitis occur infrequently. Pulmonary fibrosis is one of the most severe, and rare, complications related to amiodarone. Baseline pulmonary function, thyroid function, and liver function tests should be obtained before initiating therapy.

Caution should also be used when prescribing amiodarone due to interactions with many other drugs. In particular, amiodarone augments the effects of digitalis and warfarin.

In low doses, amiodarone may suppress atrial fibrillation or flutter. Higher doses are useful for ventricular tachycardia suppression. The intravenous formulation is helpful in treating recurrent episodes of ventricular tachycardia and fibrillation. Unlike other antiarrhythmic drugs, amiodarone very rarely causes proarrhythmia, and if it occurs, it is almost always associated with hypokalemia.

Sotalol is another potassium blocker with beta-blocking properties that is used in the treatment of life-threatening arrhythmias. It is a nonselective beta-adrenergic antagonist introduced for the treatment of hypertension. By prolonging the action potential duration, it has antiarrhythmic effects in humans. It also causes an increase in refractory period of human atria, ventricles, AV nodes, Purkinje fibers, and accessory pathways.

Side effects of sotalol include an increase in bronchospasm, fatigue, impotence, depression, and headache, as well as sinus node slowing, AV block, hypotension, and worsening of congestive heart failure. This medication also exhibits dose-related proarrhythmia. On the brighter side, significant drug interactions are infrequent. This medication is useful for the treatment of atrial fibrillation and flutter, and may be helpful in patients with ventricular tachycardia and implantable defibrillators.

Dofetilide has the ability to block only the ion channel carrying the rapid component of the delayed rectifier potassium current, while having no effect on sodium channels, alpha receptors or beta receptors. It increases the duration of action potentials in a predictable, concentration-dependent manner, primarily due to

Table 11.2: Algorithm for Dofetilide Prescribing and Dosing (Copyright Pfizer Inc.; reproduced with permission). PfizerLab. (2004, March). Tikosyn [Pamphlet]. United States of America: Pfizer. Retrieved August 12, 2008, from http://www.pfizer.com/files/products/ uspi_tikosyn.pdf.

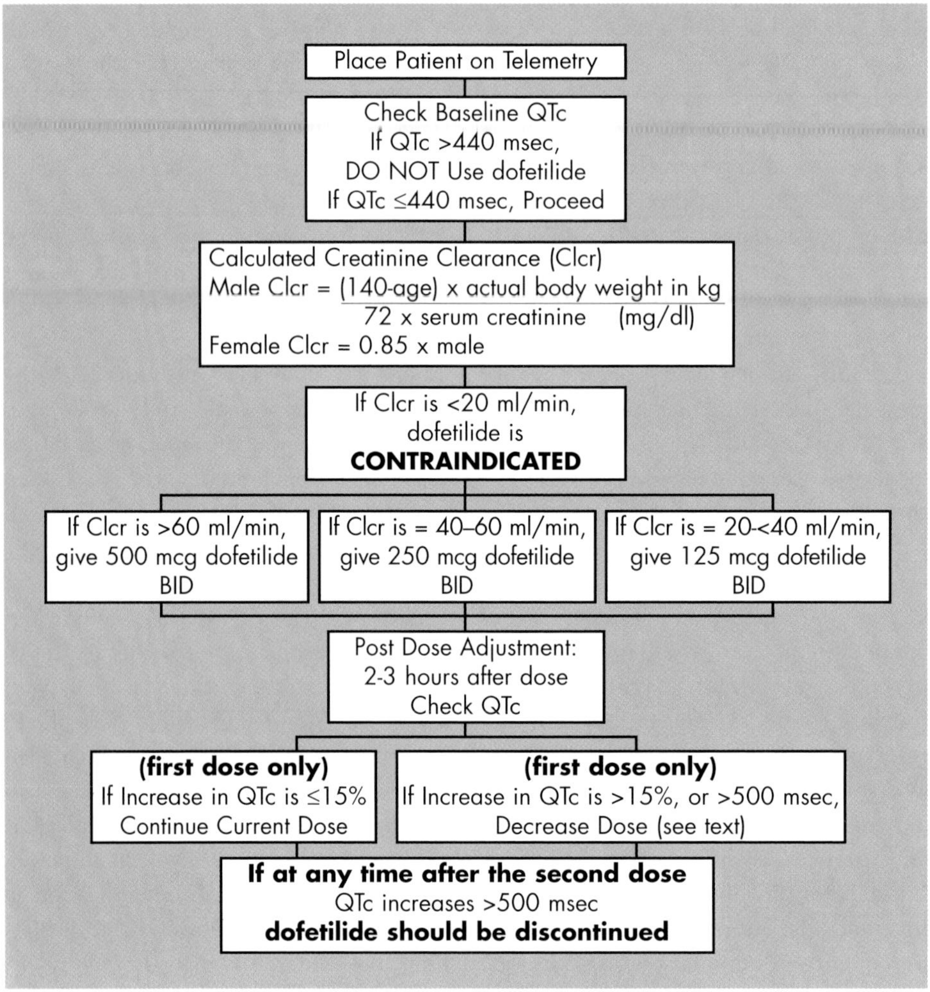
Place Patient on Telemetry
Check Baseline QTc
If QTc >440 msec,
DO NOT Use dofetilide
If QTc ≤440 msec, Proceed
Calculated Creatinine Clearance (Clcr)
Male Clcr = (140-age) x actual body weight in kg
72 x serum creatinine (mg/dl)
Female Clcr = 0.85 x male
If Clcr is <20 ml/min,
dofetilide is
CONTRAINDICATED
If Clcr is >60 ml/min,
give 500 mcg dofetilide
BID
If Clcr is = 40–60 ml/min,
give 250 mcg dofetilide
BID
If Clcr is = 20-<40 ml/min,
give 125 mcg dofetilide
BID
Post Dose Adjustment:
2-3 hours after dose
Check QTc
(first dose only)
If Increase in QTc is ≤15%
Continue Current Dose
(first dose only)
If Increase in QTc is >15%, or >500 msec,
Decrease Dose (see text)
If at any time after the second dose
QTc increases >500 msec
dofetilide should be discontinued

delayed repolarization, while increasing the effective refractory period of both atria and ventricles.

Dofetilide can cause ventricular proarrhythmia, primarily torsades de pointes, associated with QT prolongation. Unfortunately, the use of dofetilide in conjunction with other drugs that prolong the QT interval is not recommended. This medication is relegated to the treatment of atrial fibrillation and flutter, and can be administered cautiously to patients with left ventricular dysfunction. Dofetilide is available only to hospitals and prescribers who have received appropriate education. Table 11.2 shows an algorithm used to prescribe and dose this medication.

Class IV Antiarrhythmic Drugs

Class IV antiarrhythmic drugs are the non-dihydropyridine calcium-channel blocking system. These medications (in particular, verapamil and diltiazem) may be useful for rate control of atrial fibrillation and flutter. In addition, they can suppress some forms of paroxysmal supraventricular tachycardia. In general, these medications are less preferable (second line) to beta blockers in patients with coronary artery disease and/or a prior myocardial infarction.

Antiarrhythmic Drugs and Devices

With the number of device implants increasing dramatically each year, it is important to understand that certain antiarrhythmic drugs may affect pacing and defibrillation thresholds. In particular, thresholds must be checked with the addition of Class I and/or III antiarrhythmic drugs. Amiodarone and mexiletene have the potential to increase pacing and defibrillation thresholds, whereas sotalol might have the opposite effect on defibrillation thresholds (but no effect on pacing thresholds).

In the Antiarrhythmic Versus Implantable Defibrillator (AVID) trial, use of the defibrillator was associated with increased survival compared to amiodarone or sotalol in patients with hemodynamically significant ventricular tachycardia and/or fibrillation. In addition, amiodarone and placebo were associated with a higher mortality compared with the implantable cardioverter-defibrillator in the Sudden Cardiac Death in Heart Failure Trial (SCD-HeFT).

In summary, implantable cardioverter-defibrillators are better than antiarrhythmic drugs in preventing sudden arrhythmic death. However, these medications do have a role in suppressing frequent and/or incessant ventricular arrhythmias in these defibrillator patients.

Chapter 12

Catheter Ablation

One of the major advances in the management of cardiac arrhythmias during the past two and a half decades has been the innovation of catheter ablation. Initially performed in the early 1980s, this technique may be attributed to the pioneering work of Dr. Melvin Scheinman.

The first technique in which catheter ablation was performed invoked the application of direct current energy from the end of a pacing catheter and attached to a skin electrode/plate to destroy focal cardiac tissue. Dr. Scheinman described a series of patients with drug-refractory supraventricular tachycardias in which a pacing catheter was placed near the His bundle (AV junction). Electrical energy was applied and resulted in complete heart block, which served to control the tachyarrhythmias. This technique is of limited clinical use, though, since the patient becomes pacemaker-dependent. Refinement of this technique has occurred over many years.

Eventually a more focal energy delivery system with radiofrequency energy was employed and described by Dr. Steven Huang. Attaching a radiofrequency generator at wavelengths of 300–500 megahertz (MHz) enables electrical energy to be delivered to large-tip, steerable electrophysiology catheters that are placed percutaneously. This technique creates focal myocardial lesions that are well circumscribed. The size of the electrode and the amount of energy delivered to that electrode determine the size of the myocardial lesion produced through resistive heating. Cooling the tip of the electrode can create larger lesions.

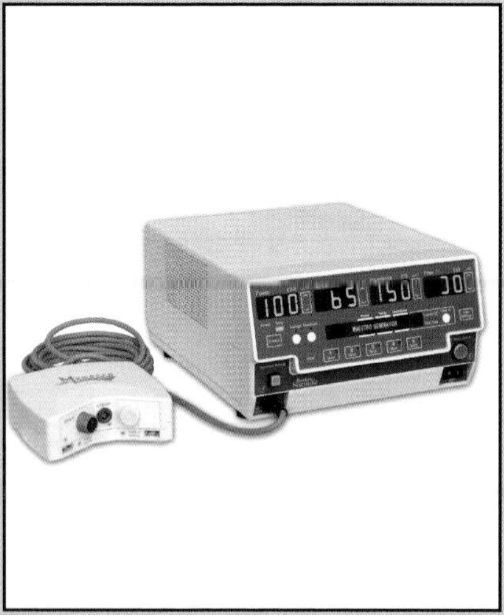

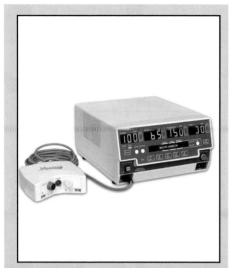

Figure 12.1: A radiofrequency catheter ablation system (Maestro 3000™ Cardiac Ablation System, courtesy of Boston Scientific, Natick, MA).

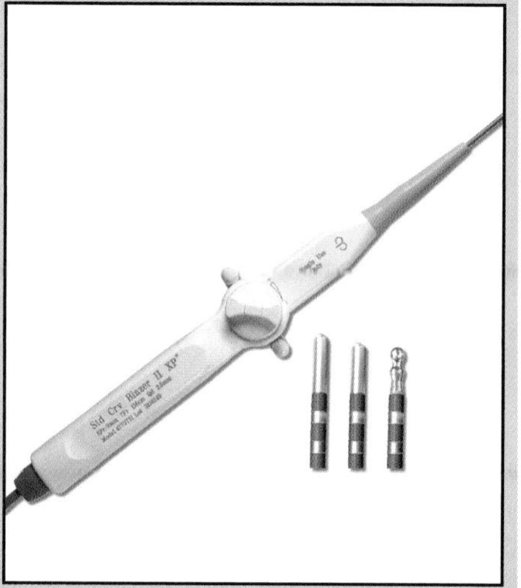

Figure 12.2: Catheters used to treat tachycardias (left- and right-sided) (Std Crv Blazer II XP, courtesy of Boston Scientific, San Jose, CA).

Figure 12.1 shows a radiofrequency catheter ablation system. A radiofrequency energy generator is hooked through a cable to a control box. The box is then attached to a grounding pad as well as to a radiofrequency ablation catheter (figure 12.2).

Table 12.1 shows a list of tachycardias in which catheter ablation may be indicated. In general, patients should be symptomatic or at risk from the hemodynamic or embolic consequences of the tachycardia. Importantly, tachycardia-induced cardiomyopathy has been described, which is reversible after tachycardia cure and/or effective rate control. Catheter ablation may be a preferable first-line alternative to drug therapy in patients with symptomatic supraventricular tachycardia and/or idiopathic ventricular tachycardia. Although not listed in table 12.1, patients with highly symptomatic drug refractory ventricular premature contractions (without nonsustained ventricular tachycardia) can be effectively cured by catheter ablation. This technique should be performed as a last resort, though, due to the benign nature of the dysrhythmia.

This technique was originally used in patients with drug-refractory atrial fibrillation, by performing AV junction ablation with implantation of a permanent pacemaker. Subsequently, the effectiveness of catheter ablations has been demonstrated with almost all types of supraventricular tachycardias (table 12.2). AV-node reentrant tachycardia, in which there is presence of two pathways in the AV node and a circus movement tachycardia, can be cured in more than 98 percent of cases.

Initially, radiofrequency catheter ablation of a fast AV nodal pathway was performed. This approach, however, resulted

Table 12.1: Catheter Ablation Indications

1. AV-node reentrant tachycardia
2. AV reentrant tachycardia (including Wolff-Parkinson-White syndrome)
3. Atrial flutter
4. Atrial tachycardia
5. Bundle branch reentrant ventricular tachycardia
6. Idiopathic ventricular tachycardia (right ventricular outflow tract or left ventricular septum)
7. Fascicular tachycardias
8. Myocardial ventricular tachycardia with prior myocardial infarction/scar
9. Surgical scar reentrant tachycardias (congenital repairs/other)
10. Symptomatic and/or drug-refractory atrial fibrillation may be treated with AV junction ablation and permanent pacemaker, or catheter ablation for cure of atrial fibrillation
11. Inappropriate sinus tachycardia

Table 12.2: Effectiveness of Catheter Ablation

Ablation Type	Anticipated Success Rate
AV-Node Reentry	98 percent
AV Reentry (WPW)	95 percent
Atrial Flutter	90 percent
Atrial Tachycardia	95 percent
Atrial Fibrillation:	
Paroxysmal	65–85 percent
Persistent	50–60 percent
Idiopathic Ventricular Tachycardia	90 percent
Coronary Disease Ventricular Tachycardia	50–75 percent
Bundle-Branch Reentrant Ventricular Tachycardia	95 percent

in complete heart block in approximately six percent of cases. Subsequently, the procedure has evolved such that the preferred approach and accepted technique is to ablate the slow pathway of the AV node, which carries a very low risk of complete heart block.

Radiofrequency catheter ablation is also highly effective in patients with Wolff-Parkinson-White (WPW) syndrome. Sixty percent of patients with WPW syndrome have left-sided bypass tracts; approximately 25 percent of patients have septal or paraseptal bypass tracts, and the remaining 15 percent have bypass tracts on the right side of the myocardium. Left-sided radiofrequency catheter ablation can be performed via either a transseptal or a retrograde aortic approach. Both are very successful for ablating left-sided bypass tracts. The success rate for ablation of accessory pathways is approximately 95 percent.

Other arrhythmias such as atrial tachycardia and atrial flutter can also be treated successfully via radiofrequency catheter ablation. Atrial flutter is a very common macro-reentrant tachycardia involving the right atrium. Flutter waves move across an area called the isthmus, between the tricuspid valve and the inferior vena cava. By creating a line of block via radiofrequency energy and electrically disrupting the connections between the tricuspid valve and the inferior vena cava, one can eliminate the ability to sustain typical atrial flutter.

Other types of atrial flutter and other tachycardias involving anatomical scars or barriers such as post-surgical repair of congenital heart disease can be ablated successfully via this method as well. A nonfluoroscopic three-dimensional mapping technique can be useful in helping elucidate these more complicated tachycardias.

The uses of a three-dimensional mapping technique and the anatomic ablation of atrial fibrillation have been well described by Dr. Carlo Pappone. Sixty-five to 85 percent of patients who have atrial fibrillation may have electrical discharges from pulmonary veins. Radiofrequency catheter ablation in which lesions are created that circumscribe and isolate the pulmonary veins on the left side (outside of the pulmonary vein openings) enables a significant number of patients with paroxysmal and even persistent atrial fibrillation to be successfully cured. Additional radiofrequency applications to the cavotricuspid isthmus and left-sided linear lesions may also be required. The success rate for chronic and/or persistent atrial fibrillation is approximately 50 to 60 percent, but many patients require repeat procedures. Patients with persistent atrial fibrillation may require additional ablation sessions, additional linear lines for catheter ablation (including a roof line and a cavotricuspid isthmus line, as well as ablation of continuous atrial fractionated electrograms). Patients with paroxysmal atrial fibrillation have a higher success rate (approximately 65 to 85 percent) and may be treated solely with pulmonary vein isolation in the majority of cases. Even in paroxysmal atrial fibrillation, additional sessions may occasionally be necessary in order to achieve a cure. Adjunctive pharmacologic therapy may also be required.

Radiofrequency catheter ablation for ventricular tachycardia can also be performed with a high success rate. Focal ventricular tachycardias such as right ventricular outflow tract ventricular tachycardia or posterior septal fascicular tachycardia can also be defined in patients with structurally normal hearts. By using a pace mapping technique in which one paces from the end of the ablation catheter and attempts to mimic the 12-lead morphology of the ventricular tachycardia, one can successfully identify the site to perform catheter ablation. Using an appropriate nonfluoroscopic three-dimensional mapping technique may facilitate catheter ablation with a success rate of as high as 90 percent. The reader should note that three-dimensional mapping can also be performed with a deployable balloon-shaped catheter which can be visualized fluoroscopically (figure 12.3).

Patients with coronary artery disease and myocardial scarring, as well as patients

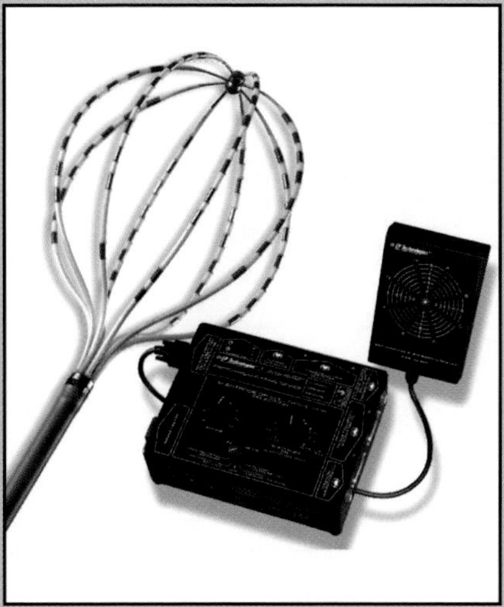

Figure 12.3: A three-dimensional mapping system using a deployable balloon-shaped catheter (courtesy of Boston Scientific, San Jose, CA).

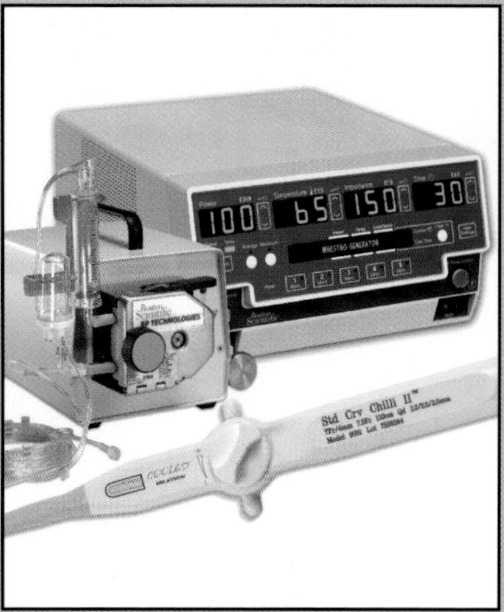

Figure 12.4: Maestro 3000™ Cardiac Ablation System, CircuCool System® v3, and standard Chilli II™ Cooled Ablation Catheter (courtesy of Boston Scientific, Natick, MA).

with a non-ischemic dilated cardiomyopathy, may have reentrant ventricular tachycardia involving scar or bundle-branch reentry. To perform a successful ventricular tachycardia ablation in a patient with coronary artery disease, it is useful to perform "concealed entrainment" to define the critical slow zone of the tachycardia circuit. The ventricle is paced faster than the tachycardia so that it entrains (gets into the circuit of the tachycardia) in order to determine whether the catheter location is in a zone critical for tachycardia maintenance. The success rate of ventricular tachycardia ablation in patients with coronary artery disease and prior myocardial infarction is approximately 50 to 75 percent. This technique may also be indicated in patients who have an implantable cardioverter-defibrillator that is frequently discharging (incessant ventricular tachycardia) and is refractory to antiarrhythmic drugs.

Patients with a dilated cardiomyopathy (ischemic or nonischemic) may have bundle-branch reentrant tachycardia, in which the tachycardia travels down one bundle branch and up the other. These patients typically have His-Purkinje disease (HV interval greater than 65 msec) and a left interventricular conduction delay or a left bundle-branch block pattern. By ablating the right bundle-branch block, one can eliminate the tachycardia.

Certain types of ablations require the creation of larger myocardial lesions. This can be achieved with large-tip electrodes (10-mm tip) and high-output 100-watt radiofrequency generators. Alternatively, irrigation of fluids through the tip of an ablation catheter during the delivery of radiofrequency energy can achieve a similar goal of creating larger lesions. Two examples are the NAVISTAR® THERMOCOOL® Catheter (Biosense Webster

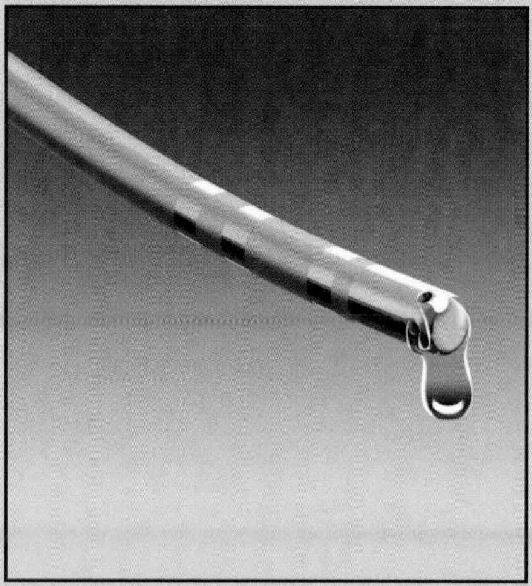

Figure 12.5: The NaviStar® ThermoCool® irrigated tip catheter (courtesy of Biosense Webster, Inc., a Johnson & Johnson company, Diamond Bar, CA).

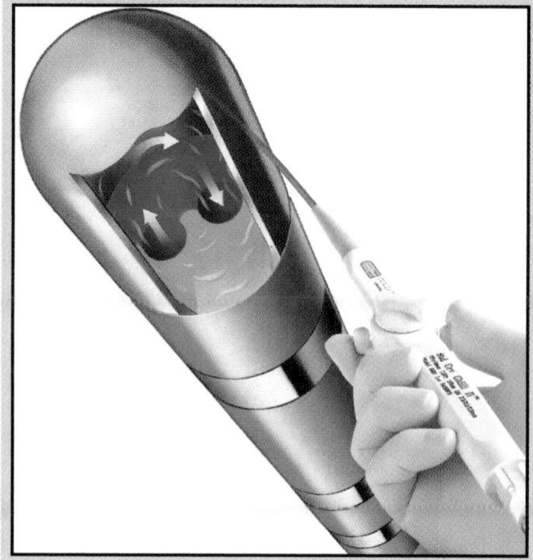

Figure 12.6: Chilli II™ internally cooled tip catheter (courtesy of Boston Scientific, San Jose, CA).

Inc., a Johnson & Johnson company, Diamond Bar, CA; figure 12.5), which has an open irrigation system in which saline is delivered from inside the catheter through the tip electrode towards the outside blood stream or myocardium, and the Chilli II Cooled Ablation Catheter (Boston Scientific, San Jose, CA; figures 12.4 and 12.6), which is a closed irrigation system in which dextrose 5 percent water is recirculated within the catheter tip and does not enter the blood stream.

Alternative modalities for catheter ablation include cryoablation, in which myocardial tissue is frozen. To produce cryotherapeutic temperatures, heat is removed from the tissue, rather than "injecting" cold energy into the tissue. During cryoablation, the removal of heat from the tissue creates a temperature gradient that extends from the catheter tip to the edge of the "cryotherapy zone". At the tip/tissue interface of the 4 mm tip ablation catheter, the cryotherapy temperature can be either -30°C or -75°C, depending on the type of intervention (cryomapping or cryoablation). Larger tip ablation catheters (6 to 8 mm tip) function under a constant N_2O flow setting, and temperatures may get as cold as -85°C. The temperature in the cryotherapy zone ranges from the sub-zero cryogenic temperature at the tip/tissue interface to body temperature at sites distant from the catheter tip. This zone is "dynamic" as it expands during freezing and shrinks upon re-warming. In living tissue, vascularity always provides a heat source and will, as a result, cause local variations in temperature (figures 12.7 and 12.8). Catheter cryoablation is a safe and clinically effective method for ablation of AV-node reentrant tachycardia. Although the acute procedural success rate of catheter

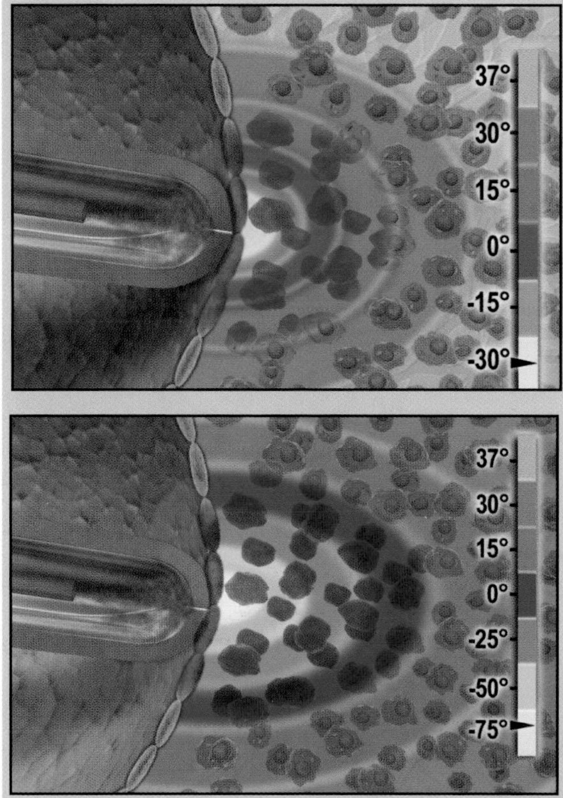

Figures 12.7 (top) and 12.8 (bottom): A cryotherapy zone can be seen in both cryomapping (top figure) and cryoablation (bottom figure) procedures with the 4 mm tip ablation catheter. The zone is thermally dynamic over time as cells that remain above a zero temperature gradient display a transient electrical effect while cells experiencing subzero temperatures are ablated. (reprinted with permission from *EP Lab Digest* 2003;3:1,6,7.)

cryoablation for this arrhythmia may be slightly lower than that reported for radiofrequency ablation, it has an excellent safety profile with no reported instances to date of inadvertent atrioventricular block requiring implantation of a permanent pacemaker. Using this technology (such as the products seen in figures 12.9 and 12.10), one can perform reversible cryomapping, which helps to identify suitable ablation targets while also identifying sites where cryoablation should be avoided. For patients with midseptal and parahisian accessory pathways, in whom the risk of producing inadvertent atrioventricular block is

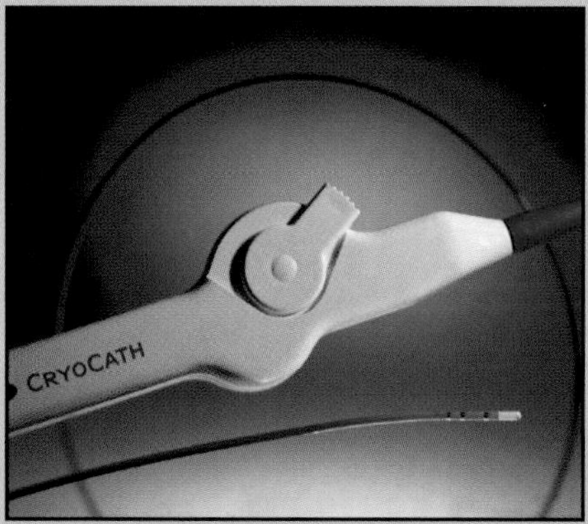

Figure 12.9: The Freezor® cryocatheter, used to treat arrhythmias during cryotherapy (Reproduced with permission of Medtronic, Inc., Minneapolis, MN).

substantial, catheter cryoablation is a safe and effective alternative to radiofrequency ablation. Catheter cryoablation of common atrial flutter causes much less patient discomfort than radiofrequency ablation, with excellent acute and long-term efficacy. It can also potentially be used to isolate the pulmonary veins during ablation of atrial fibrillation. Presently the techniques are being applied during concurrent open-heart surgery (initial valve repair, for example).

Please note that catheter ablation is also discussed in each of the following chapters that are titled for specific arrhythmias: Chapter 15: Atrial Fibrillation, Chapter 16: AV-Node Reentrant Tachycardia, Chapter 17: Atrial Tachycardia, Chapter 18: Atrial Flutter, Chapter 20: Accessory Pathways, and Chapter 21: Ventricular Tachycardia.

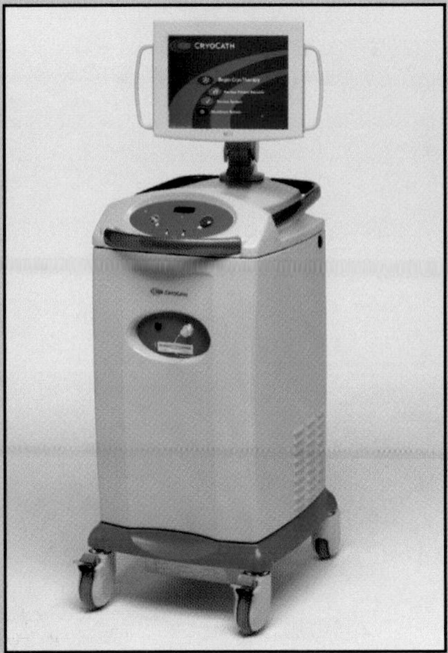

Figure 12.10: The CryoTherapy Console (Reproduced with permission of Medtronic, Inc., Minneapolis, MN).

Chapter 13

Nonfluoroscopic Three-Dimensional Mapping and Intracardiac Imaging

Nonfluoroscopic three-dimensional mapping of the myocardium has been very helpful for isolating focal and nonfocal tachycardias. The technique is very similar to localization using the global positioning system. Using reference electrodes in the XYZ planes, one can identify the location of catheters and tachycardias within the heart. The catheters themselves or the surface electrodes can be used in setting the reference coordinates for mapping a tachycardia.

The two most common mapping systems are produced by Johnson and Johnson Inc. (CARTO® XP System, Biosense Webster, Inc.) and St. Jude Medical, Inc. (EnSite® System).

The CARTO® solution (figures 13.1–13.3) uses a surface electrode as a reference and a special reference mapping catheter to enable point-to-point three-dimensional reconstruction of the myocardium. Visualization of the catheters is performed using an electromagnetic source (underneath the table). In addition, the catheter can be helpful in mapping the electrical depolarization (voltage maps of the myocardium). This technique can be useful for mapping a variety of tachycardias and has been especially helpful in patients who have atrial fibrillation and warrant a pulmonary vein isolation procedure. This system uses specially-designed ablation catheters and surface electrodes.

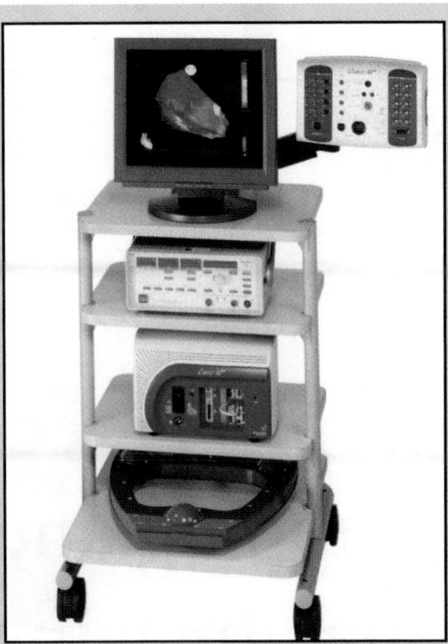

Figures 13.1: The CARTO® XP three-dimensional mapping system. The computer screen shows right-heart 3-D construction (courtesy of Biosense Webster, Inc., a Johnson & Johnson company, Diamond Bar, CA).

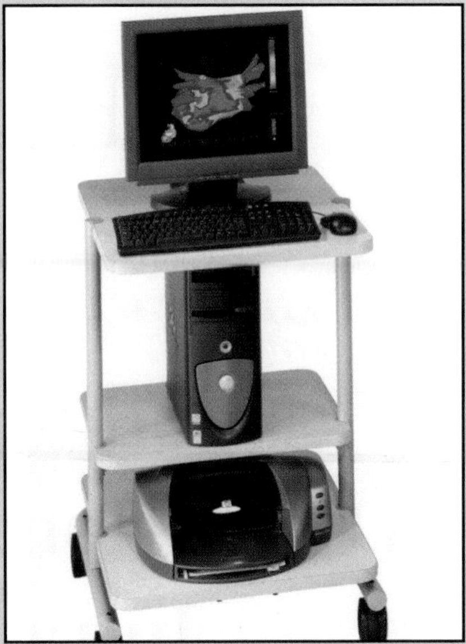

Figures 13.2: The CARTO® XP 3-D mapping system. The computer screen shows left atrial 3-D construction; this method can be used for pulmonary vein isolation procedures (atrial fibrillation ablation). (Courtesy of Biosense Webster, Inc., a Johnson & Johnson company, Diamond Bar, CA.)

The EnSite System offers two methods of cardiac mapping. One is a non-contact method in which a 64-pole balloon-configured array catheter is deployed in the chamber of the heart where the arrhythmia is suspected (figures 13.4–13.8). Virtual (unipolar) electrograms can be calculated to identify focal and reentrant tachycardias. The latter tachycardias are illustrated via the breakthrough points seen in the myocardium and the image. The other method collects data from up to 64 electrodes on 12 standard EP catheters in a single heartbeat, to provide voltage and activation maps.

In addition to these two common mapping systems, another system has been developed. The LocaLisa system by Medtronic (no longer commercially available) is an anatomic point-mapping system that does not provide information related to electrical activities. It merely tags three-dimensional positions of the catheter with limited graphic capabilities.

Intracardiac echocardiography (ICE) (figures 13.9 and 13.10) is an imaging tool in which an ICE catheter is inserted percutaneously into the heart and planar echocardiographic images are obtained. This technique can directly visualize endocardial structures such as the crista terminalis, coronary sinus vein, and foramen ovale. Anatomic ablations, transseptal procedures, and identification

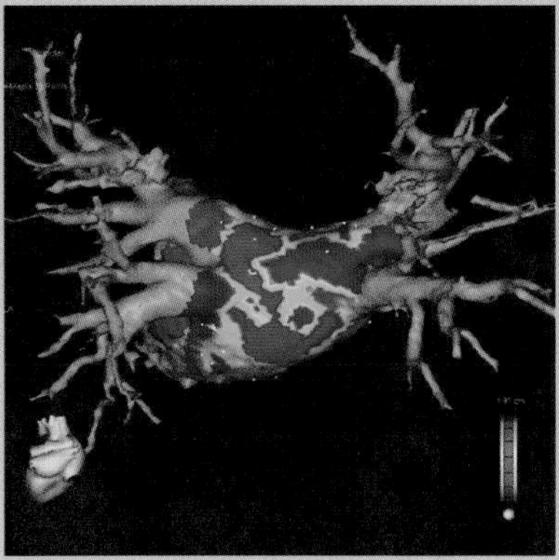

Figure 13.3: The CARTO® XP System with the CARTOMERGE® Image Integration Software Module. Registered CT image of a left atrium with a projected electrical activation on its shell (courtesy of Biosense Webster, Inc., a Johnson & Johnson company, Diamond Bar, CA).

of cardiac perforations can all be facilitated via ICE.

In our experience, three-dimensional mapping using a nonfluoroscopic system (such as the EnSite System) has been very helpful, predominantly in mapping focal tachycardias such as atrial tachycardias and idiopathic ventricular tachycardias, and in patients with recurrent atrial flutter. The system makes it very easy to see and locate breakthrough conduction across the cavotricuspid isthmus (the point in which all flutter waves travel in typical atrial flutter). This is particularly

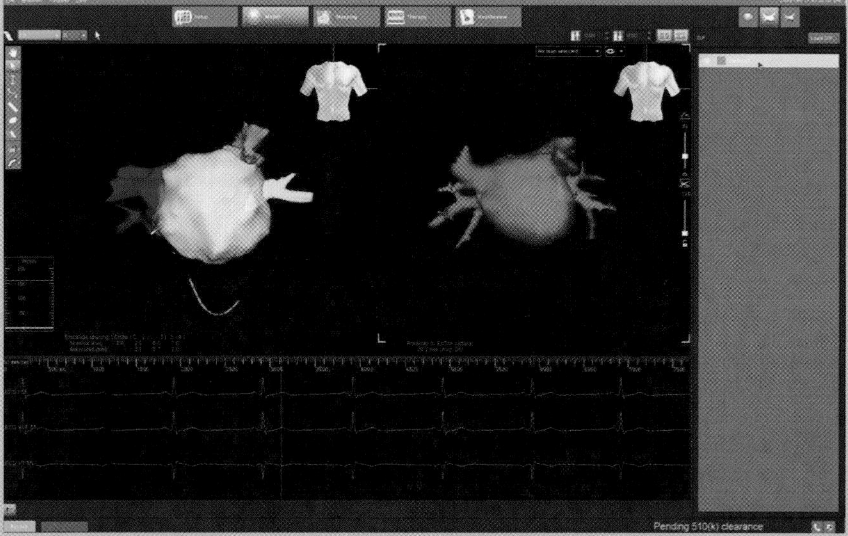

Figure 13.4: Side by side view of EnSite NavX™ left atrial chamber model and a segmented 3-D CT chamber model created in EnSite Velocity™ Cardiac Mapping System (courtesy of St. Jude Medical, Inc., St. Paul, MN).

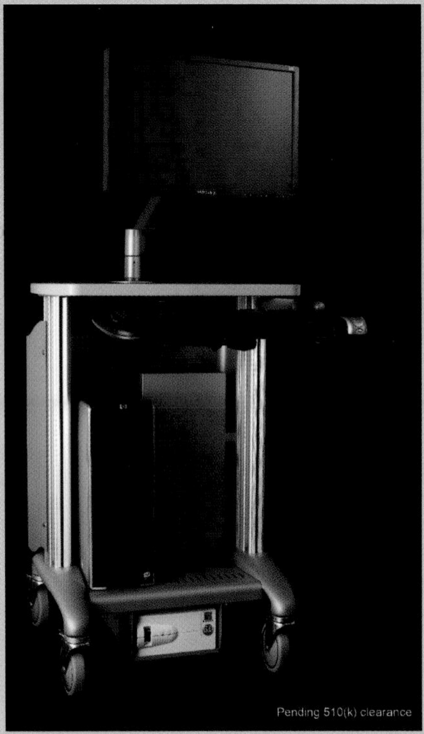

Figure 13.5: EnSite Velocity™ Cardiac Mapping System display work station shown on a mobile cart (courtesy of St. Jude Medical, Inc., St. Paul, MN).

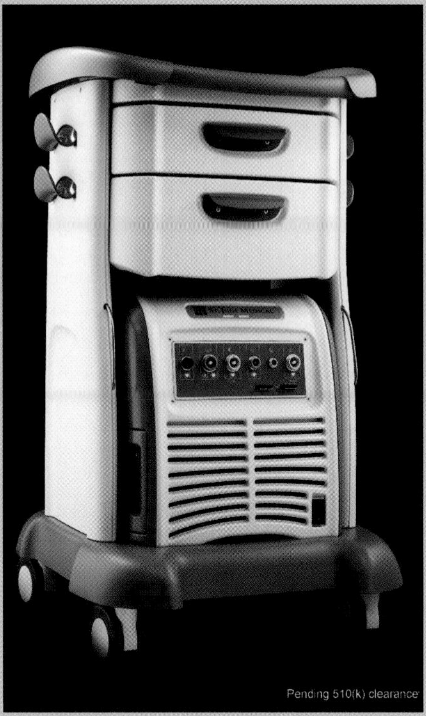

Figure 13.6: EnSite Velocity™ Cardiac Mapping System amplifier cart shown in a mobile configuration (courtesy of St. Jude Medical, Inc., St. Paul, MN).

helpful in cases of recurrent atrial flutter following an initial successful atrial flutter ablation (performed with or without nonfluoroscopic three-dimensional mapping). Mapping examples can be seen in ablation of atrial tachycardia (Chapter 17), atrial flutter (Chapter 18), and ventricular tachycardia (Chapter 21).

It is important to know the traditional method of point-to-point mapping using standard EP catheters without a three-dimensional mapping system. If an operator depends exclusively on a three-dimensional mapping system to perform all ablative services, he or she may be in trouble if the system is not available or breaks down during a procedure. Although these systems are helpful, they should be used as a tool in conjunction with standard electrophysiology practices and not solely to analyze tachycardias.

The three-dimensional mapping systems described here have been a great asset to complicated radiofrequency catheter ablation procedures. These systems help localize the focus, provide the operator with a target, and permit placement of the catheters nonfluoroscopically in an appropriate location in order to produce a successful radiofrequency catheter ablation procedure.

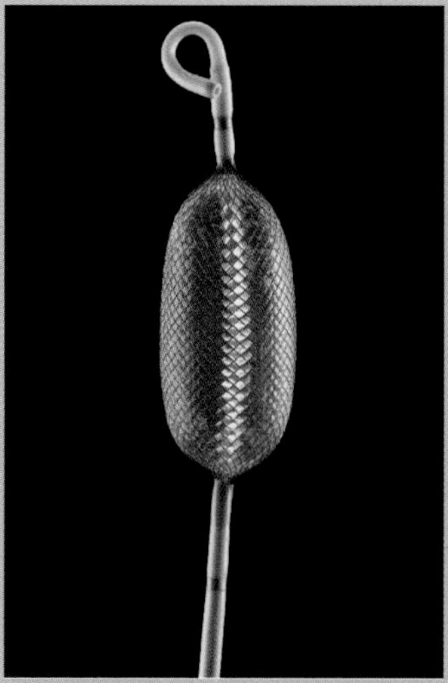

Figure 13.7: EnSite Array™ noncontact catheter (courtesy of St. Jude Medical, Inc., St. Paul, MN).

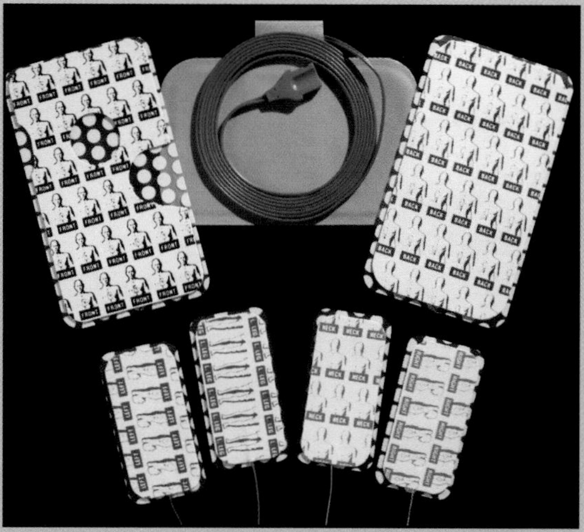

Figure 13.8: EnSite NavX™ Visualization and Navigation Technology surface electrode patches (courtesy of St. Jude Medical, Inc., St. Paul, MN).

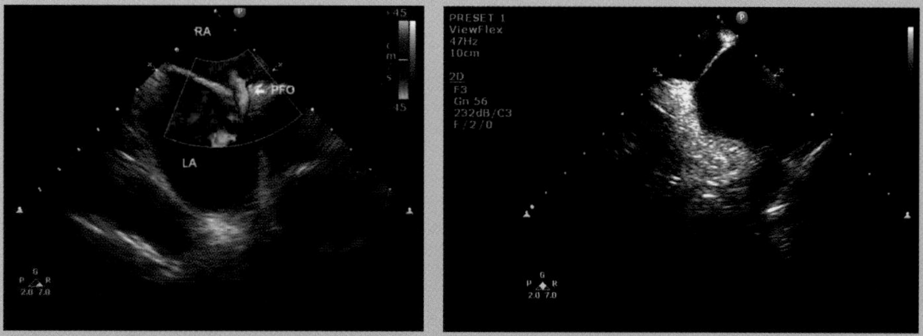

Figure 13.9: ViewMate™ II Intracardiac Echocardiography System (ICE) provides real-time imaging of cardiac structures and blood flow within the heart (courtesy of St. Jude Medical, Inc., St. Paul, MN).

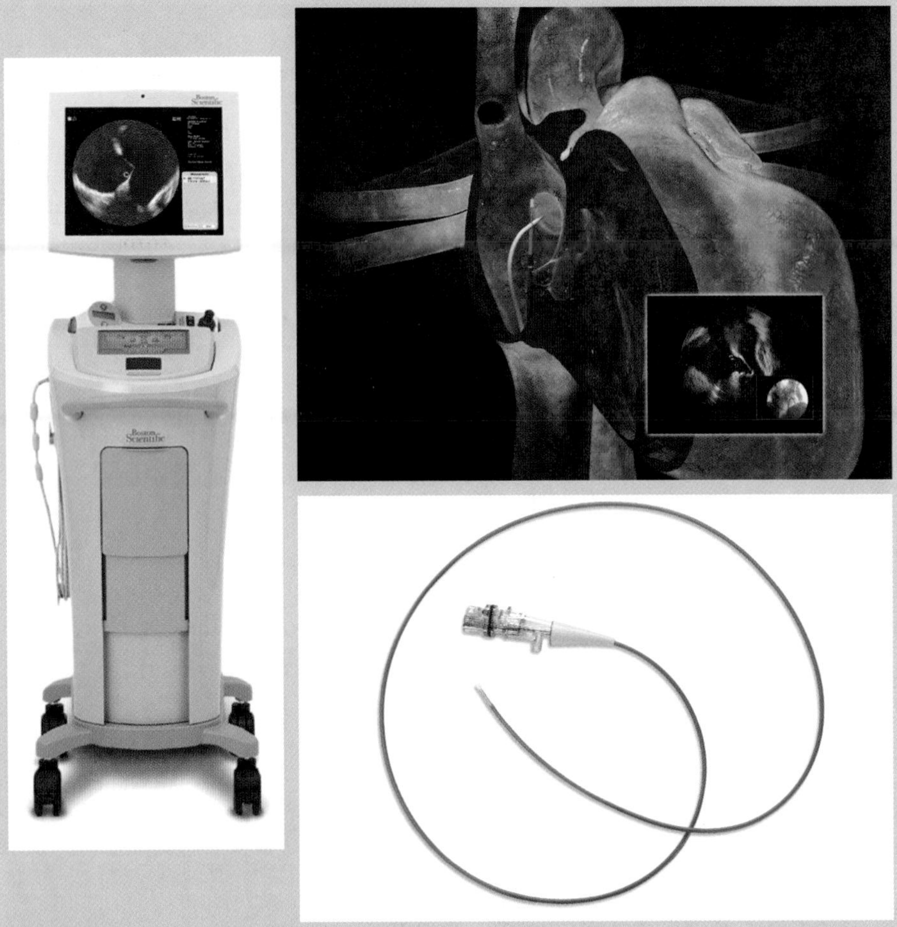

Figure 13.10: Another nonfluoroscopic method that uses intracardiac ultrasound to identify endocardial structures (courtesy of Boston Scientific, San Jose, CA).

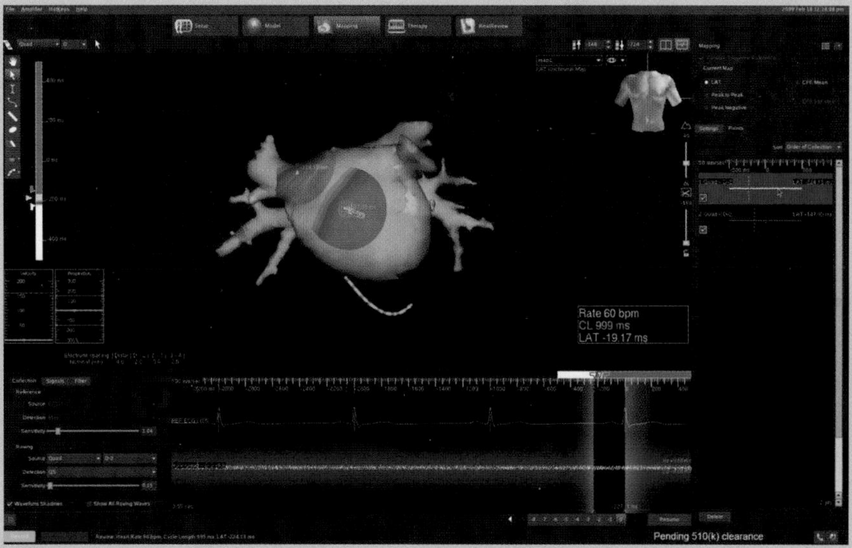

Figure 13.11: Local activation timing map created in EnSite Velocity™ Cardiac Mapping System new user interface (courtesy of St. Jude Medical, Inc., St. Paul, MN).

Chapter 14

Programmed Electrical Stimulation

To induce arrhythmias, a technique known as programmed electrical stimulation is performed. Programmed electrical stimulation uses standard pacing of the atrium or ventricle at a predetermined heart rate or cycle length with the placement of premature extrastimuli. The premature extrastimuli start at a preset interval and get progressively more premature.

Generally, programmed stimulation starts at a drive cycle length faster than the sinus cycle length. Standard pacing typically occurs at a drive cycle length of 8 beats to 10 beats at 600 msec, 500 msec, or 400 msec. This drive cycle length is followed by a single premature stimulus that is often 100 msec to 200 msec shorter than the drive cycle length.

The interval between the last drive cycle length and the first premature beat is called the coupling interval. This coupling interval is shortened by intervals of 10 msec to 20 msec after each drive train until the paced stimulus fails to capture the myocardium. Subsequently, a second stimulus can be added. The cycle length of the first stimulus should be increased by 30 msec or 40 msec from the refractory period, and the second stimulus could be the same as or slightly less than the coupling interval of the first stimulus. There may be stylistic differences amongst the various EP operators with respect to how programmed electrical stimulation is performed.

For nomenclature, the stimulus recorded for the drive cycle length is called S1. Each subsequent premature stimulus is labeled sequentially: S2, S3, S4, etc. In other words, S2 is the first extrastimulus, S3 is the second extrastimulus, and S4 is the third extrastimulus. The coupling

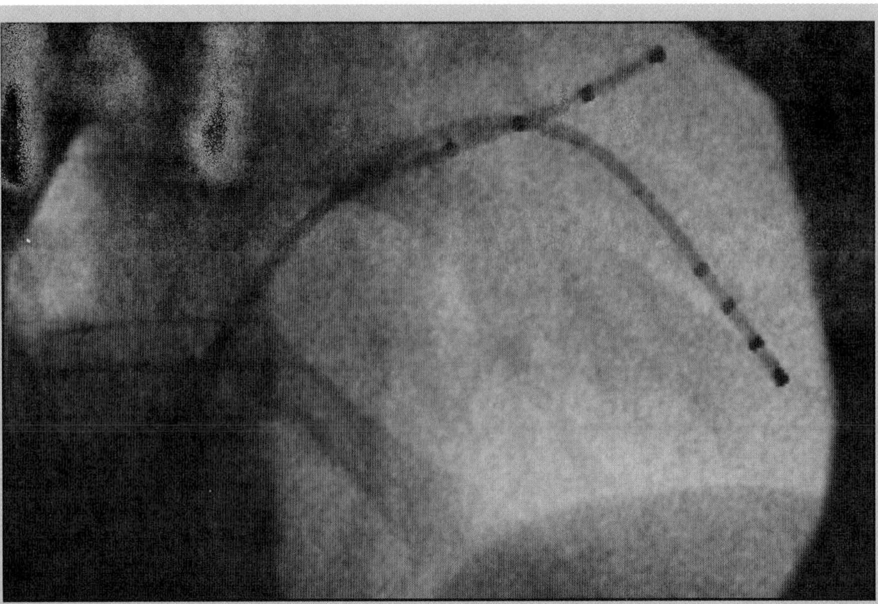

Figure 14.1: A fluoroscopic image of two catheters positioned in the right ventricle. One is near the right ventricular apex, the other is near the right ventricular outflow tract.

intervals for these premature stimuli should not go below 180 msec; lower than 180 msec may induce a nonspecific arrhythmia such as atrial fibrillation (during atrial stimulation) or ventricular fibrillation (during ventricular stimulation).

The method of ventricular program electrical stimulation is similar to that of atrial program electrical stimulation. Figure 14.1 shows two catheters positioned in the right ventricle. Programmed electrical stimulation traditionally is performed from two ventricular sites. In some institutions, programmed stimulation begins with one extrastimulus and progresses to two extrastimuli and then three extrastimuli at a given cycle length. This is then repeated at a different drive cycle length. In our lab, we often use an accelerated protocol, beginning with triple extrastimuli, to save time.

The standard ventricular programmed electrical stimulation is performed from two right ventricular sites, often the RV apex and RV outflow tract, at two different drive cycle lengths for up to three extrastimuli. Stimulation can also be performed from the left ventricle, which can be helpful in inducing arrhythmias that are noninducible from the right side. Also, the use of ventricular burst pacing (typically at cycle lengths of 220 msec to 350 msec for two to five seconds), occasionally with the addition of isoproterenol or other stimulants, can be helpful during arrhythmia induction.

Figure 14.2 shows an induced sustained monomorphic ventricular tachycardia. Note the consistent pattern of the arrhythmia. Figure 14.3 shows a sustained polymorphic ventricular tachycardia induced by S1, S2, S3, and S4. Note the chaotic, nonconsistent polymorphic (many-shaped)

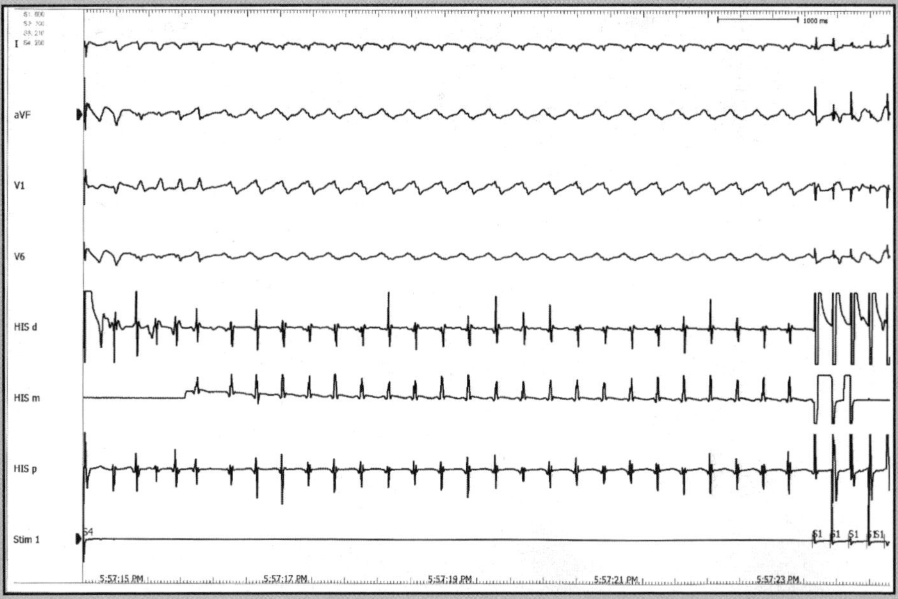

Figure 14.2: An inducible sustained monomorphic ventricular tachycardia.

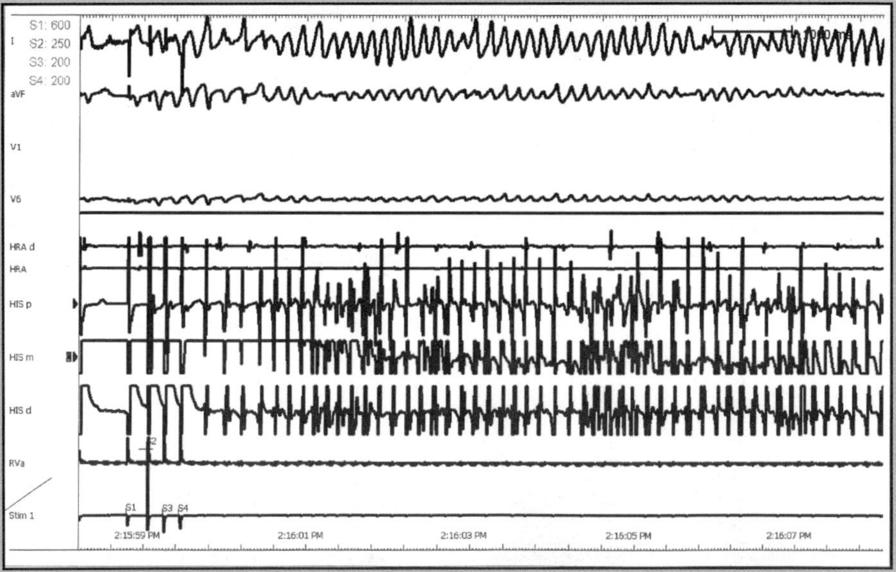

Figure 14.3: A sustained polymorphic ventricular tachycardia induced by S1, S2, S3, and S4.

Table 14.1: Electrophysiology Study Indications

1. Syncope of unknown etiology
2. Supraventricular tachycardia (diagnosis and treatment)
3. Ventricular tachycardia/ventricular fibrillation not in setting of a myocardial infarction (diagnosis and treatment)
4. Nonsustained ventricular tachycardia in patients with:
   (a) a prior myocardial infarction and ejection fraction of less than or equal to 40 percent;
   (b) dilated cardiomyopathy with symptoms;
   (c) right ventricular dysplasia
5. Unexplained palpitations
6. Evaluation of hereditary conditions such as Brugada syndrome and long QT syndrome
7. Evaluation of conduction disease and determination of the need for a permanent pacemaker (in a patient with sick sinus syndrome, unspecified AV block, or bifascicular/trifascicular block)

pattern of the ventricular tachycardia. Monomorphic ventricular tachycardia is a more specific finding; polymorphic ventricular tachycardia may be nonspecific (*i.e.*, meaningless), and must be taken in context with the patient's history, physical state, ECG, and cardiac substrate.

In summary, an assessment of conduction and refractoriness (see Chapter 9) and programmed electrical stimulation, with or without the addition of pharmacologic agents (atropine, isoproterenol, aminophylline, procainamide, and adenosine) comprise the essential components of a routine electrophysiology study. In addition to what is described in this chapter, programmed electrical stimulation can also be performed from the atrium (in particular, for studying supraventricular tachycardia). Premature extrastimuli can also be delivered without a drive train (by sensing the intracardiac activity and delivering a stimuli to the particular myocardial site at a predetermined coupling interval) and may be useful in differentiating AV-node reentrant tachycardia from AV reentrant tachycardia (which utilizes a bypass tract). Table 14.1 lists the indications for an electrophysiology study.

Chapter 15

Atrial Fibrillation

Atrial fibrillation is one of the most common arrhythmias. According to the American Heart Association, approximately 2.2 million people in the United States are living with atrial fibrillation. The most commonly associated cardiac condition of this arrhythmia is hypertension, although it is also common to find atrial fibrillation in patients with other types of cardiac abnormalities such as myocardial infarction and ischemia, valvular disease, and hypertrophic cardiomyopathy.

Atrial fibrillation is diagnosed as an irregular rhythm in which the atrial depolarization occurs in a very fast, chaotic manner (figure 15.1). The mechanism may be related to abnormal stretch and/or foci in the myocardium at areas such as the pulmonary veins, the coronary sinus, and the right atrial appendage.

Atrial fibrillation may be classified based on two criteria: 1) episode frequency; and 2) the ability to convert spontaneously back into normal sinus rhythm. If a patient presents with two or more episodes, this is called *recurrent* atrial fibrillation. Recurrent atrial fibrillation may be *paroxysmal* (terminates spontaneously) or *persistent* (does not terminate spontaneously, but only after pharmacologic or electrical cardioversion). Long-standing persistent atrial fibrillation may also be called *chronic* atrial fibrillation. When this tachyarrhythmia is unable to be cardioverted successfully, it is called *permanent* atrial fibrillation.

The importance of maintaining sinus rhythm has been investigated by a number of studies. One of the most important studies was the

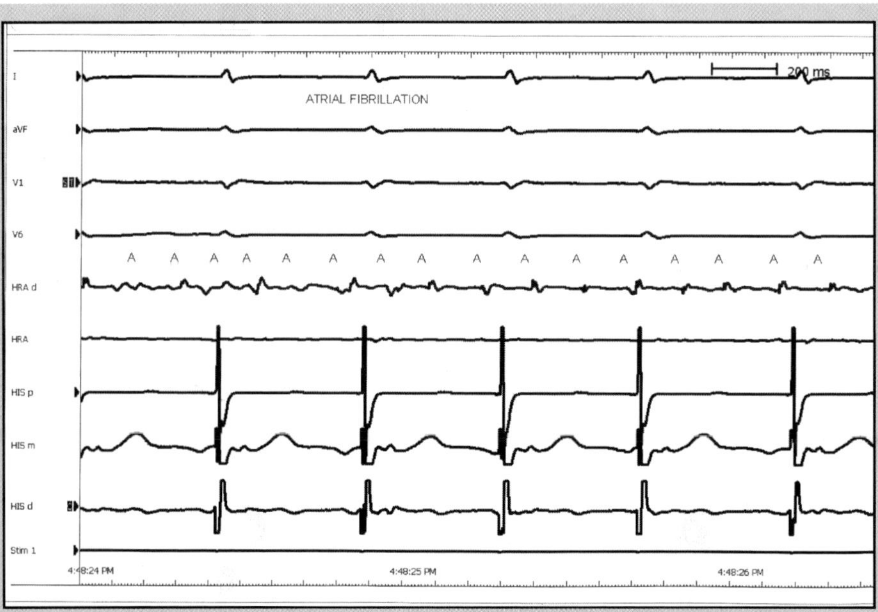

Figure 15.1: Atrial fibrillation, observed during an electrophysiology study.

Atrial Fibrillation Follow-up Investigation of Rhythm Management (AFFIRM) trial, in which patients with atrial fibrillation were treated by either antiarrhythmic drug therapy or rate control and anticoagulation. Antiarrhythmic drug therapy showed no benefit over rate control and anticoagulation.

The best antiarrhythmic drug for suppression of atrial fibrillation is amiodarone, based on the Canadian Trial of Atrial Fibrillation, which compared amiodarone to propafenone and sotalol. Amiodarone may be very effective when taken in a low dosage (200 mg orally daily) and may have limited though progressive toxicity over time. More recently, dofetilide has also been shown to be useful for atrial fibrillation; however, this drug has a higher potential for producing proarrhythmia than amiodarone, and requires hospitalization for initiation.

Our standard approach to patients with atrial fibrillation is as follows: If it is the first episode of atrial fibrillation, the patient warrants an evaluation of thyroid function as well as a two-dimensional echocardiogram to determine whether he or she has any structural myocardial abnormality, such as left ventricular hypertrophy or valvular disease. In addition, the patient may benefit from an attempt at electrical or pharmacologic cardioversion. The author believes that every patient deserves at least one attempt at conversion if spontaneous conversion does not occur.

Should the patient revert back into atrial fibrillation, rate control and anticoagulation should be considered. Antiarrhythmic drug therapy and/or catheter ablation alternatives should be considered based on the patient's symptoms.

Table 15.1: Indications and Recommendations for Atrial Fibrillation Ablation*

1. Highly symptomatic patients who fail at least one antiarrhythmic drug therapy
2. Testing of endpoints including demonstration of pulmonary vein isolation as well as testing for complete conduction block for any lines created

*Adapted from Calkins H, Brugada J, Packer DL, et al. HRS/EHRA/ECAS expert Consensus Statement on catheter and surgical ablation of atrial fibrillation: Recommendations for personnel, policy, procedures and follow-up. A report of the Heart Rhythm Society (HRS) Task Force on catheter and surgical ablation of atrial fibrillation. *Heart Rhythm* 2007;4:816-861.

There are two strategies regarding radiofrequency catheter ablation for atrial fibrillation. The first is an ablate-and-pace strategy in which one ablates the AV junction and implants a permanent pacemaker. This can be considered if rate control is difficult to achieve despite multiple negative chronotropic agents. It is important to remember that ventricular pacing in this circumstance is more physiologic from the right ventricular outflow tract as compared with the right ventricular apex. Right ventricular outflow tract or biventricular pacing should be considered in some patients (particularly those with significant initial mitral regurgitation and/or heart failure) in order to optimize ventricular synchronization. A rare complication in which acute pulmonary decompensation following AV junction ablation and RV apical pacing has been described and is most likely the result of exacerbation of preexisting significant mitral regurgitation.

The second strategy is atrial fibrillation ablation, involving an anatomic ablation around the pulmonary veins. Additional linear applications (right- and left-sided) might also be useful. This should be considered in patients who are highly symptomatic despite drug refractory therapy. A higher success rate is achieved in patients with paroxysmal atrial fibrillation and structurally normal hearts than in patients with persistent atrial fibrillation and structural myocardial abnormalities. The risks, benefits, and alternatives to atrial fibrillation ablation should be discussed at length with the patient, since there is significant comorbidity associated with the procedure. These risks include bleeding, infection, vascular injury, cardiac tamponade, air and thromboembolism resulting in transient ischemic attack and/or cerebrovascular accident, damage to the phrenic nerve, pulmonary vein stenosis resulting in pulmonary hypertension, and an atrial-esophageal fistula.

Generally accepted indications for atrial fibrillation ablation include symptoms that persist despite treatment with at least one antiarrhythmic drug. Differences in approaches and treatment results have been reported for paroxysmal and persistent atrial fibrillation. Success rates in the order of 65 to 85 percent have been reported via pulmonary vein isolation in patients with paroxysmal atrial fibrillation. Lower success rates (in the order of 50 to 60 percent) have been reported in patients with chronic and/or persistent atrial fibrillation using

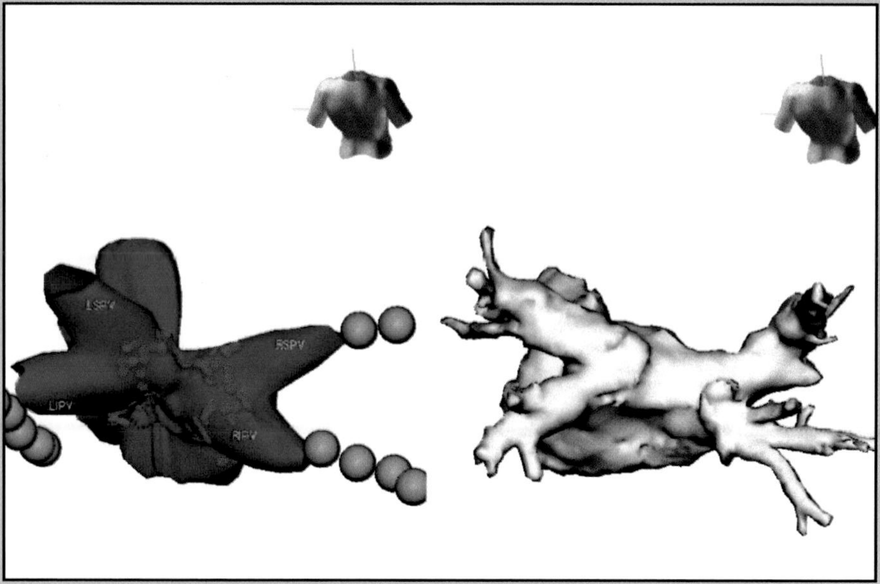

Figure 15.2: Shows nonfluoroscopic electroanatomic images of a pulmonary vein isolation procedure (courtesy of John Fisher, M.D., at Montefiore Medical Center, New York).

pulmonary vein isolation, ablation of continuous atrial fractioned electrograms, and additional linear lines. Importantly, the new guidelines for atrial fibrillation ablation stress the importance for distinguishing endpoints. For example, if a line is created in order to isolate pulmonary veins, testing should be performed via the electrophysiologist to demonstrate the inability for conduction to traverse that line. Table 15.1 shows the generally accepted indications for an atrial fibrillation ablation procedure. In addition, the table emphasizes the importance of testing for complete conduction block for any lines created.

Figure 15.2 shows nonfluoroscopic electroanatomic images of a pulmonary vein isolation procedure (courtesy of John Fisher, M.D., at Montefiore Medical Center, New York). Radiofrequency applications were delivered outside the pulmonary veins in order to achieve pulmonary vein isolation. The right superior and inferior pulmonary veins are circumscribed by a single circle of ablation lesions. Similarly, the left superior and inferior pulmonary veins are also circumscribed. An additional radiofrequency ablation line is drawn between both circular lesions, thereby creating an "eyeglass" configuration. Interventional electrophysiologists should be aware of the close proximity of the esophagus to the left atrium, thereby creating the potential for an esophageal atrial fistula (a serious and usually fatal complication post atrial fibrillation ablation).

Chapter 16

AV-Node Reentrant Tachycardia

One of the most common types of supraventricular tachycardias is AV-node reentrant tachycardia. As the name indicates, this is a micro-reentrant tachycardia that involves the AV node. In approximately 25 percent of patients, there is more than one AV nodal pathway. These patients often have a fast (alpha) pathway and a slow (beta) pathway (figure 16.1).

In these patients, a premature beat occurs and blocks in the alpha pathway and travels down the slower beta pathway. Recovery in the alpha limb will permit retrograde conduction back

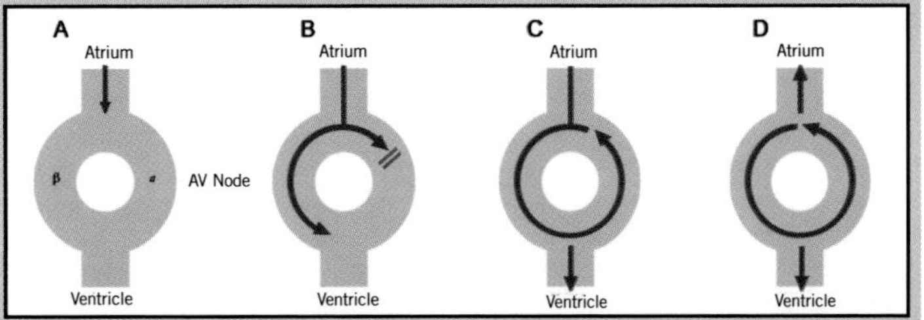

Figure 16.1: (A) Shows an atrial premature impulse approaching the dual pathways (fast α and slow β) needed to satisfy the criteria for AV-node reentrant tachycardia. (B) The premature impulse finds the fast pathway refractory and travels down the slow pathway. (C) The impulse then can travel to the ventricle and return up the fast pathway, which is no longer refractory. (D) A circus movement tachycardia sending impulses nearly simultaneously to the atria and ventricles.

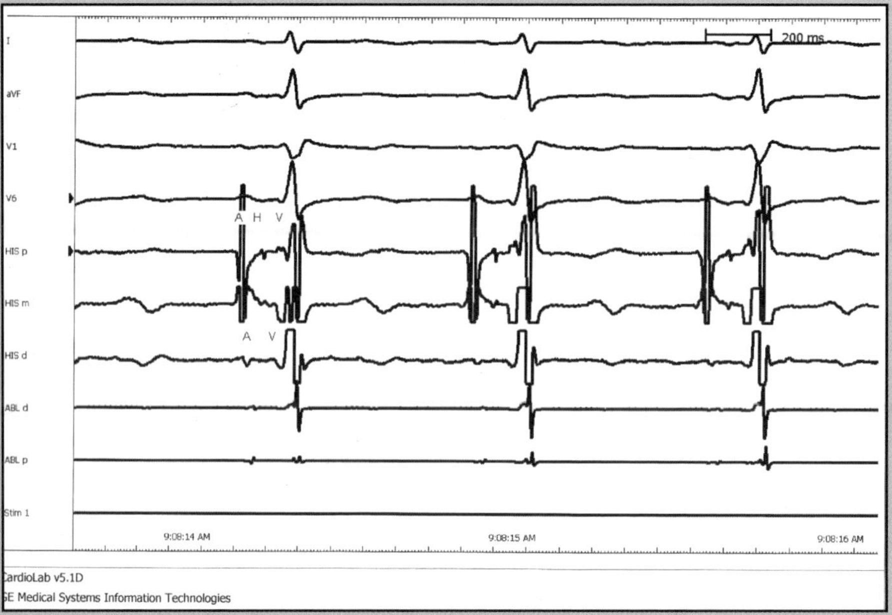

Figure 16.2: Baseline recordings in a patient with AV-node reentrant tachycardia.

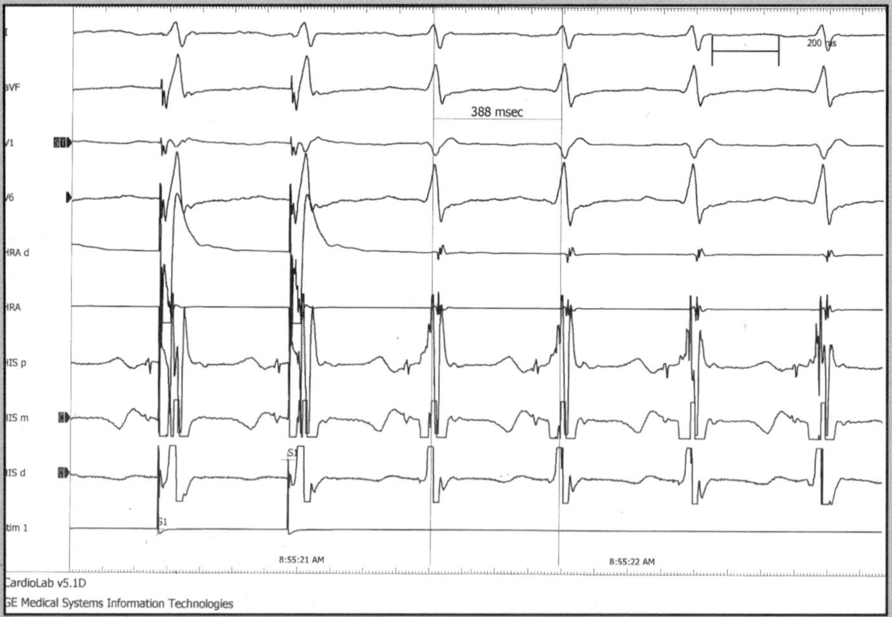

Figure 16.3: The induction of AV-node reentrant tachycardia during atrial overdrive pacing.

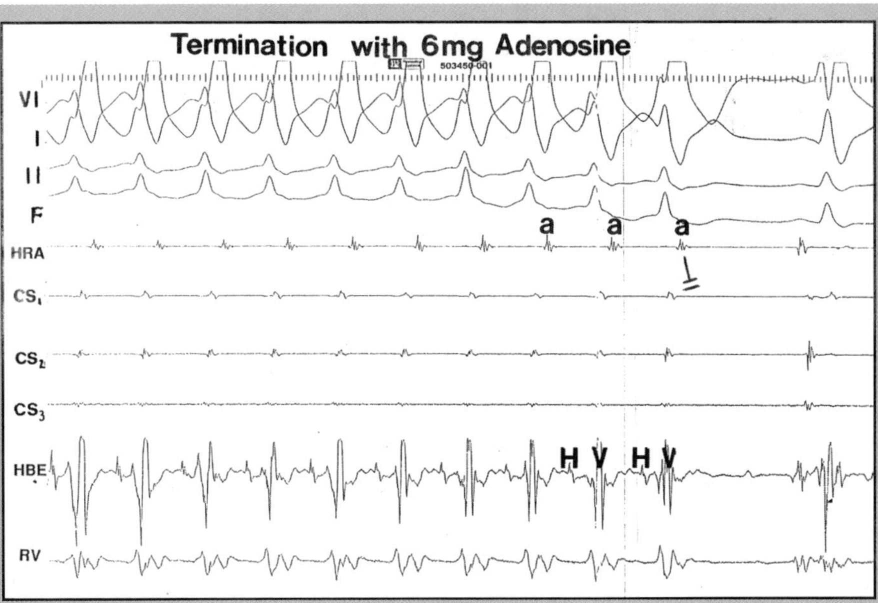

Figure 16.4: The termination of the tachycardia ending with an atrial electrogram helps to rule out an atrial tachycardia.

toward the atrium. This tachycardia satisfies the Mines postulate for reentry, resulting in a circus movement tachycardia.

In AV-node reentrant tachycardia, the atrial electrogram is typically encompassed within or at the tail end of the QRS complex. Figure 16.2 demonstrates baseline recordings in a patient who has AV-node reentrant tachycardia. In this patient, the AH and HV intervals are normal. Subsequently, during atrial overdrive pacing, AV-node reentrant tachycardia is induced (figure 16.3). An atrial electrogram is seen in the high right atrial recording, at the latter part of the QRS complex. In typical AV-node reentrant tachycardia, conduction occurs down a slow AV nodal pathway and up a fast AV nodal pathway.

These tachycardias can easily be terminated with the infusion of adenosine (6 mg initially and 12 mg if they fail to respond). The tachycardias can also be terminated with carotid sinus massage. The termination of the tachycardia ending with an atrial electrogram helps to rule out an atrial tachycardia (figure 16.4).

Programmed atrial stimulation (A1A2) typically reveals the presence of a "jump" in which progressive earlier extrastimuli (decrements of 10 msec) demonstrate a jump in the A2H2 interval (greater than or equal to 50 msec) indicative of refractoriness in the fast AV nodal pathway (figure 16.5). Elimination of the slow pathway (postablation) reveals no evidence of a jump and only a single curve (see the bottom of figure 16.5).

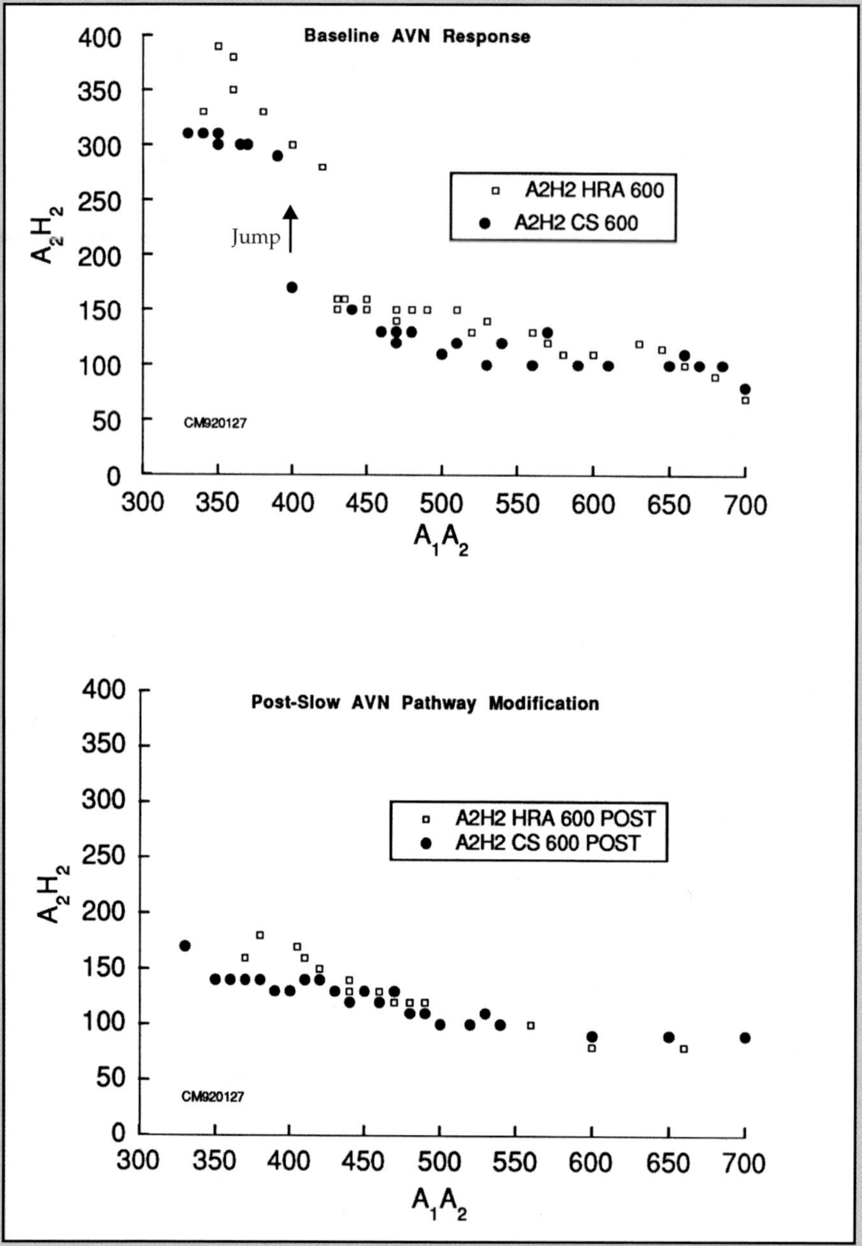

Figure 16.5: Programmed atrial stimulation (A1A2) typically recalls the presence of a "jump" in which progressive earlier extrastimuli (decrements of 10 msec) demonstrate a jump in the A2H2 interval (by greater than or equal to 50 msec) indicative of refractoriness in the fast AV nodal pathway (top figure). After ablation of the slow AV nodal pathway, there is no evidence of a "jump" (bottom figure).

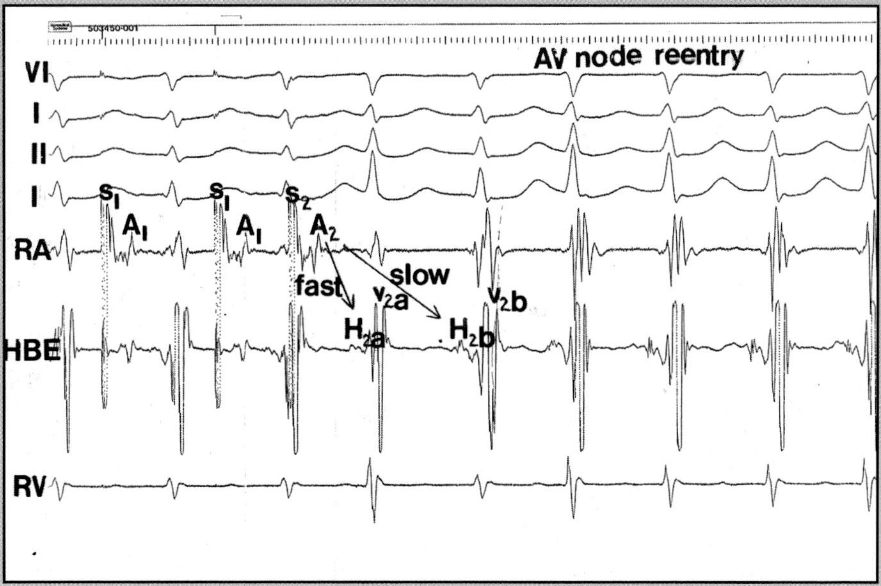

Figure 16.6: Simultaneous conduction over both the fast and slow AV nodal pathways and resultant double firing (H2aV2a and H2bV2b).

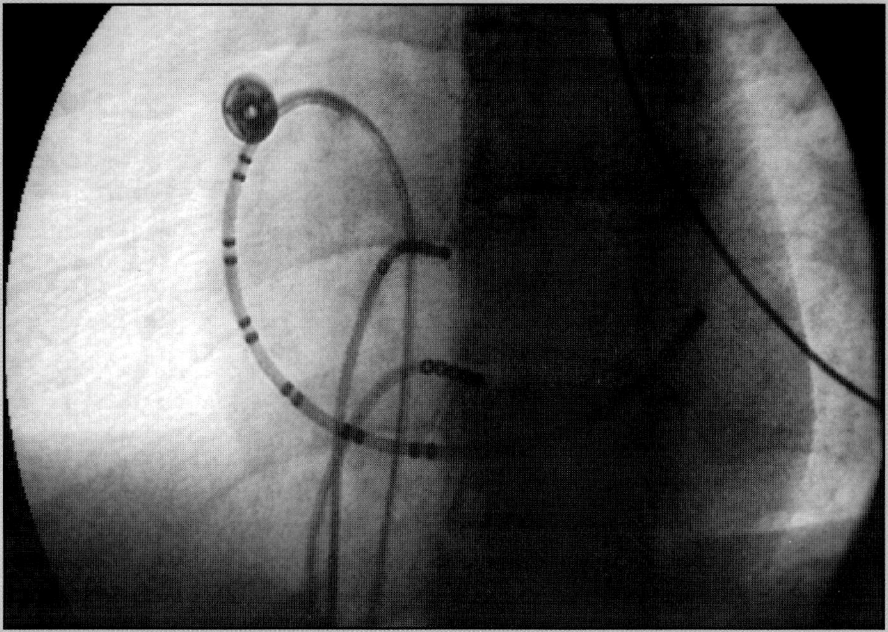

Figure 16.7: A left anterior oblique view of a slow AV nodal pathway ablation. A 20-pole catheter is placed in the coronary sinus vein. The ablation catheter is slightly above the coronary sinus and against the septum to ablate the slow AV nodal pathway. The catheter above the ablation catheter records the His bundle.

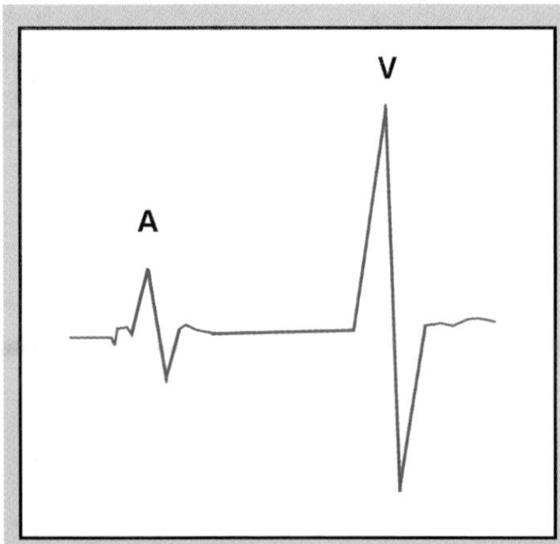

Figure 16.8: The electrogram recorded at the site of a slow pathway ablation showing an optimal A:V amplitude ratio of 1:4.

A rarer occurrence in patients with dual AV nodal pathways is dual conduction via a single atrial extrastimulus (A2). Figure 16.6 shows simultaneous conduction over both the fast and slow AV nodal pathways and resultant double firing (H2aV2a and H2bV2b).

Fluoroscopically, the AV junction can be divided into two components: a fast pathway and a slow pathway. In figure 16.7, a 20-pole coronary sinus catheter, typical quadripolar catheter (His bundle catheter), and the ablation catheter can be seen. In the left anterior oblique projection in which the catheter is toward the septum, the large-tip ablation catheter is located near the slow AV nodal pathway (mid-septum). Most slow AV nodal pathway ablations are performed slightly inferior to this location (posterior septal location). This is where the radiofrequency catheter ablation is typically performed with an electrogram in which the V is approximately four times the size of the A (figure 16.8). As the catheter is moved in a cephalic direction (toward the His bundle), the fast pathway of the AV node is identified.

In figure 16.9, an application of radiofrequency energy results in a junctional rhythm. Occasionally, an accelerated junctional rhythm may also occur (figure 16.10). Subsequent induction of AV-node reentrant tachycardia was not accomplished after an isoproterenol infusion.

In general, radiofrequency catheter ablation to treat AV-node reentrant tachycardia (via slow pathway ablation) can be accomplished with an immediate success rate of approximately 98 percent. There is a 5 percent recurrence rate in these patients. Ablation of the slow pathway as the primary approach has a complete heart block incidence of less than 1 percent. Inadvertent ablation of the fast pathway has a 6 percent incidence of complete heart block.

Other types of AV-node reentrant tachycardias include atypical AV-node reentrant tachycardia, also known as fast-slow AV-node reentrant tachycardia. In this case, there is a long RP tachycardia, with the P wave more than halfway between the two QRS complexes. The circuit is such that electrical pulses travel down the fast pathway of the AV node and retrograde up the slow pathway of the AV node.

Since the AV node itself is a separate entity between the atrium and the ventricle, it is possible to dissociate (in both typical and atypical AV-node reentrant tachycardia) the ventricle or the atrium. Upper final common pathway block during the tachycardia can demonstrate atrial dissociation; lower final common pathway block during the tachycardia can demonstrate AV block. These occurrences are relatively uncommon, though. Figure 16.11 shows AV-node reentrant tachycardia with 2:1 infrahisian block.

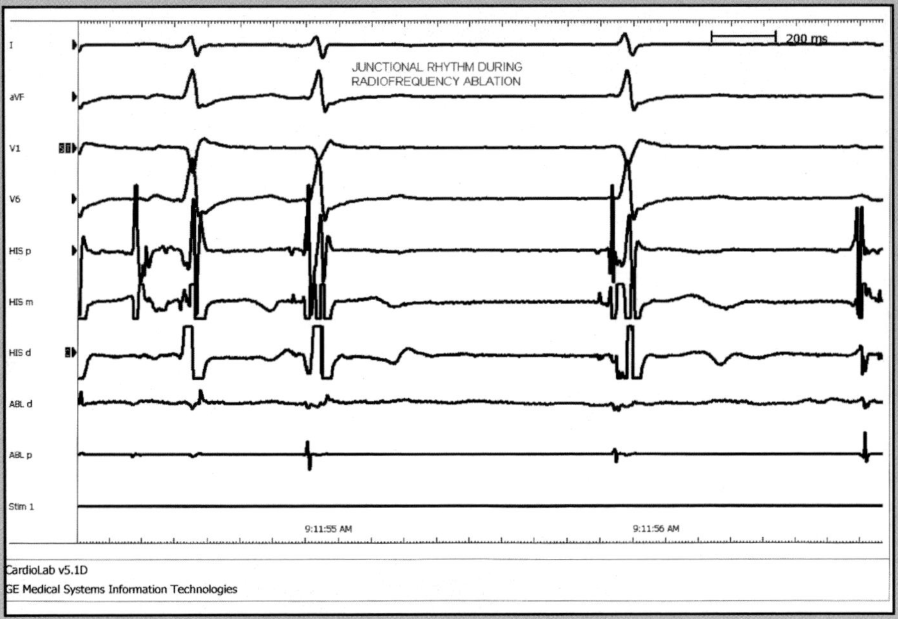

Figure 16.9: This figure demonstrates a junctional rhythm which occurred following the delivery of radiofrequency energy to the slow pathway of the AV node.

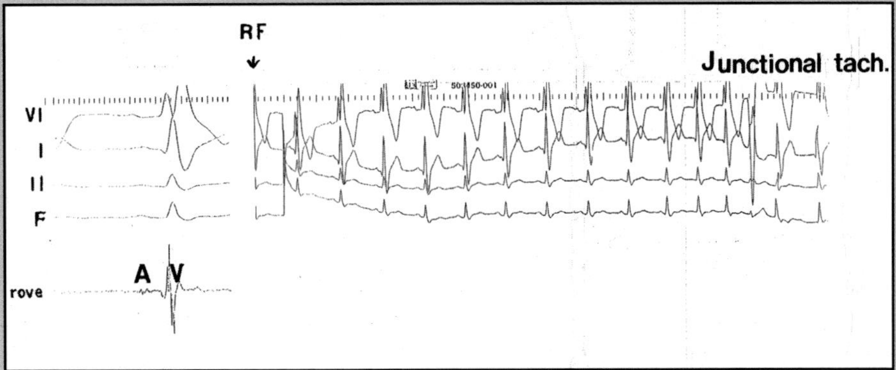

Figure 16.10: An accelerated junctional rhythm may also occur as the result of radiofrequency ablation of the slow AV nodal pathway.

In summary, the ablation of the slow AV nodal pathway to treat AV-node reentrant tachycardia is a technically simple procedure that can successfully be performed in the vast majority of patients with a very low complication rate. It should be considered as a primary therapy in patients who are highly symptomatic and choose not to undergo pharmacologic therapy.

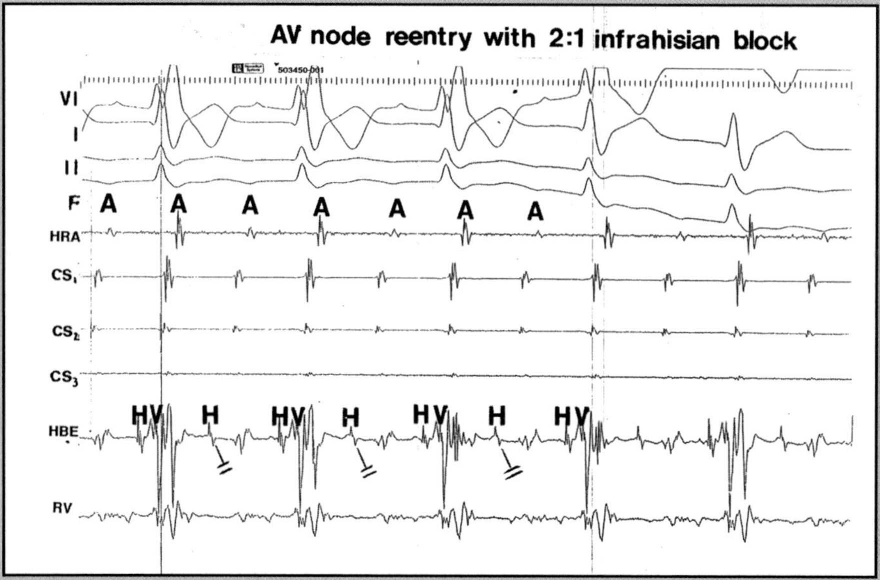

Figure 16.11: AV-node reentrant tachycardia with 2:1 infrahisian block.

Chapter 17

Atrial Tachycardia

Atrial tachycardia is a common atrial arrhythmia seen in individuals who have valvular disease or other structural heart disease; it is sometimes seen in people who have a structurally normal myocardium as well. Less common than atrial fibrillation and AV-node reentrant tachycardia, it is probably more common than AV reciprocating tachycardias (those that use an accessory pathway).

It is often difficult to determine whether an atrial tachycardia is of an automatic or a triggered mechanism. The focality of this arrhythmia, however, is pivotal to its management. In making the diagnosis of an atrial tachycardia, it is often important to dissociate the atrium from the ventricle and show that the ventricle is not a critical component of the circuit.

Figure 17.1 shows an atrial tachycardia with AV block present with more atrial electrograms than ventricular electrograms. In addition, when adenosine (an AV nodal blocking agent) is given to patients in atrial tachycardia, the tachycardia may at times terminate; however, it almost never terminates with an atrial electrogram. The termination of the tachycardia with an atrial electrogram almost certainly rules out an atrial tachycardia as a diagnosis during an electrophysiology study.

Initially, the diagnosis and management of an atrial tachycardia via radiofrequency catheter ablation was performed using multipolar catheters and point-by-point mapping in the myocardium to locate the site of earliest activation. In such instances, it was often

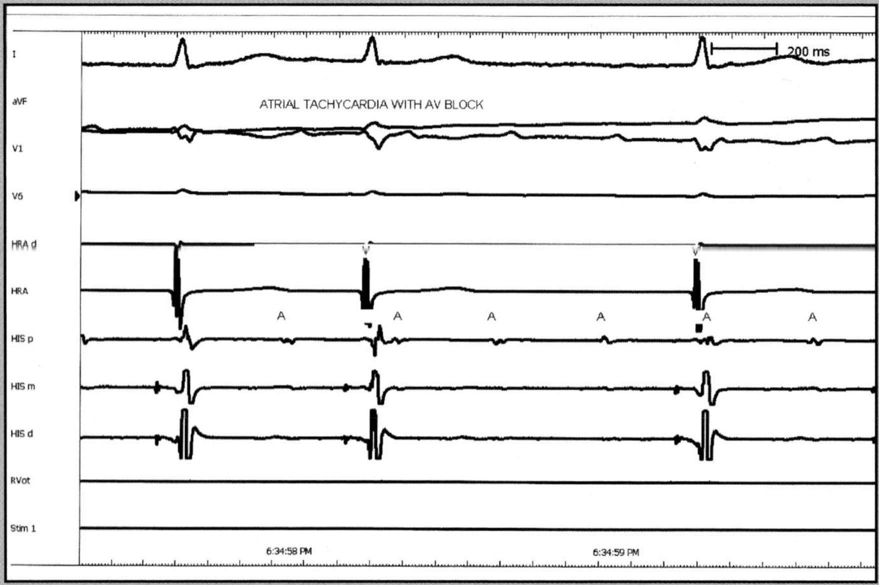

Figure 17.1: An atrial tachycardia with AV block present.

necessary to place a coronary sinus catheter or a right atrial catheter near the crista terminalis, and a radiofrequency mapping ablation catheter (in which one would map either the right atrium or the right ventricle) at critical points.

Atrial tachycardias often live in certain areas such as near the crista terminalis (often referred to as a "hot zone" or "trigger zone" for atrial tachycardias), the right atrial appendage, the tricuspid or mitral annulus, the coronary sinus, and the pulmonary veins. Other areas of the myocardium may also be triggers for these atrial tachycardias. More recently, nonfluoroscopic three-dimensional mapping techniques have been very helpful in isolating and mapping atrial tachycardias.

In figure 17.2, one can see sinus tachycardia in a patient on isoproterenol and atropine. A coronary sinus catheter placed from T1 to T10 (distal to proximal) shows the normal activation sequence from the sinus node.

A right atrial tachycardia induced by programmed electrical stimulation can be seen in figure 17.3. The right atrial tachycardia shows a subtle difference in its activation sequence, though it exhibits similarities to the sequence of the sinus tachycardia. The cycle length is considerably shorter for the right atrial tachycardia: 280 msec versus 380 msec.

In figure 17.4, a left atrial tachycardia was induced. The earliest activation point is seen in T4, on the left side of the heart.

Figure 17.5 shows a nonfluoroscopic three-dimensional map of the sinus tachycardia after radiofrequency catheter ablation. One can see the tachycardia initiating from the sinus node; it appears quite different from the darker images, which

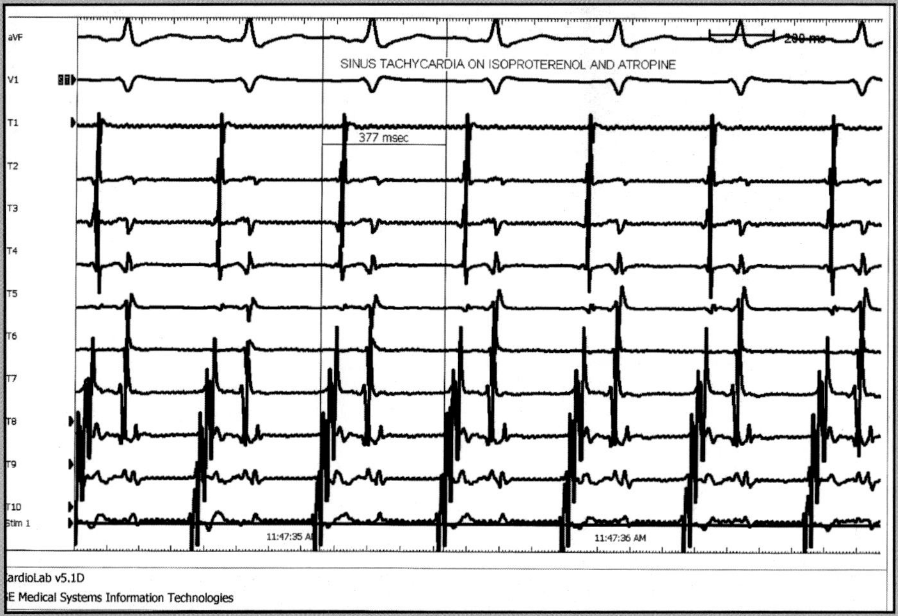

Figure 17.2: Sinus tachycardia in a patient on isoproterenol and atropine. A coronary sinus catheter placed from T1 to T10 (distal to proximal) shows the normal activation sequence from the sinus node.

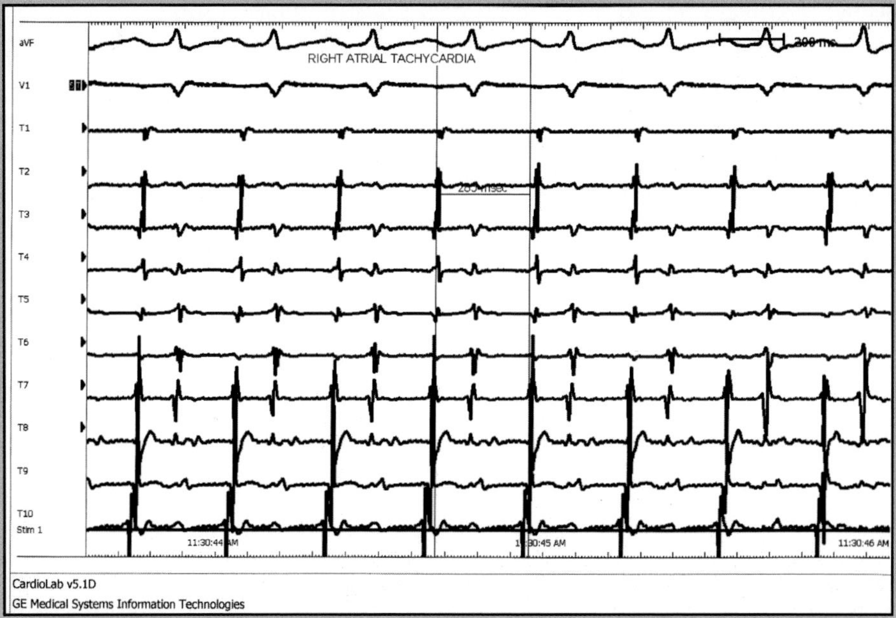

Figure 17.3: A right atrial tachycardia induced by programmed electrical stimulation.

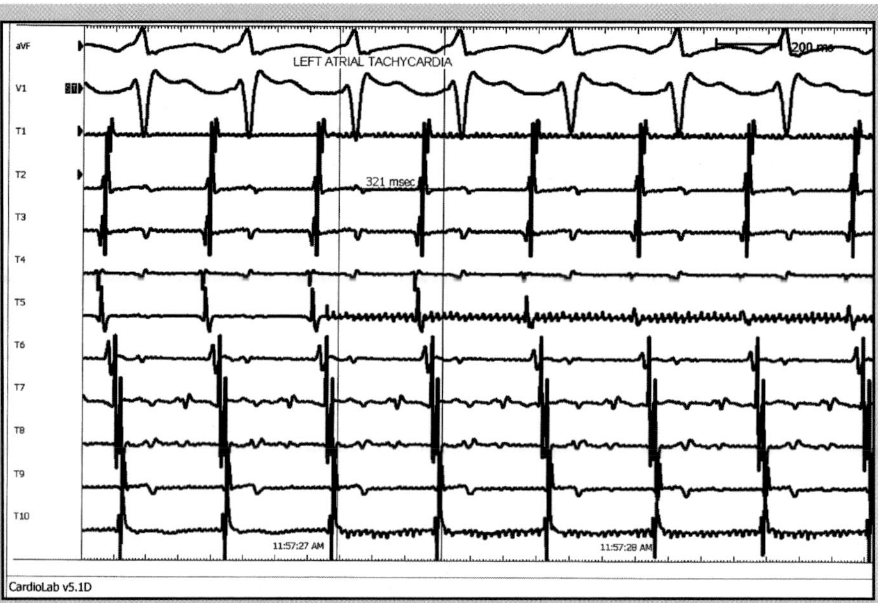

Figure 17.4: An induced left atrial tachycardia. The earliest activation point is seen in T4, on the left side of the heart. The coronary sinus catheter T1 (distal), T10 (proximal) was deep within the coronary sinus vein.

indicate where radiofrequency catheter ablation occurred.

In figure 17.6, one sees a right atrial tachycardia with activation sequence inferior to that of the sinus tachycardia along the crista terminalis.

Figure 17.7 shows a left atrial tachycardia (recorded from the right side) breaking through from the septum near the coronary sinus, which was also identified via mapping. Radiofrequency energy was applied to the right atrial tachycardia in the middle portion of the crista terminalis, with disruption of the tachycardia. A full repeat study failed to demonstrate any tachycardias. Follow-up of this patient and evidence of a recurrent tachycardia would perhaps lead to a transseptal procedure in order to tackle the left atrial tachycardia.

In another patient, a symptomatic atrial tachycardia was identified as mapped near the His bundle (parahisian atrial tachycardia). Figure 17.8 shows a map of the His bundle region, which was just superior to a right atrial tachycardia (seen in figure 17.9). Complete mapping of the tachycardia focus and the His bundle may be helpful for avoiding complete heart block in atrial tachycardias close to the His bundle.

Patients who have multiple atrial tachycardias that are not amenable to very complex mapping techniques and are refractory to pharmacologic therapy may benefit from an AV junction ablation and permanent pacemaker.

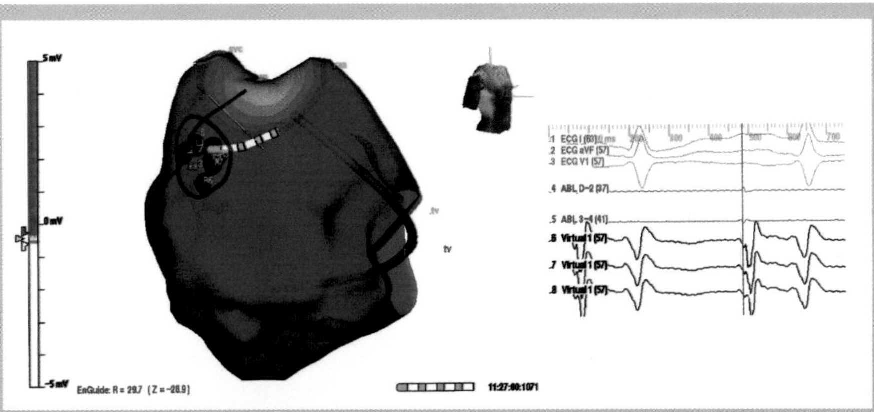

Figure 17.5: A three-dimensional mapping of the sinus tachycardia after radiofrequency catheter ablation. The tachycardia, initiating from the sinus node, appears quite different from the darker images, where radiofrequency catheter ablation occurred.

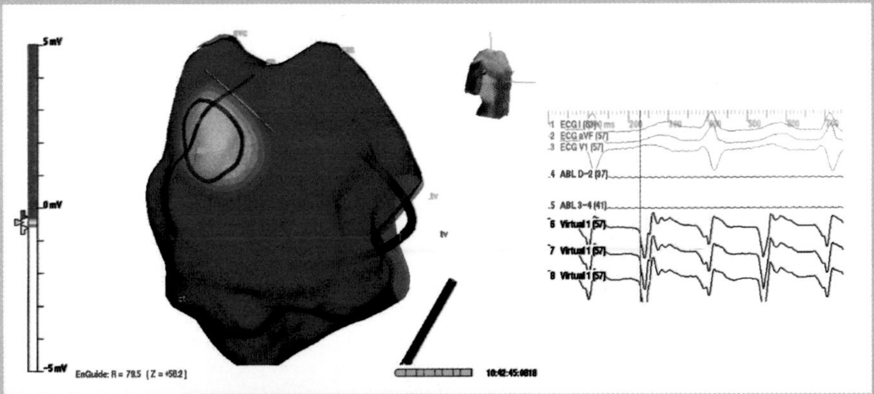

Figure 17.6: A right atrial tachycardia with activation sequence inferior to that of the sinus tachycardia along the crista terminalis.

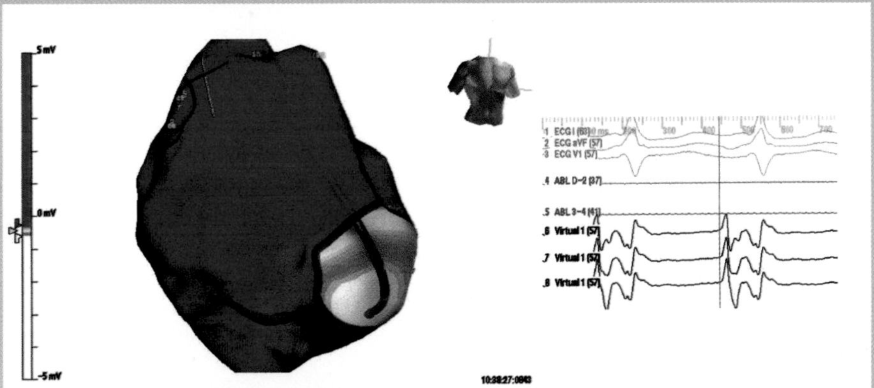

Figure 17.7: A left atrial tachycardia (recorded from the right side) breaking through from the septum near the coronary sinus.

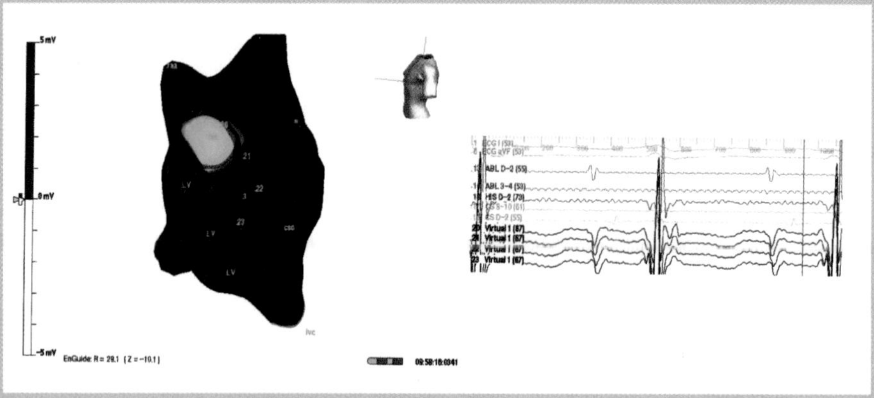

Figure 17.8: A map of the His bundle region.

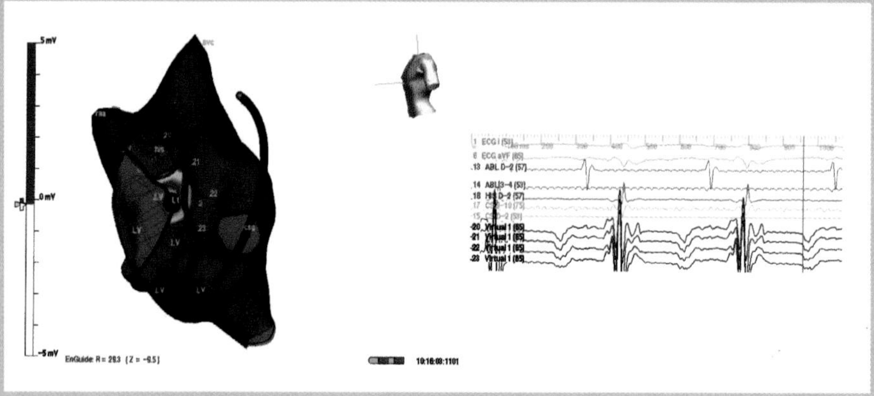

Figure 17.9: A map of a parahisian atrial tachycardia, slightly below the His bundle.

Chapter 18

Atrial Flutter

Typical atrial flutter is a macro-reentrant tachycardia. It differs from an atrial tachycardia (which emanates from a discrete focus) by its continuous electrical activity around a relatively large anatomic structure, such as the right tricuspid valve. It is principally a right atrial disease, but can occasionally occur in the left atrium or around surgical scars. Classic atrial flutter most frequently moves counterclockwise around the right atrial structures, but occasionally may move clockwise. Figure 18.1 shows a 12-lead ECG in a patient with typical atrial flutter. Note the sawtooth flutter waves seen in the inferior leads (II, III, and aVF).

To diagnose atrial flutter and its mechanism, it is useful to position a multipolar electrode catheter from the femoral vein and cross the isthmus into the coronary sinus. This can be seen in figure 18.2. The catheter traverses the isthmus and records continuous atrial conduction, as observed in the figure at an atrial cycle length of 259 msec. One can pace directly on the isthmus in a critical zone of the tachycardia and entrain (get into the circuit of) the tachycardia. Typically, a large (10-mm) ablation tip catheter is placed across the tricuspid valve in order to record a large ventricular electrogram with a small atrial electrogram. In the left anterior oblique fluoroscopic projection at approximately 45 degrees, the tricuspid valve is open and resembles a clock facing right at the operator (figure 18.3). The ablation is performed from that viewpoint, and the catheter tip serves as the small hand of the clock for location purposes. The operator typically performs a cavotricuspid isthmus ablation with the catheter

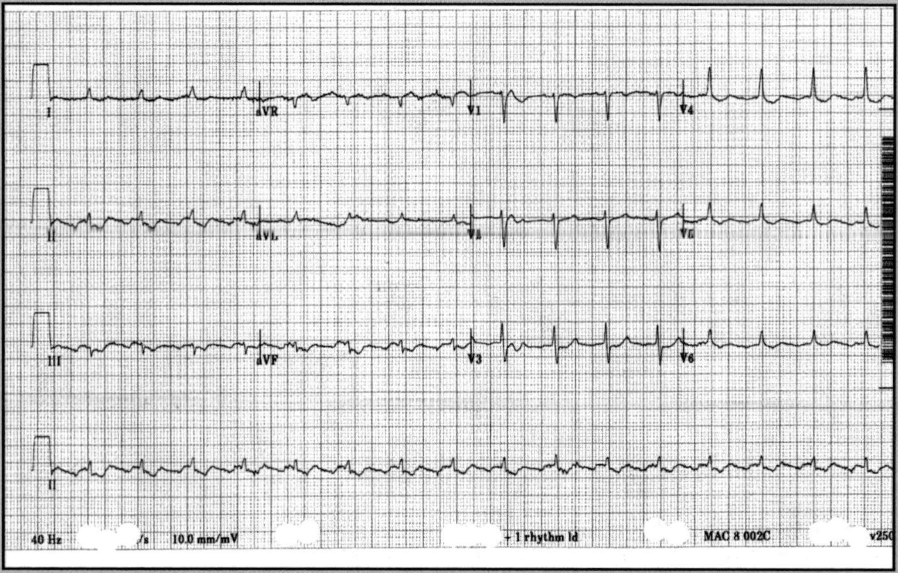

Figure 18.1: A 12-lead ECG in a patient with typical atrial flutter. Note the sawtooth waves in the inferior leads II,III, and aVF.

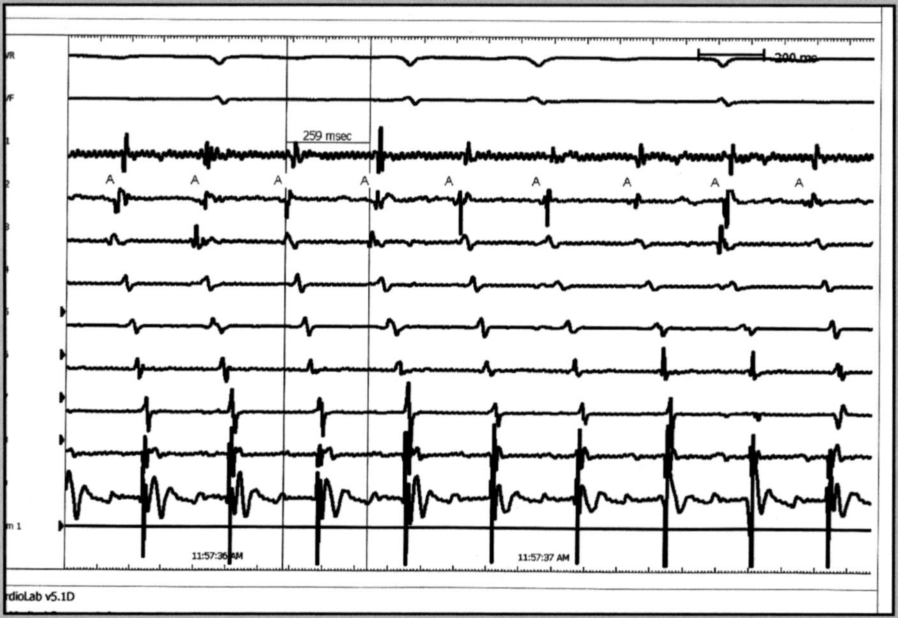

Figure 18.2: A coronary sinus multipoled pacing catheter is placed up from the femoral vein across the isthmus.

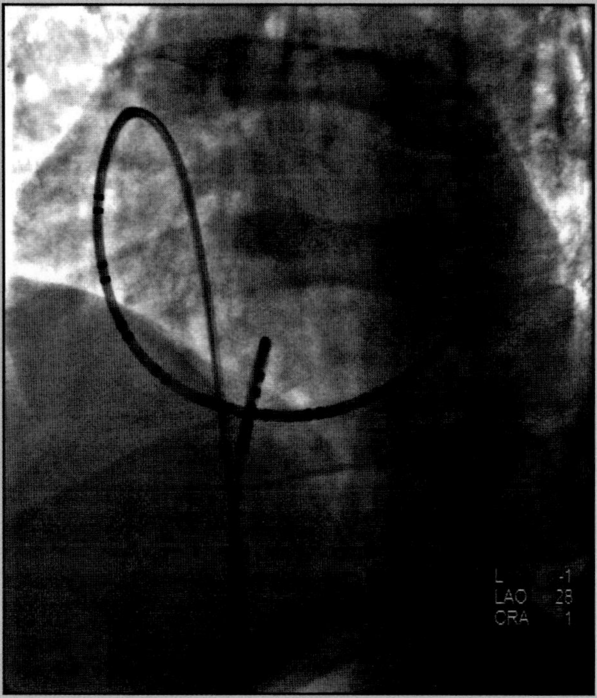

Figure 18.3: Shows the typical catheter locations for an atrial flutter ablation using just two catheters (a multipolar coronary sinus catheter and a large-tip ablation catheter) as viewed fluoroscopically in the left anterior oblique projection. The large loop of the coronary sinus catheter forms a circle largely resembling a clock. The tip of the catheter, if it were the small hand, would be located at 6 o'clock. The catheter is pulled back slowly in this view (between ablation applications), maintaining a 6 o'clock position.

at 6 o'clock, as viewed in the left anterior oblique projection. The author typically delivers 45 seconds of radiofrequency energy at 100 watts and a temperature of 55 degrees centigrade. Other operators may have subtle variations of the precise power, temperature, and duration of the particular radiofrequency energy applications.

A complete line of block is created across the isthmus with a technique that is similar to and often called "spot welding": applying discrete lesions to the isthmus and then pulling back the catheter and applying additional lesions. Alternatively, the "drag and burn" strategy, in which the catheter is very slowly pulled back during the ablation, can also be used. By applying either technique and pulling back the catheter from the tricuspid valve all the way down to the inferior vena cava, one can create a complete line of block across the isthmus.

Figure 18.4 shows pacing from the distal end of the coronary sinus and continuous conduction across the isthmus from T2 (the more distal end of the coronary sinus) to T9 (the more proximal end of the catheter). There is continuous conduction across the isthmus.

By performing a radiofrequency ablation as described above, complete isthmus block was created, as illustrated in figure 18.5. Atrial pacing from both sides of the catheter ablation line demonstrated inability for an impulse to directly traverse that line.

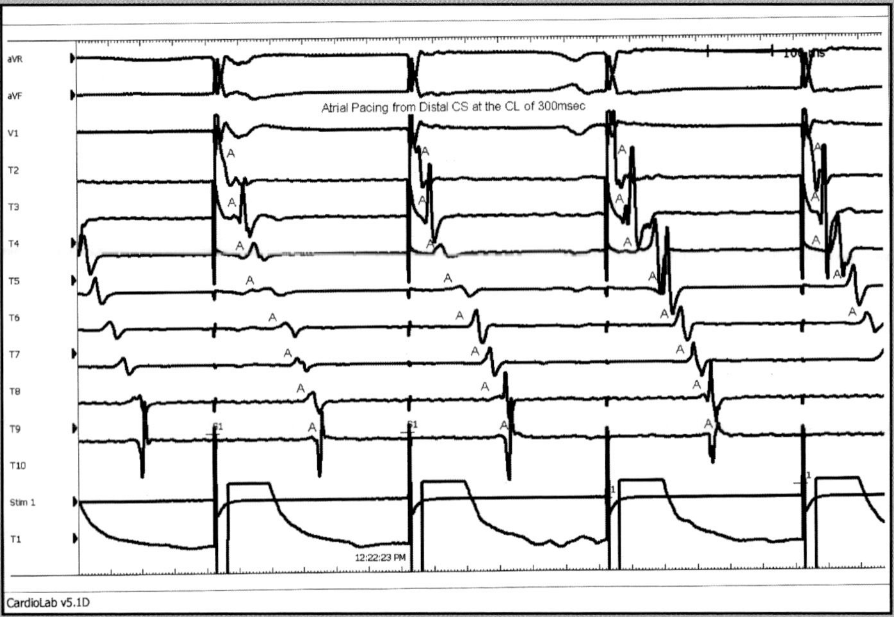

Figure 18.4: Pacing from the distal end of the coronary sinus and continuous conduction across the isthmus from T2, the more distal end of the coronary sinus, to T9.

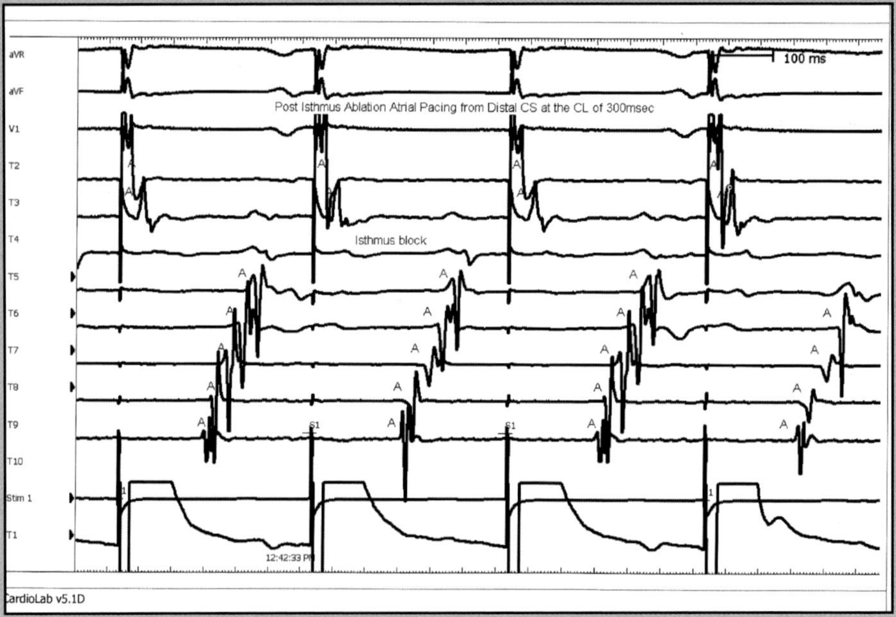

Figure 18.5: A complete isthmus block resulting from a radiofrequency ablation.

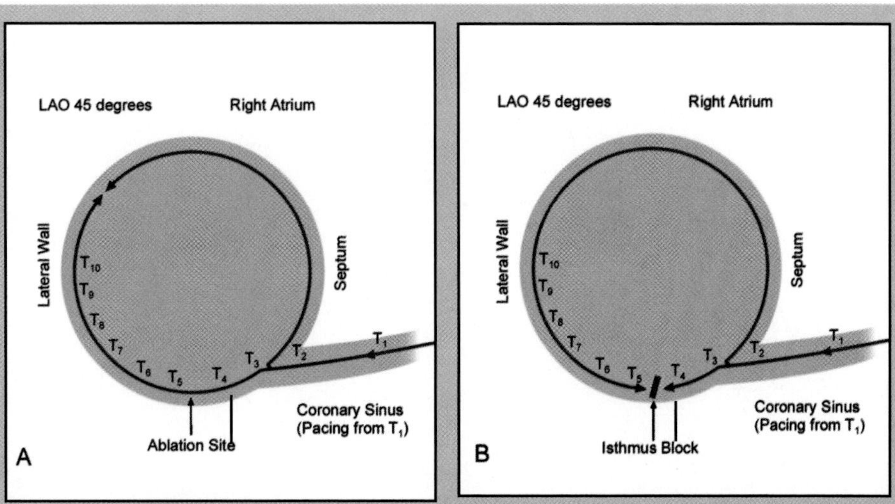

Figure 18.6: A diagram showing the progression of conduction and waveform of depolarization in patients while pacing from the coronary sinus. The figure at left (A) shows typical fusion due to unimpeded conduction across the isthmus. This corresponds to figure 18.4. (B) shows complete isthmus block after coronary sinus pacing (indicated by the double line). This corresponds to figure 18.5. Electrical impulses cannot cross the isthmus, and conduction can only reach the other side of the block from a counterclockwise direction despite pacing from the coronary sinus.

Radiofrequency energy was delivered at the T4 bipole of the coronary sinus, and by pacing from the distal end of the coronary sinus, conduction traveled from T2 to T3 and then T4. Thereafter, complete conduction block occurs such that atrial activation must travel all the way around the right atrium to T9 progressing down to reach T5. This is characteristic of complete isthmus block.

Figure 18.6 shows the progression of conduction and waveform of depolarization in patients while pacing from the coronary sinus. Figure 18.7a and 18.7b show two fluoroscopic images during the ablation in the right anterior oblique projection. Figure 18.7a shows the catheter near the tricuspid valve. The catheter is pulled back only a few millimeters following each discrete radiofrequency application (spot-welding technique). Finally, an application is delivered just before the inferior vena cava (figure 18.7b), where an atrial electrogram is still recorded. The catheter is located at 6 o'clock while directly facing the tricuspid valve in the 45-degree left anterior oblique projection. The operator pulls back the catheter from the tricuspid valve to the inferior vena cava in order to achieve complete isthmus block. If a 6 o'clock catheter ablation fails, a second ablation line can be performed in a similar manner, slightly to the left or right of that line.

Nonfluoroscopic three-dimensional mapping can be useful at demonstrating whether complete isthmus block is present. It is important to note, however, that patients who undergo initial catheter ablation of typical atrial flutter using nonfluoroscopic three-dimensional mapping have

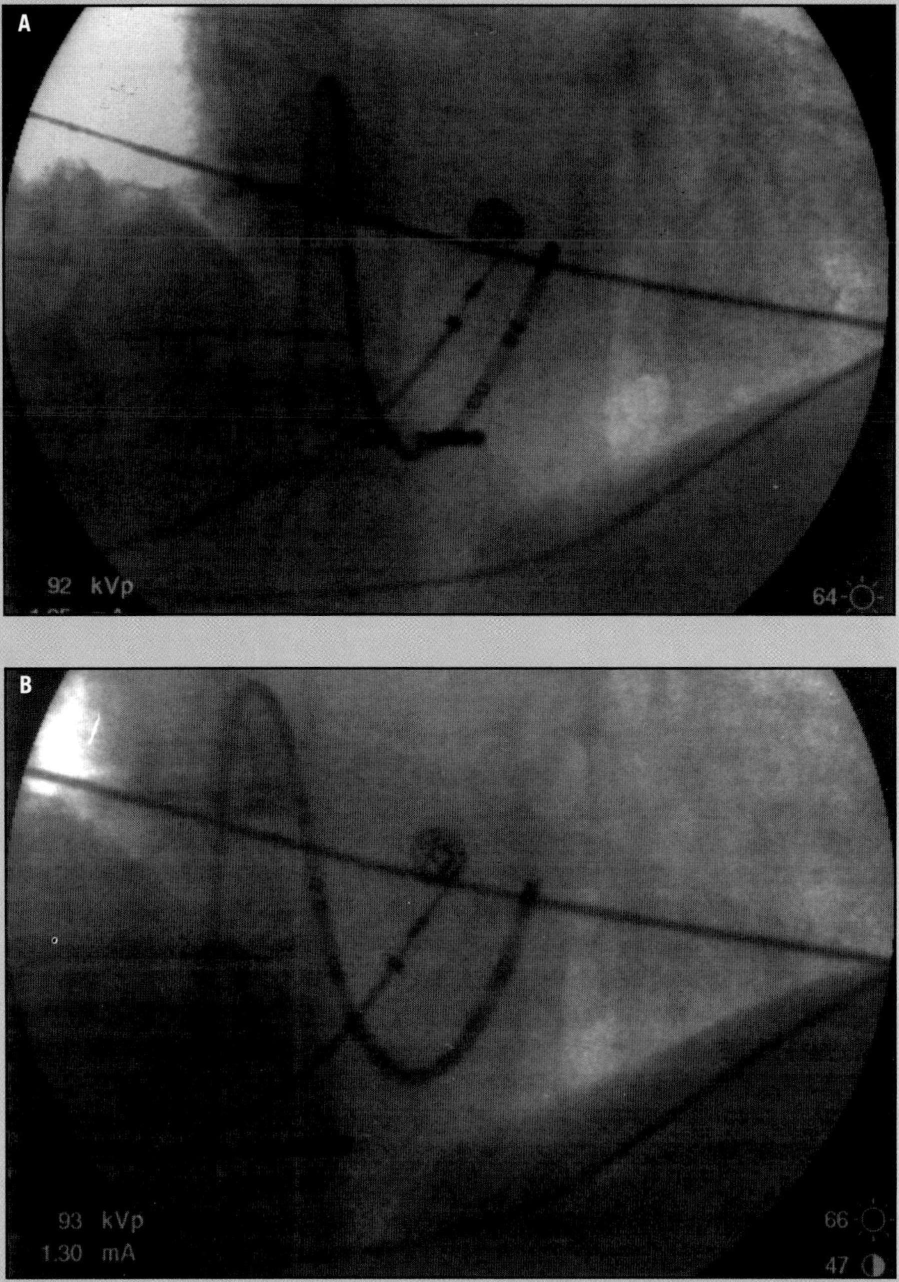

Figure 18.7: Two right anterior oblique fluoroscopic images during the ablation; the catheter was placed across the ventricle at 6 o'clock while directly facing the tricuspid valve in the 45-degree left anterior oblique projection.

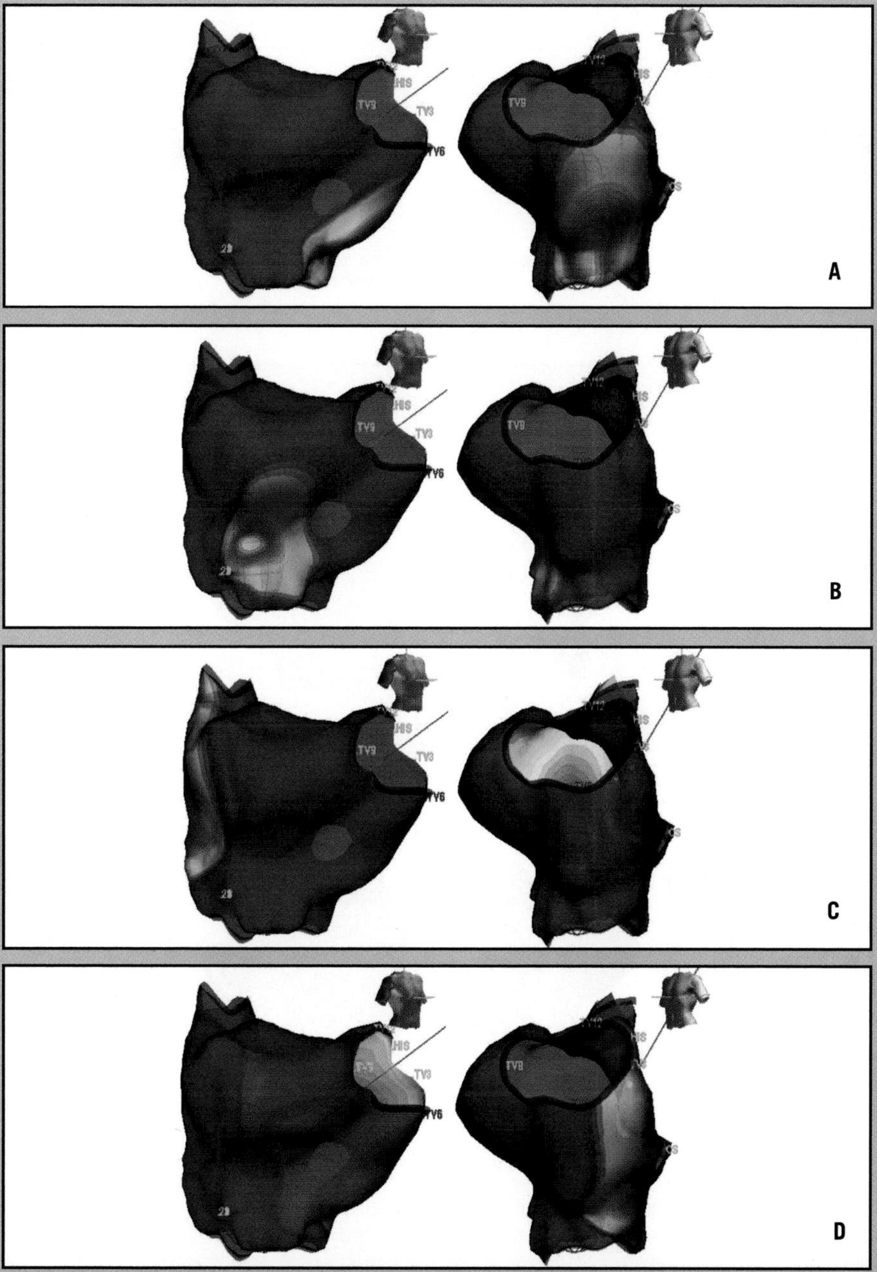

Figure 18.8: Shows right and left anterior oblique projections of a nonfluoroscopic mapping procedure showing clockwise atrial flutter. (A) Shows passage of atrial flutter through the isthmus. (B) Shows propagation of atrial flutter up the lateral right atrial wall. (C) Shows propagation across the posterior right atrial wall. (D) Shows eventual propagation across the right atrial septum.

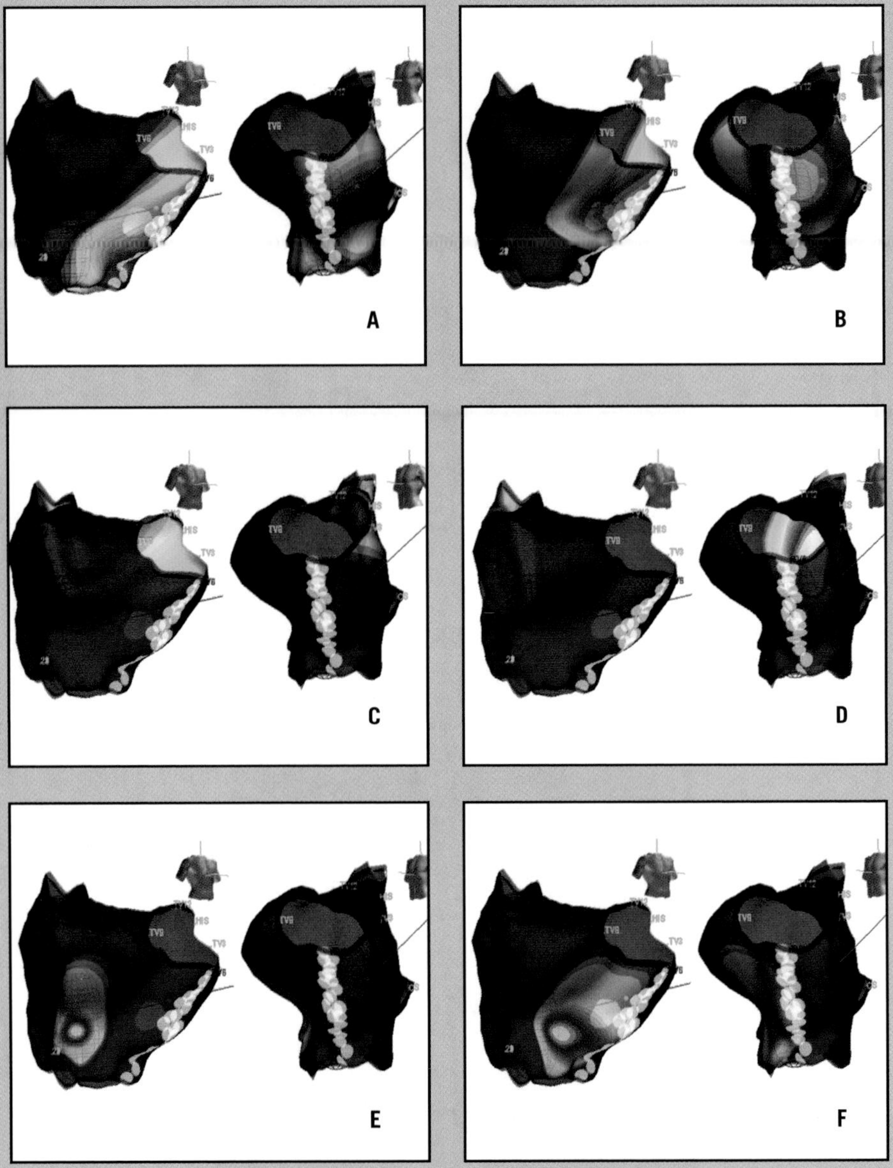

Figure 18.9: (A) Demonstrates right and left anterior oblique views of coronary sinus pacing, medial to the line of isthmus block created by catheter ablation. (B) Shows propagation up to the line of isthmus block (activation does not cross this line, *i.e.*, complete medial isthmus block). (C) Shows propagation away from the ablation line, toward the septum. (D) Shows propagation across the posterior right atrial wall. (E) Shows propagation to the lateral right atrial wall. (F) Shows propagation to the lateral aspect of the ablation line.

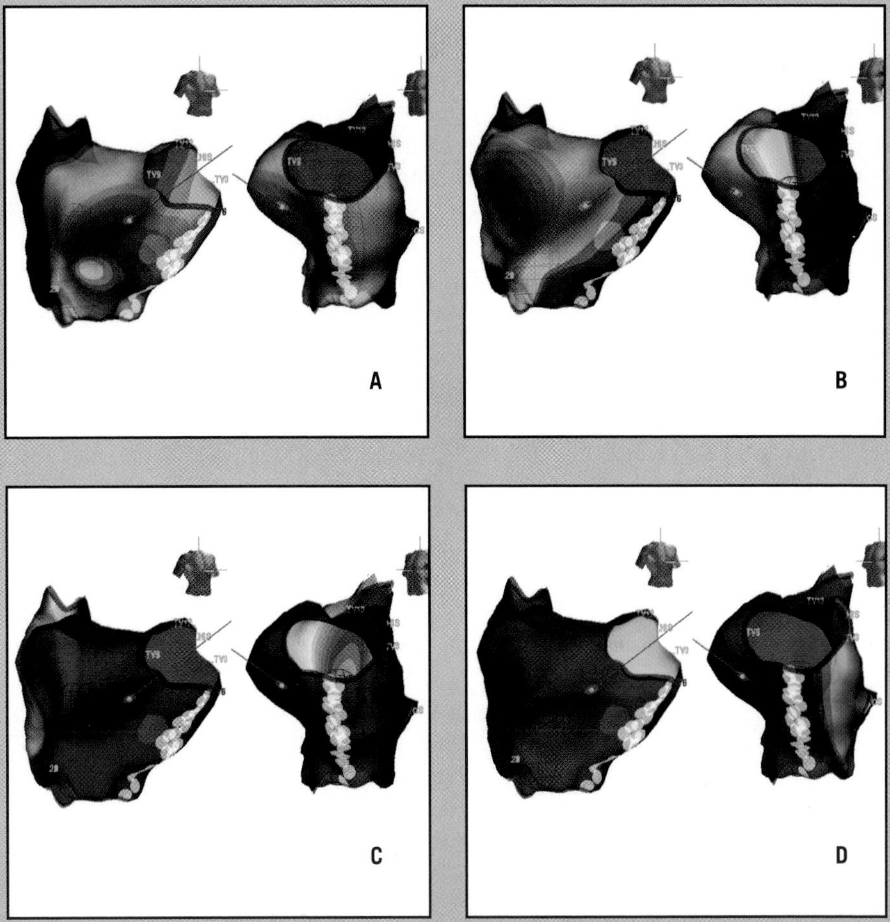

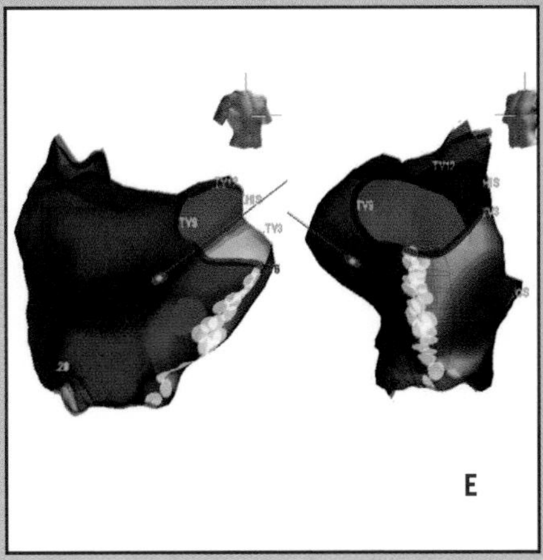

Figure 18.10: (A) Demonstrates right and left anterior oblique views of right atrial pacing, lateral to the line of isthmus block created by catheter ablation (activation does not cross this line, *i.e.*, complete lateral isthmus block). (B) Shows posterolateral propagation in the right atrium. (C) Shows posterior propagation in the right atrium. (D) Shows septal right atrial propagation. (E) Shows propagation medial to the ablation line.

equivalent outcomes when compared to more traditional fluoroscopic mapping with only a multi-poled catheter placed across the cavotricuspid isthmus and an ablation catheter. Nonfluoroscopic mapping is often particularly useful in cases of recurrent atrial flutter following a successful atrial flutter ablation. Figures 18.8a–18.8d show sequential right and left anterior oblique nonfluoroscopic three-dimensional mapping projections of clockwise atrial flutter with conduction across the isthmus. Figures 18.9a–18.9f show sequential images demonstrating coronary sinus pacing and complete medial isthmus block. Figures 18.10a–18.10e show lateral right atrial pacing and complete lateral isthmus block. In particular, nonfluoroscopic three-dimensional mapping can demonstrate electrical conduction across a catheter ablation line indicative of incomplete isthmus block. The catheter then could be guided to that region and additional applications could be delivered, in order to complete the line of block and prevent recurrent atrial flutter.

In addition to the atrial flutter circuits described herein, other flutter circuits have been described. These include upper loop reentry, septal flutter, and mitral annular/post atrial fibrillation ablation flutter. Nonfluoroscopic three-dimensional mapping is also useful for defining these circuits and guiding catheter ablation.

Chapter 19

External Cardioversion and Defibrillation

Cardioversion is synchronized delivery of direct current energy (typically to the chest), but potentially directly to the myocardium by internal catheters. Unlike its asynchronous counterpart, defibrillation, cardioversion delivers direct current energy synchronously to the R-wave of the electrogram (or electrocardiogram) in order to prevent inadvertent discharge during the vulnerable cycle and resultant ventricular fibrillation.

It is important to know how to perform an external cardioversion for the treatment of hemodynamically stable tachycardias. The most frequent cardioversion indication is for conversion of atrial fibrillation or atrial flutter. During these arrhythmias, the rapid atrial rhythm must be disrupted and reset into a more normalized sinus rhythm.

In order to perform an electrical cardioversion, the patient must be connected to an external monitor and cardioverter-defibrillator device. Either through such a device or separately, an electrocardiogram is monitored or recorded. It is also optimal for the cardioverter-defibrillator to have external pacing capabilities should the patient become profoundly bradycardiac. If this procedure is performed electively, the patient should be administered oxygen via nasal cannula and should have an intravenous line inserted. The intravenous line could be used for intravenous fluids, conscious sedation, antiarrhythmic drugs, and if necessary, resuscitation medications. Occasionally during a cardioversion, the patient may become bradycardiac, making it necessary to give epinephrine and/or atropine.

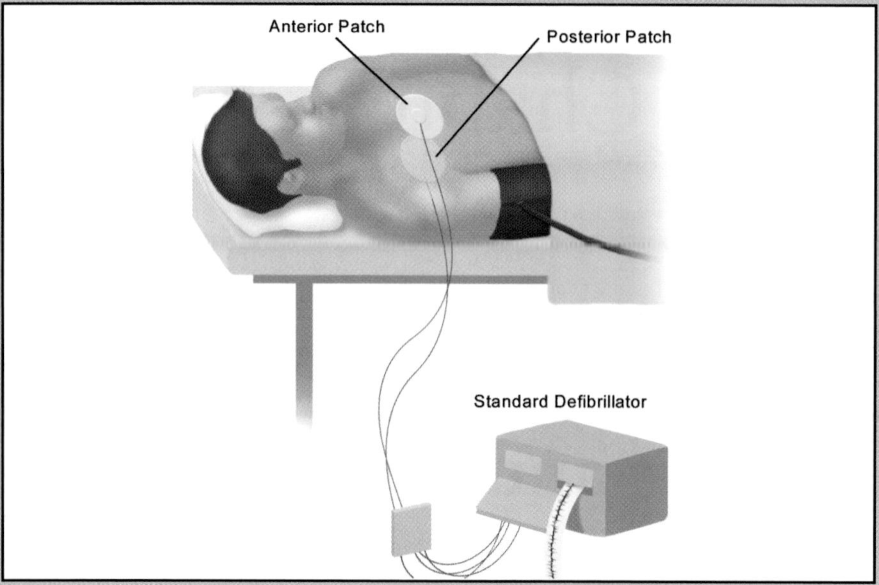

Figure 19.1: Placement of the skin patches in a midsternal anterior; intrascapular posterior location is in order to perform "hands off" electrical cardioversion of atrial fibrillation.

For an elective cardioversion of an atrial dysrhythmia (atrial fibrillation, flutter, or tachycardia), the procedure can be performed with external paddles, though it is preferable to use large external skin patches connected to the external defibrillator. This latter method provides for a hands-off ability to cardiovert the patient (figure 19.1). For cardioversion, the patches are placed directly midsternum anteriorly and posteriorly between the scapula in order to encompass a sufficient amount of atrial tissue in the wave of depolarization.

It is necessary to obtain written informed consent if the procedure is elective. In the compromised patient in whom it is necessary to stabilize the arrhythmia (resulting from ongoing ischemia and/or infarction, congestive heart failure or hemodynamic compromise), the patient can be cardioverted urgently without informed written consent.

In elective cardioversions, conscious sedation for the patient is preferred. This can be performed by cardiologists and/or electrophysiologists who are certified in conscious sedation with the administration of midazolam, fentalyl and/or morphine sulfate. The patient is sedated until drowsy in an effort to produce not only sedation but also an amnestic effect. In addition, the heart rate, blood pressure, and an ECG are continuously monitored. Oxygen saturation is measured via standard oximetry and should be adequate during the procedure. It is important to have a crash cart and intubation material nearby as well as reversing agents (naloxone and flumazenil). Alternatively, an anesthesiologist can administer propofol to achieve deep sedation.

After conscious sedation is achieved, the defibrillator should be charged to the

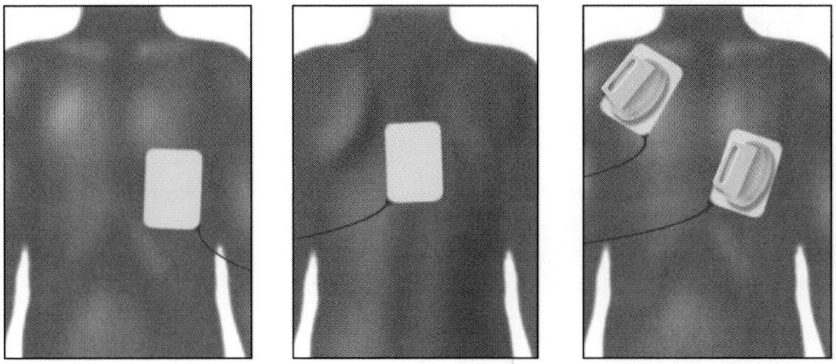

Figure 19.2: The placement of the patches for ventricular tachycardia. The first and third figures are anterior, and the second figure is posterior.

desired level. A biphasic defibrillator is used, up to 360 joules of output, which is then synchronized to the R wave in order to cardiovert the patient. The maximum output is used only in atrial fibrillation patients who are morbidly obese or have significant chronic obstructive pulmonary disease. If the patient has a slender cardiac silhouette, one should routinely start at 150 joules for synchronous biphasic cardioversion, although advanced cardiac life support suggests lower energies. This operator uses higher energies because of the statistically improved probability of conversion and the need for fewer additional shocks delivered to the patient.

An alternative to failed electrical cardioversion is the application of pressure directly anterior on top of the patch during the synchronized cardioversion. It is important that while applying pressure the operator uses an insulated material and does not have any contact directly with the patient or any electrically-conducted material. The pressure is applied at the 20-lb. to 40-lb. range directly over the chest during the delivery of direct current energy. Paddles (either not connected to the defibrillator directly applied over the patches or used without patches) allow for pressure. A recording strip should be obtained during and after the cardioversion procedure. Should the patient experience a significant bradycardia, external pacing should be considered along with atropine and epinephrine.

In some instances, failed cardioversion can be facilitated with the infusion of ibutilide. It is important to note that ibutilide prolongs the QT interval, and three hours of monitoring post-ibutilide infusion is essential

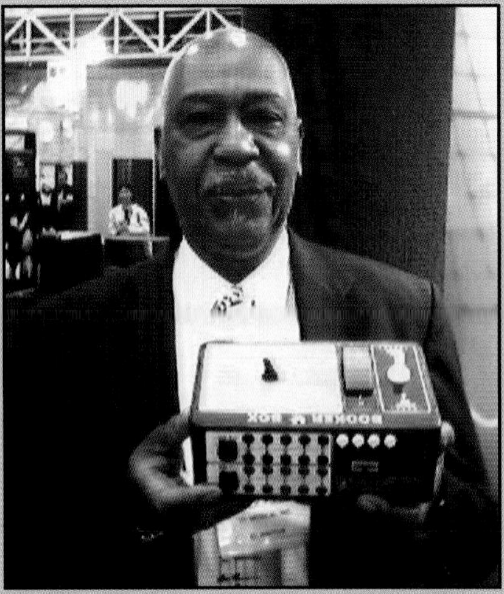

Figure 19.3: Photo of Booker Pullen holding the Booker Box, which he developed.

to make sure that latent proarrhythmia (torsades de pointes) does not occur.

In hemodynamically stable patients with a stable ventricular arrhythmia such as ventricular tachycardia, a synchronized defibrillation (*i.e.*, cardioversion) can be performed. The energy level we routinely use for these patients is 360 joules of synchronous biphasic energy. For failed elective cardioversion of ventricular tachycardia, we will again use pressure to decrease the transthoracic impedance and to facilitate the defibrillation.

Please note that the patch positions for cardioversion or defibrillation of ventricular tachycardia are quite different than those used for atrial fibrillation. For ventricular tachycardia (figure 19.2), one patch is placed anteriorly on the lateral chest (under the left breast) and one posteriorly between the two scapulae (or slightly to the right). If paddles are utilized, one is placed slightly to the right of midsternum, and one slightly to the left of the midaxillary line of the patient, below the point of maximum impulse of the heart.

For unstable patients, nonsynchronized defibrillation (not cardioversion) is performed. It is important not to press the synchronize button, in order to minimize any delays for delivering the electrical energy. The highest energy output possible is employed, and if the patient fails three high-energy shocks, increased pressure to the sternum should be administered. Pressure during defibrillation of ventricular tachycardia is applied over the sternal edge patch.

Another option is a method of internal cardioversion or defibrillation using an internal pacing catheter and a switch box (figure 19.3; Booker Box, TZ Medical, Portland, Oregon), in which one can switch from standard pacing and sensing from the catheter to internal cardioversion or defibrillation. This has proven very helpful in the setting of refractory ventricular tachycardia and ventricular fibrillation in the electrophysiology laboratory. In addition, low-energy internal cardioversion during an atrial fibrillation ablation might also be facilitated via this method.

Chapter 20

Accessory Pathways

Wolff-Parkinson-White (WPW) syndrome is defined by a short PR interval on ECG (less than 120 msec) with the presence of a delta wave (slurred segment between the P wave and QRS complex) and a history of palpitations/supraventricular tachycardia. Preexcitation (a delta wave on an ECG) exists in approximately 0.15 percent of the general population. Accessory pathways (or bypass tracts) are embryonic remnants between the atria and ventricles that are found in the atrioventricular groove.

Supraventricular tachycardia as a result of accessory pathways in children younger than six years old may be a temporary phenomenon. Subsequently, as the child develops, the accessory pathway may become nonfunctional (*i.e.*, disappear). Therefore, it may be reasonable to hold off on catheter ablation in those children unless absolutely necessary.

Accessory pathways may be evident from a 12-lead ECG (figure 20.1). This is called a manifest bypass tract, in which the presence of a delta wave is readily observed. In some instances (left lateral bypass tracts, for example), preexcitation is not evident except during AV nodal blockade (via carotid sinus massage and/or infusion of adenosine). This is called a latent bypass tract.

In other instances, the bypass tract conducts only in a retrograde direction (from the ventricle to the atrium). This is called a concealed bypass tract, where there is no risk for rapid conduction of atrial fibrillation down the bypass tract.

The presence of an accessory pathway with the potential for rapid conduction in an antegrade direction (from the atrium to the ventricle)

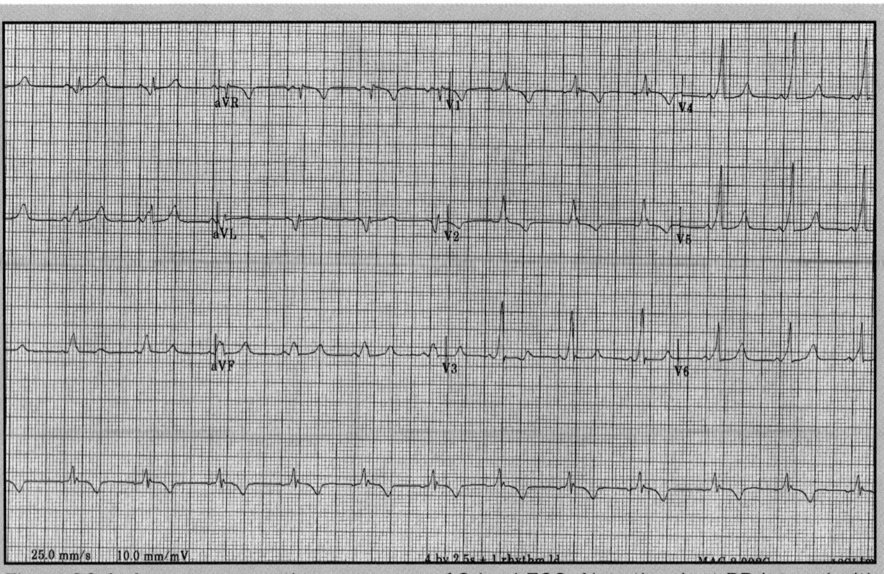

Figure 20.1: An accessory pathway seen on a 12-lead ECG. Note the short PR interval with slurred segment between the P wave and QRS complex (delta wave) consistent with the WPW pattern on ECG.

may place the patient at risk for sudden death. For example, atrial fibrillation can conduct very rapidly down the bypass tract and degenerate into ventricular fibrillation. In addition, the patient may have a rapid AV-reciprocating tachycardia in which conduction travels either down the bypass tract and up the AV node (antidromic tachycardia) or down the AV node and up the bypass tract (orthodromic tachycardia). These patients may be highly symptomatic due to the high ventricular rate of the tachycardia, which may result in hemodynamic collapse, due to decreased ventricular filling and diminished cardiac output.

The electrophysiology study can help define high-risk bypass tracts by measuring the tachycardia cycle length, the accessory pathway refractory period, and the shortest R-to-R interval during atrial fibrillation. If the latter two are less than 250 msec, this raises concern over the malignant potential of the pathway. Intermittent or loss of pre-excitation during a stress test is not a useful variable in determining the malignant potential of the bypass tract.

In the past, patients with accessory pathway-mediated tachycardia were managed with pharmacologic means or open-heart surgery. The development of radiofrequency catheter ablation has since become very helpful for isolating the accessory pathways. During an electrophysiology study involving accessory pathways, catheters are generally placed in the high right atrium, the His bundle, and the right ventricle. In addition, a 20-pole coronary sinus catheter is helpful in mapping accessory pathways.

Approximately 60 percent of accessory pathways are located on the left side of the heart. Roughly 25 percent of accessory pathways may be paraseptal in origin (in the middle of the heart, in or near the septum that separates the right and left

Accessory Pathway Localization

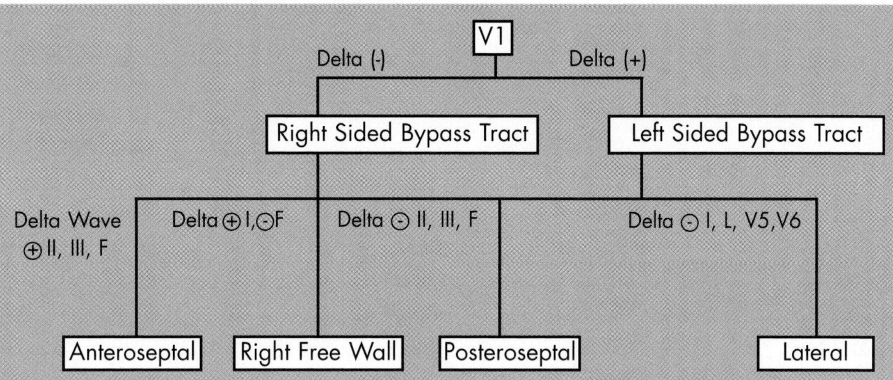

Figure 20.2: Accessory pathways localized (roughly) using the preexcitation pattern observed on the 12-lead ECG. The polarity of the delta wave (upright is positive and inverted is negative) and their ECG position can help determine the location of the accessory pathway.

ventricles), and the remaining 15 percent are right sided.

Accessory pathways can be localized (roughly) using the preexcitation pattern observed on the 12-lead ECG (figure 20.2). In addition, the transition zone is also useful in helping to determine the location of the bypass tract. Transition in precordial leads are helpful, *i.e.*, transition R > S in V2 identifies a septal accessory pathway. A left-sided accessory pathway is diagnosed if transition R > S is present in V1. One should first examine the delta wave polarity (when the delta wave is up it is called positive; when it's down, it is called negative) in lead V1. If the delta wave is negative in V1, the bypass tract is right sided. If the delta wave is positive in V1, the bypass tract is left sided.

Next, one should examine the inferior and lateral ECG leads. If the patient has a right-sided bypass tract and the delta wave is positive in the inferior leads, the patient may have a right-sided anteroseptal bypass tract. On the other hand, if the patient has a right-sided bypass tract and the delta waves are negative in the inferior leads, a posteroseptal bypass tract may be present. These patients typically have a negative delta wave in V1 that becomes positive in V2.

Right-sided bypass tracts with the delta waves having a left-axis deviation (delta waves positive in leads I and aVF) are most consistent with a right free wall bypass tract. Negative delta waves in the inferior leads suggest a posterior pathway. For example, positive delta waves in leads I and aVF plus negative delta waves inferiorly indicates a right posteroseptal bypass tract. Positive delta waves in V1 (*i.e.*, left-sided bypass tracts) with negative delta waves in the inferior leads are consistent with a left posteroseptal bypass tract. Positive delta waves in V1 with negative delta waves in lead I, aVL, V5, and V6 are consistent with a left lateral bypass tract.

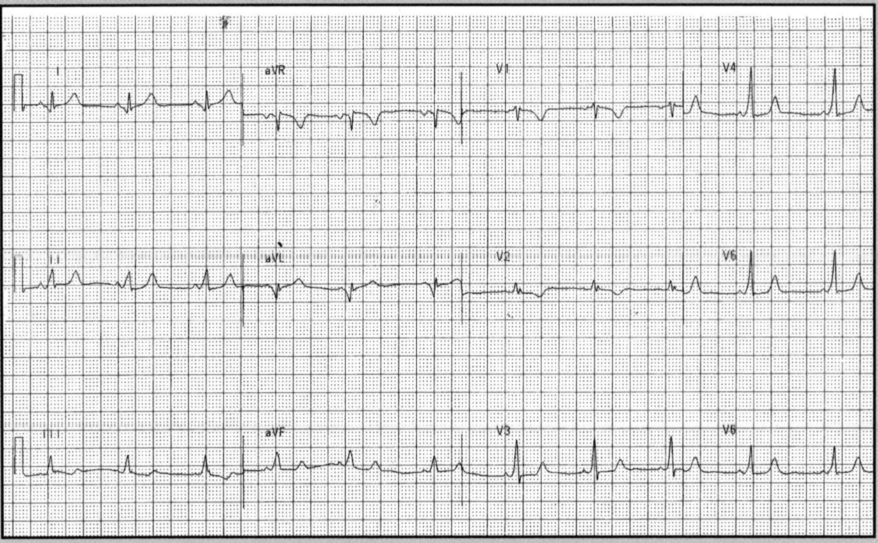

Figure 20.3. Another 12-lead ECG in the same patient with less preexcitation. Note the PR segment is slightly longer, and the QRS width is slightly shorter than that seen in Figure 20.1.

The location of left-sided accessory pathways is easily diagnosed and precisely localized using a 20-pole steerable mapping coronary sinus catheter. The coronary sinus vein runs in the atrioventricular groove, therefore, the accessory pathways themselves may be identified by the specific bipoles that bracket the bypass tract.

Left-sided bypass tracts can be mapped and ablated via the retrograde aortic approach or the transseptal approach. In the retrograde aortic approach, the ablation catheter is inserted in the femoral artery and then placed retrograde across the aortic valve. Careful prolapsing of the catheter across the aortic valve can minimize the risk of coronary artery dissection.

The transseptal approach uses the femoral vein. A needle is carefully advanced from the right atrium into the left atrium, during which time the patient's intracardiac pressures and blood oxygen saturation are monitored. Once across the atrial septum, an introducer sheath is carefully advanced so that the ablation catheter can be delivered. In about 25 percent of patients, there may be a "probe" patent foreman ovale (an embryonic flap between the right and left atrium), in which one can place the catheter directly from the right atrium into the left atrium without a transseptal needle puncture.

Careful anticoagulation for all left-sided procedures is mandatory, with activated clotting times (ACTs) measured at least every 20 minutes. In our laboratory, we try to achieve ACTs in the range of 250 to 350 seconds. Initially 5,000 units of heparin are given as soon as the interarterial septum or aortic valve is crossed by the catheter or the sheath (see Appendix D for ACT Record Sheet). Additional heparin is given based on the ACT.

Paraseptal bypass tracts (anteroseptal, midseptal, right posteroseptal, and left

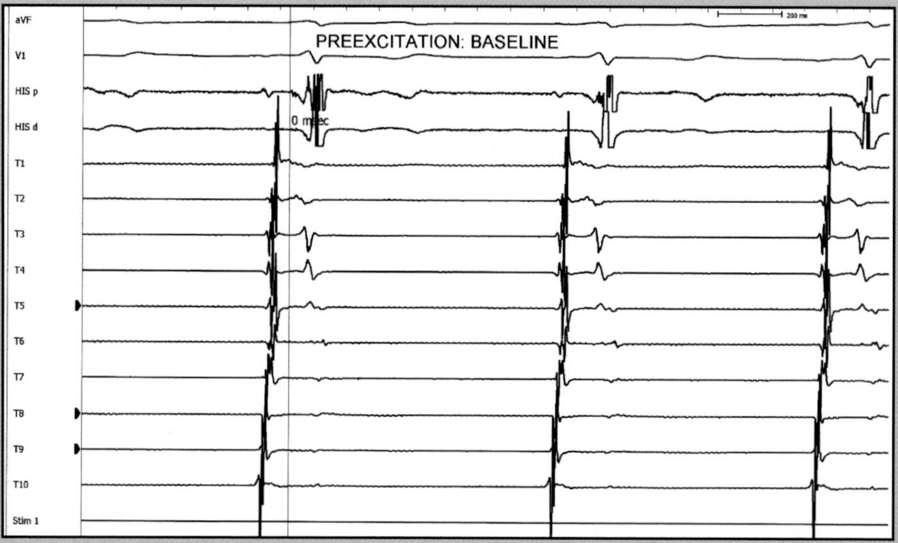

Figure 20.4: A His-bundle recording showing an HV interval of 0 msec.

posterior paraseptal locations) and parahisian bypass tracts near the His bundle require careful catheter mapping and ablation in order to eliminate the bypass tract and avoid damage to the normal conduction system. The use of long curved sheaths to gain catheter stability can be very helpful. In addition, using cryoablation, it is possible to freeze and thaw the tissues so that heart block, if it occurs, is reversible.

Right-sided bypass tracts can be mapped around the tricuspid valve annulus. In most cases, the use of a right coronary artery mapping wire is unnecessary; however, in patients with Ebstein's anomaly, in which there is an atrialized ventricle, this technique may be helpful. By carefully mapping the right side and the right annulus, possibly with long curved sheaths, one can successfully identify the presence of the bypass tract.

Case 1: Left Lateral Accessory Pathway Ablation

Figure 20.1 shows a 12-lead electrocardiogram of a patient with WPW syndrome. In this ECG, you can see that the patient has a short PR interval and no definable segment between the P waves and the QRS complex. A PR interval shorter than 120 msec is typical in patients with WPW syndrome. The ECG shows an upright delta wave in V1 as well as inverted delta waves (which may appear as Q waves) in leads I, V5, and V6, consistent with a left lateral bypass tract. Figure 20.3 shows another 12-lead ECG in the same patient with less preexcitation.

In an electrophysiology study of the same patient (figure 20.4), the His-bundle recording shows an abnormally short HV interval of 0 msec; normal HV is 35 msec to 55 msec. A 20-pole catheter was placed in the coronary sinus vein (T1 is distal; T10 is proximal).

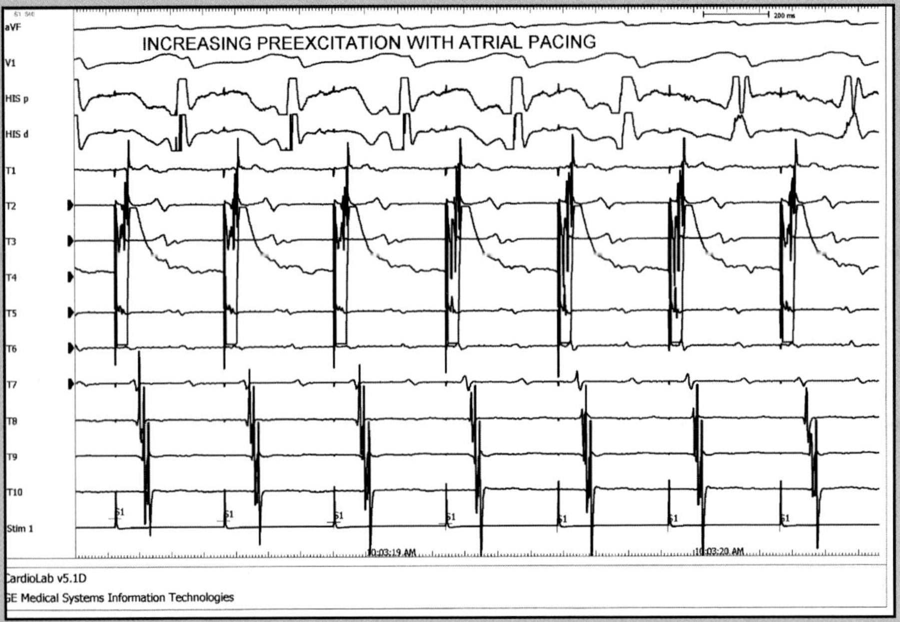

Figure 20.5: Atrial pacing at a cycle length of 340 msec. Progressively faster pacing leads to increasing preexcitation and widening of the QRS complex.

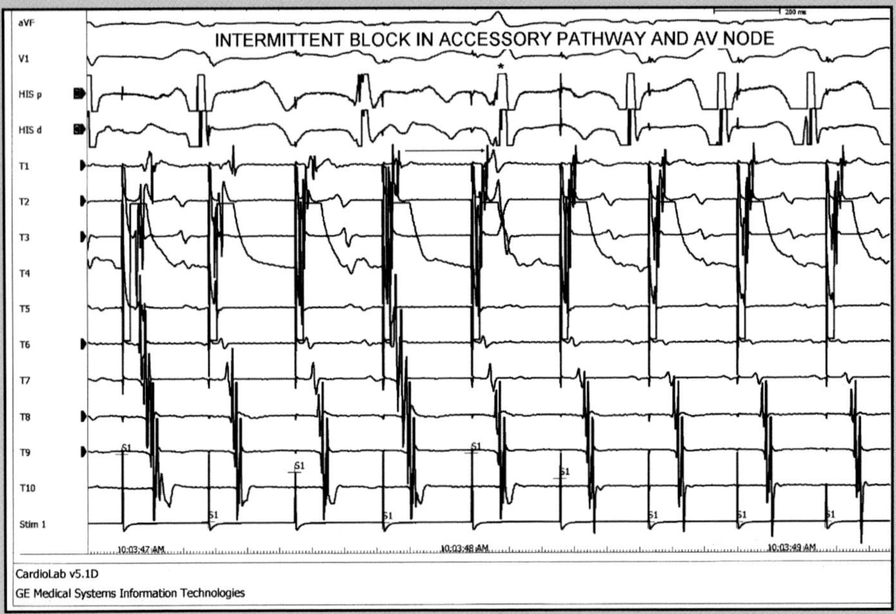

Figure 20.6: Intermittent block in the accessory pathway and the AV node during atrial pacing.

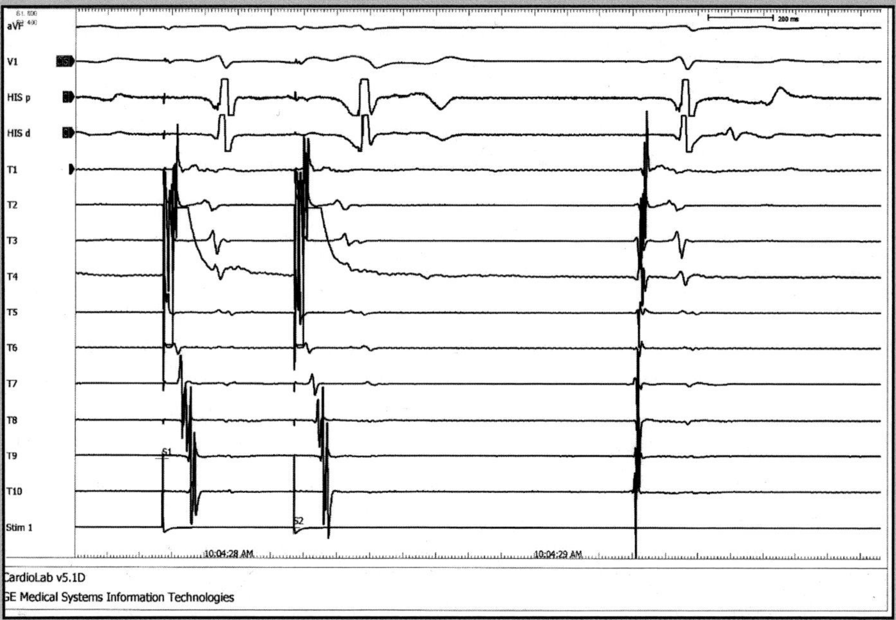

Figure 20.7: Atrial programmed electrical stimulation at a drive cycle length of 600 msec. Preexcitation is present in the first premature beat at 400-msec coupling interval.

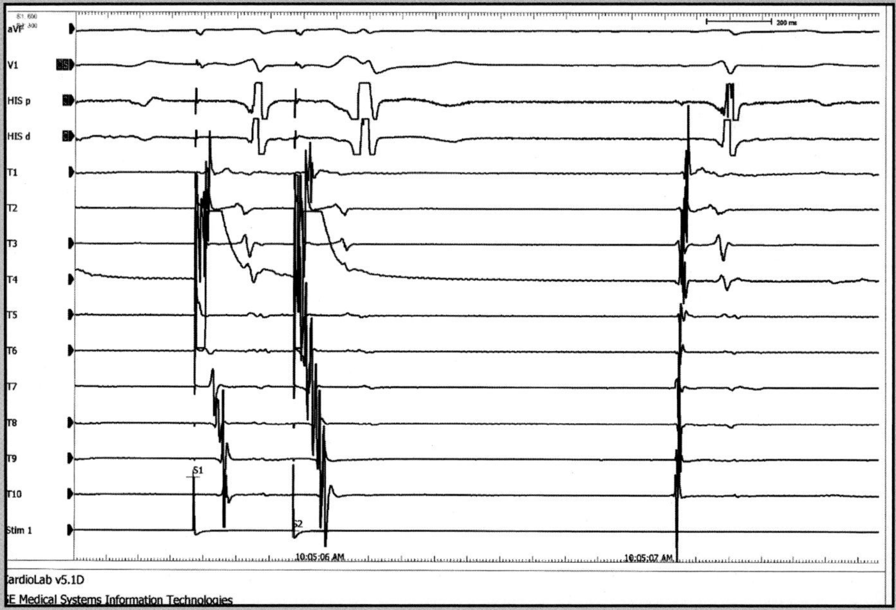

Figure 20.8: This figure shows greater preexcitation than in figure 20.7 due to a more premature atrial extrastimuli.

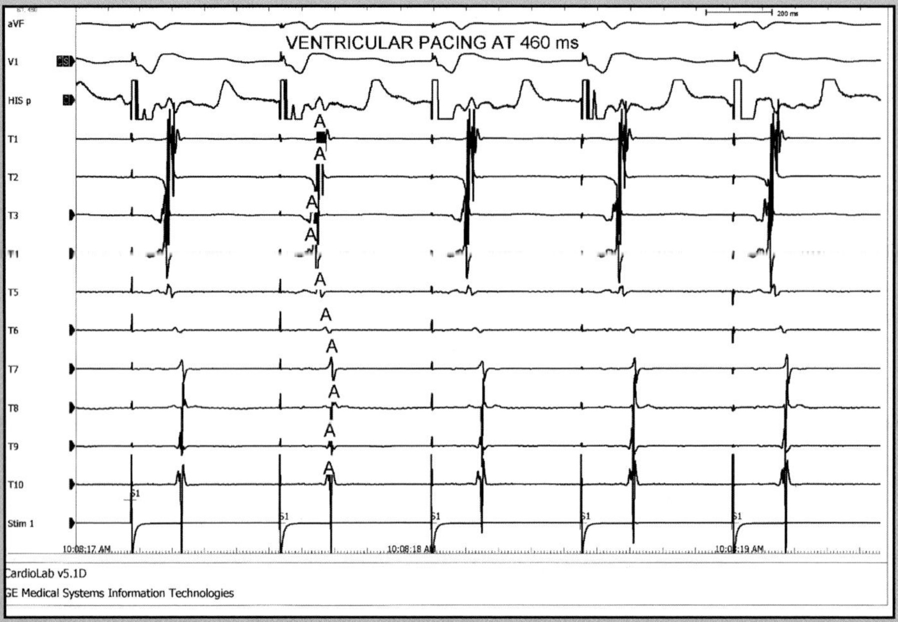

Figure 20.9: Ventricular pacing at a cycle length of 460 msec. Note the eccentric retrograde atrial conduction (T_4 is left-sided).

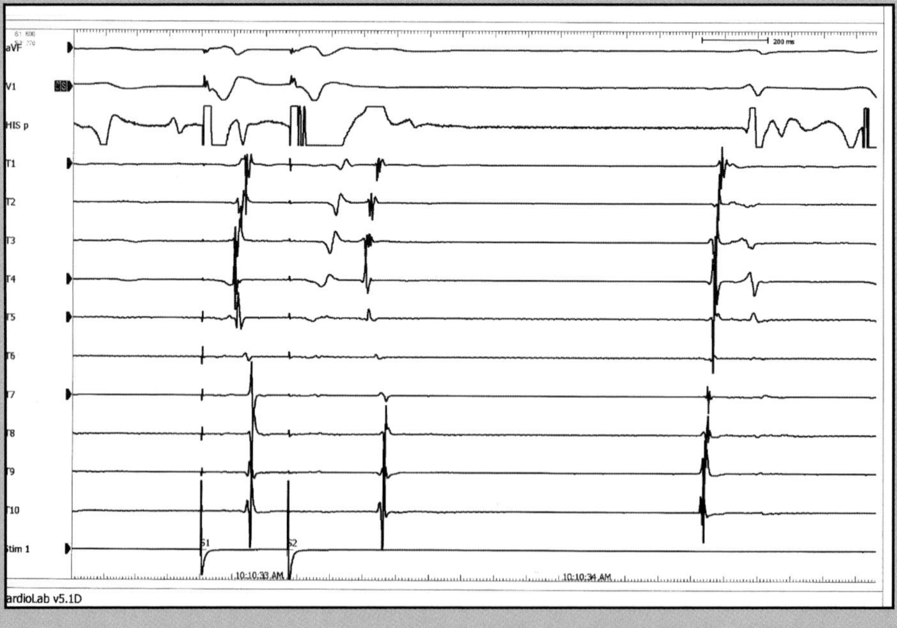

Figure 20.10: A ventricular premature contraction at a coupling interval of 270 msec. Note the retrograde atrial conduction and compare it to figure 20.11.

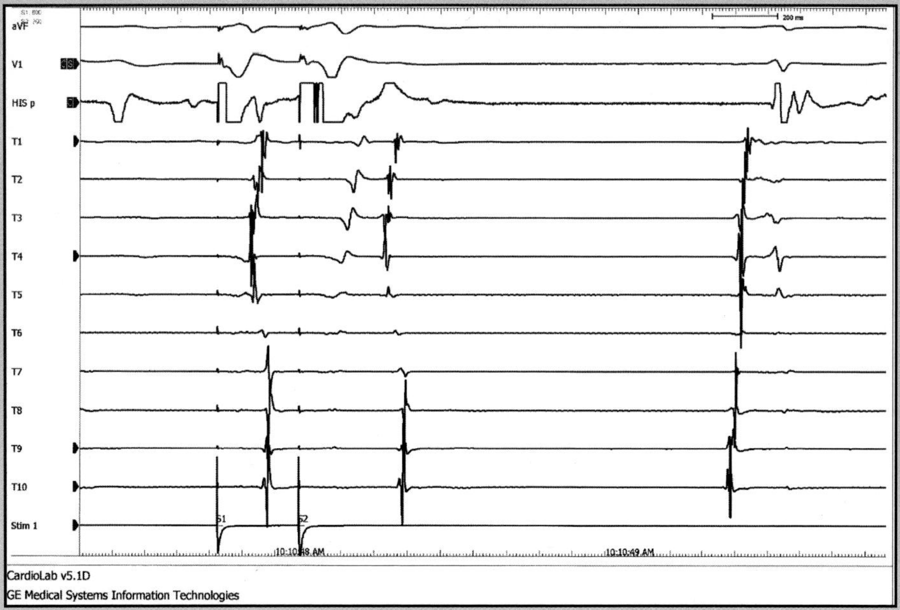

Figure 20.11: A premature ventricular contraction at a coupling interval of 250 msec exhibits identical retrograde atrial conduction, confirming the "all or none" bypass tract behavior.

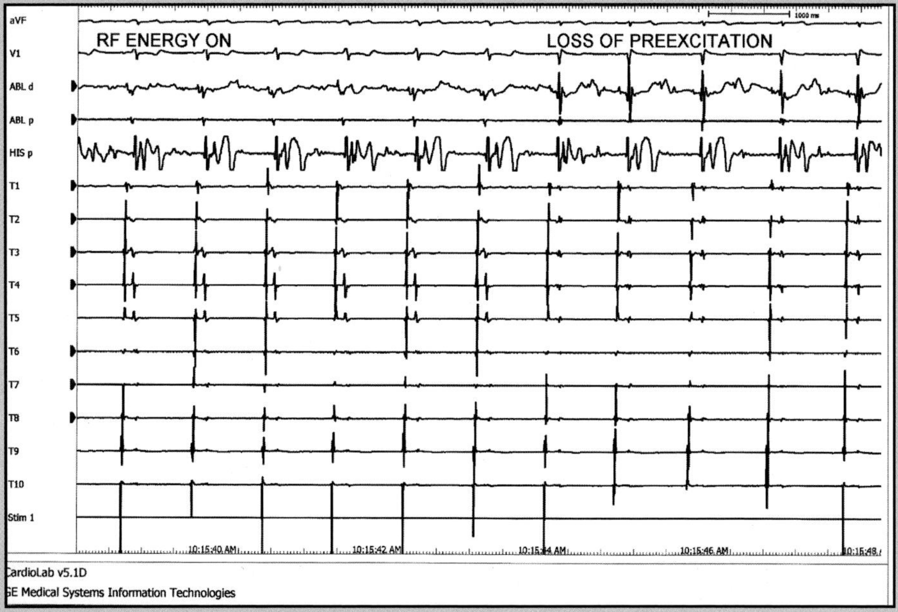

Figure 20.12: Radiofrequency catheter ablation performed via the retrograde aortic approach in a left lateral bypass tract position.

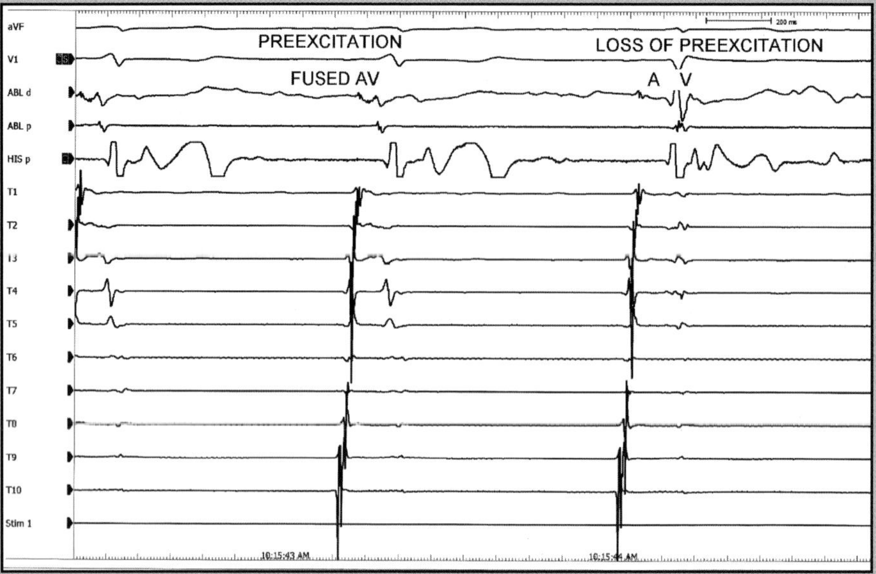

Figure 20.13: The electrogram recorded at the precise catheter location in which the bypass tract was successfully ablated.

Figure 20.5 shows atrial pacing at a cycle length of 340 msec. As the atrium is progressively paced faster, there is increasing preexcitation (with widening of the QRS complex). Figure 20.6 demonstrates intermittent block in the accessory pathway and the AV node. The first blocked atrial paced beat (second atrial paced complex) demonstrates no conduction via the bypass tract and the AV node. The second blocked atrial paced beat (fourth atrial paced complex), however, demonstrates conduction down the AV node, but not to the bypass tract. This is indicative of the accessory pathway block cycle length. An accessory pathway block cycle length of less than 250 msec is suggestive of a very rapidly conducting bypass tract, and may portend a higher risk of atrial fibrillation degenerating into ventricular fibrillation.

In addition, during atrial programmed electrical stimulation at a drive cycle length of 600 msec, preexcitation is present in the first premature atrial paced beat at 400-msec coupling interval (figure 20.7). The earlier an atrial extrastimuli, the greater the preexcitation (figure 20.8). Figure 20.9 shows ventricular pacing at a cycle length of 460 msec. The ventricular premature extrastimuli demonstrates the "all or none" behavior of the bypass tract that distinguishes it from the decremental (or delaying) behavior seen with AV nodal conduction. In figure 20.10, the retrograde atrial conduction following a ventricular premature contraction at a coupling interval of 270 msec is indistinguishable from a ventricular premature contraction at a coupling interval of 250 msec (figure 20.11).

In figure 20.12, radiofrequency catheter ablation was performed via the retrograde

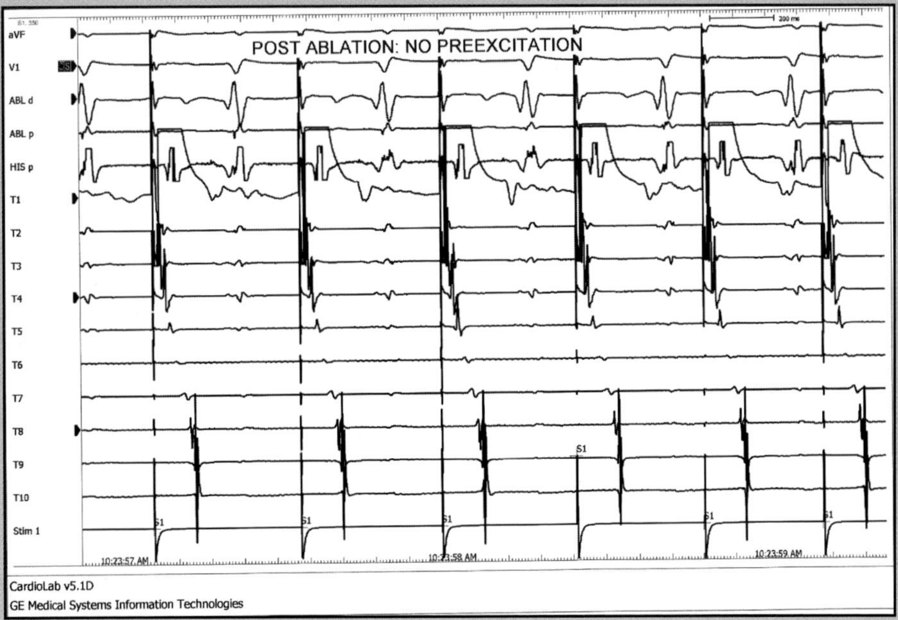

Figure 20.14: Post radiofrequency catheter ablation, there is no evidence of preexcitation (normal atrioventricular conduction through the AV node).

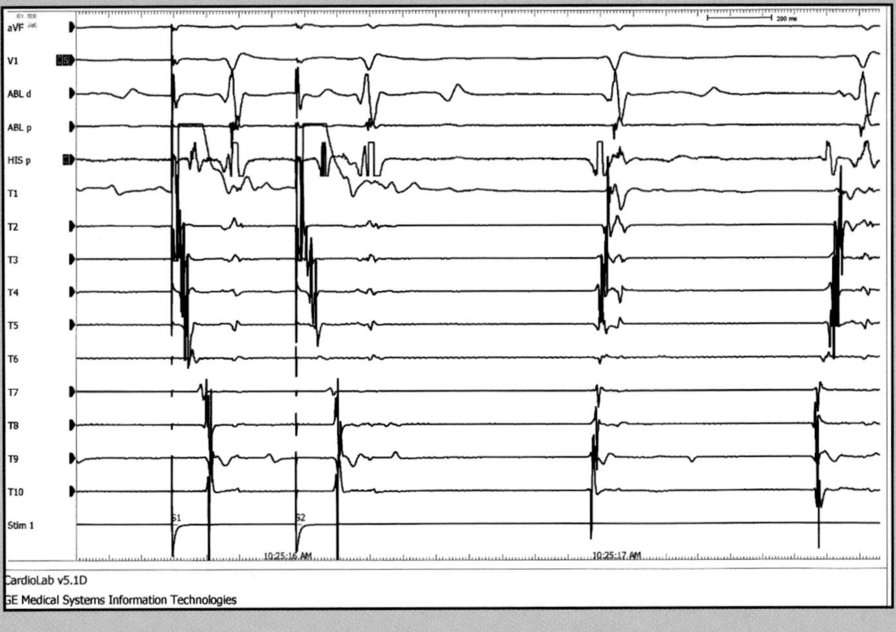

Figure 20.15: The atrial premature complexes failed to provoke preexcitation.

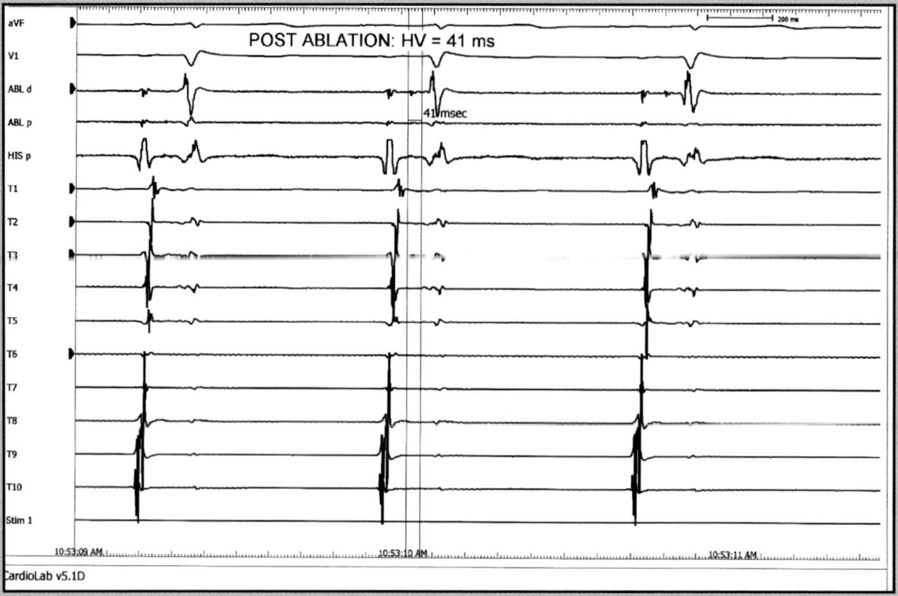

Figure 20.16: A His-bundle electrogram demonstrates normal HV interval (41 msec) and no preexcitation post successful catheter ablation.

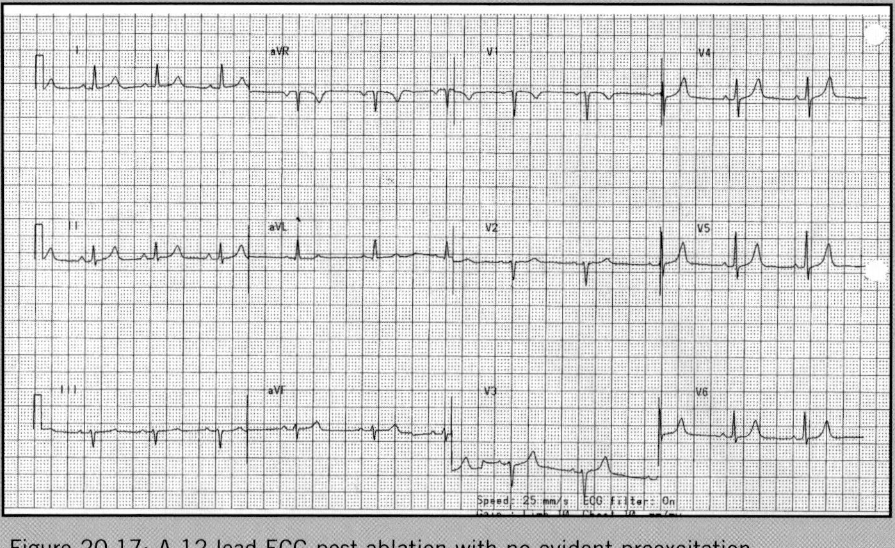

Figure 20.17: A 12-lead ECG post ablation with no evident preexcitation.

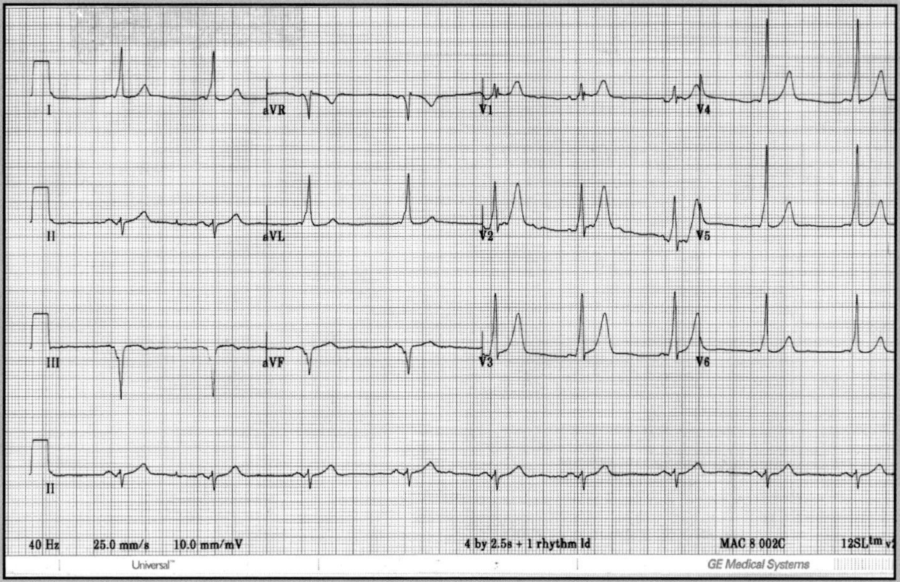

Figure 20.18: A 12-lead ECG from another patient with symptomatic Wolff-Parkinson-White syndrome in which the delta wave is positive in V1 and V2.

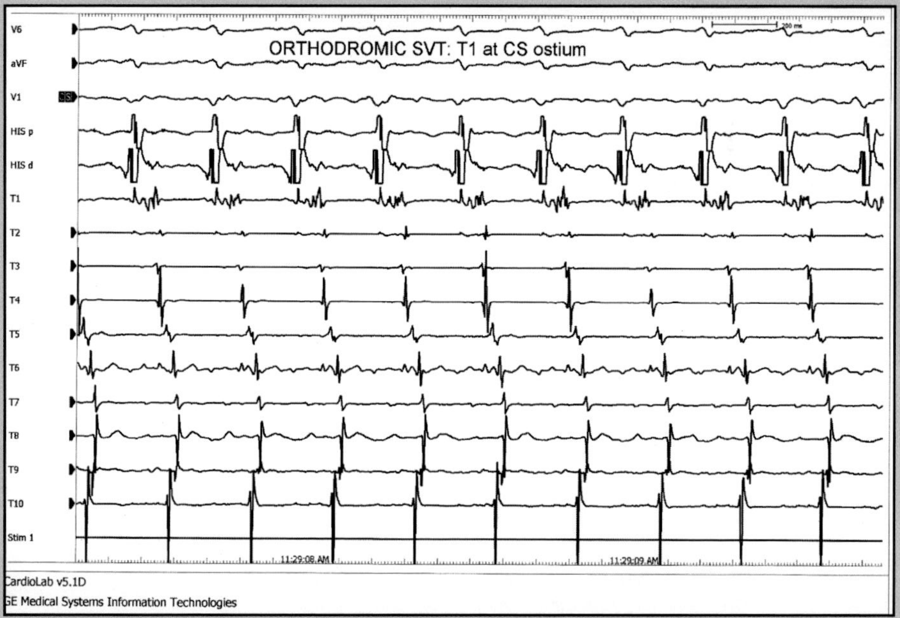

Figure 20.19: Orthodromic supraventricular tachycardia (conduction down the AV node and up a bypass tract) induced during programmed electrical stimulation.

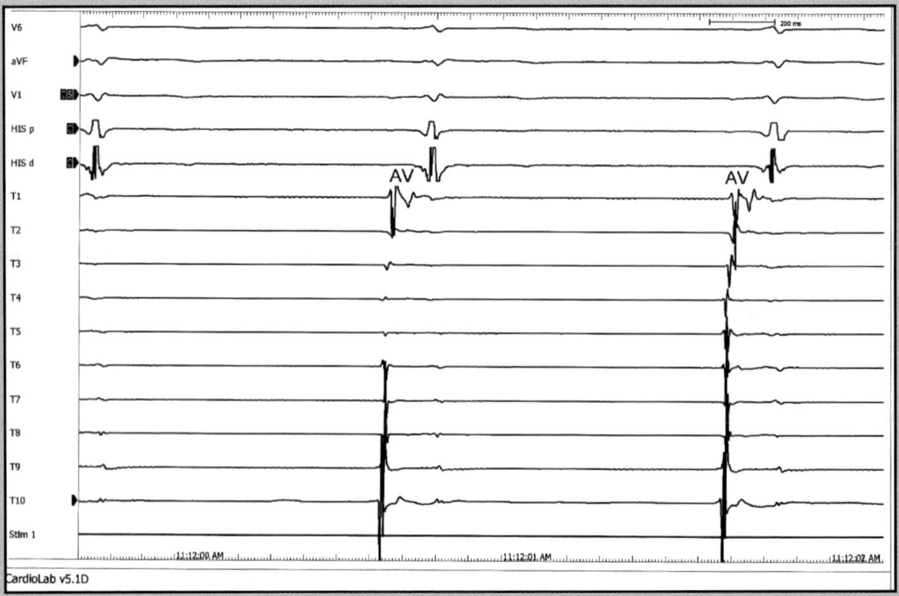

Figure 20.20: Fused atrioventricular electrogram near the coronary sinus ostium after termination of the tachycardia.

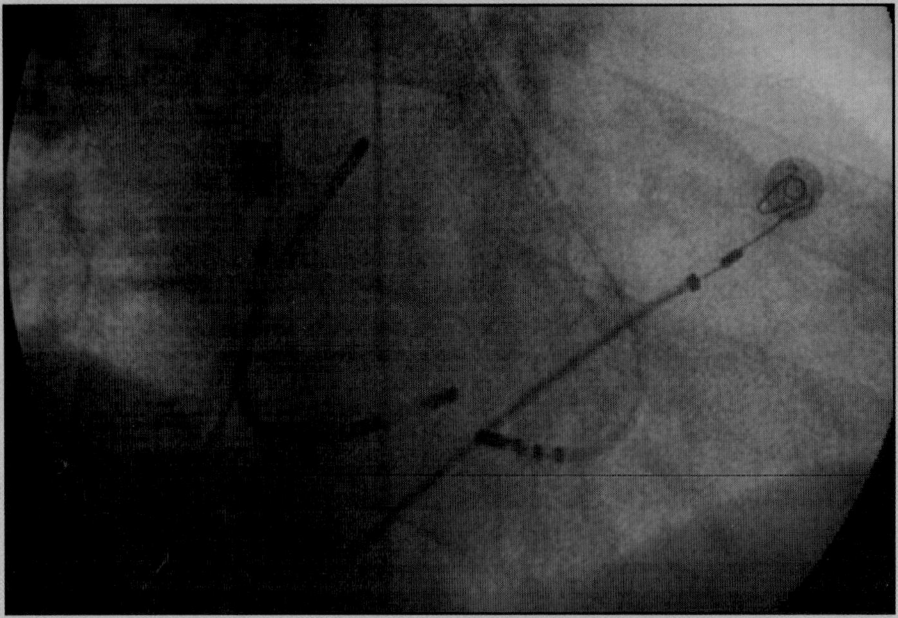

Figure 20.21: Shows the right anterior oblique fluoroscopic image of a 20-pole catheter and the ablation catheter (placed retrograde to the left posterior septum).

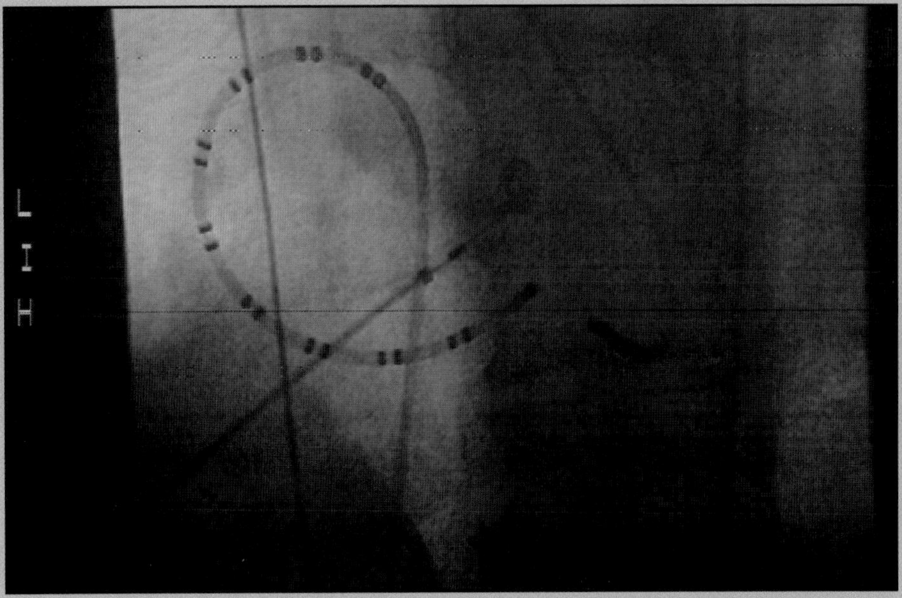

Figure 20.22: Shows the catheter locations from figure 19.21 in the left anterior oblique fluoroscopic projection.

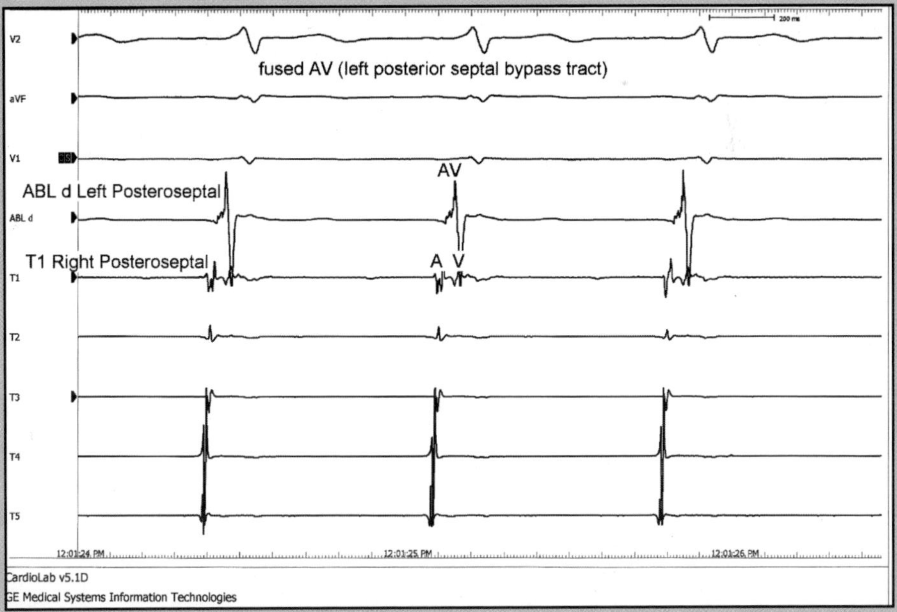

Figure 20.23: By placing a radiofrequency ablation catheter retrograde across the aortic valve and against the left posterior septum, a fused atrioventricular electrogram was recorded.

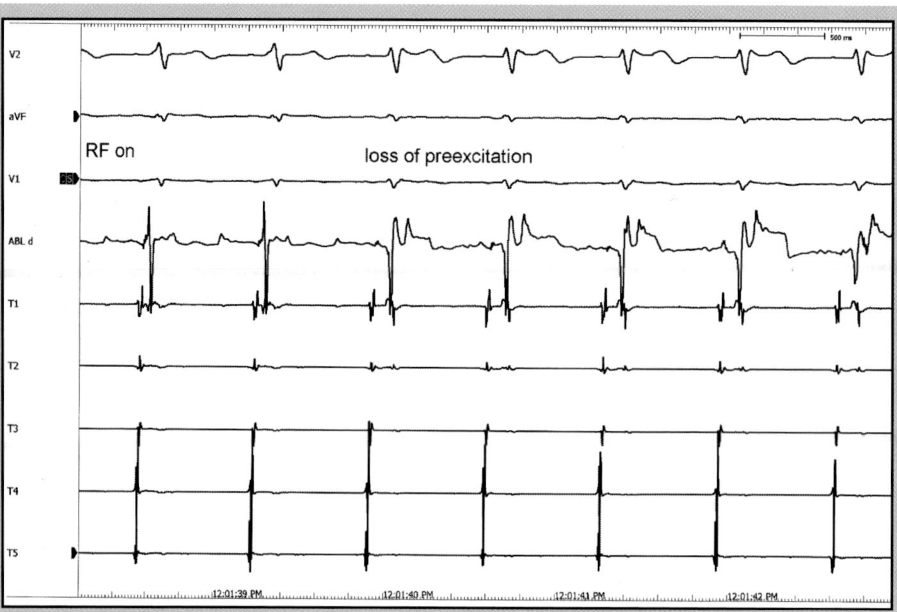

Figure 20.24: The application of radiofrequency energy to this location resulted in loss of preexcitation.

aortic approach in a left lateral bypass tract position. Within five seconds, there was loss of preexcitation and elimination of the bypass tract. Figure 20.13 shows the intracardiac electrogram recorded from the precise catheter location in which we successfully ablated the bypass tract. Please note the fused atrioventricular conduction and evident preexcitation. Immediately after initiating radiofrequency catheter ablation, there was loss of preexcitation (no delta waves) and a widening of the space between the atrial and ventricular electrograms recorded from the ablation catheter.

Figure 20.14 shows that post radiofrequency catheter ablation, there is no evidence of preexcitation (normal atrioventricular conduction through the AV node). In addition, the atrial premature complexes, as seen in figure 20.15, failed to provoke preexcitation. A His bundle electrogram, as seen in figure 20.16, demonstrates a normal HV interval (41 msec) and no preexcitation present. Figure 20.17 shows a 12-lead ECG post ablation with no evident preexcitation.

Case 2: Left Posterior Septal Accessory Pathway Ablation

In figure 20.18, a 12-lead ECG from another patient with symptomatic WPW syndrome is observed in which the delta wave is positive in V1 and V2. There are negative delta waves in leads III and aVF. Figure 20.19 shows orthodromic supraventricular tachycardia (conduction down the AV node and up a bypass tract) that was induced during programmed electrical stimulation. The retrograde atrial electrogram (conducting via the bypass tract) is earliest at T1, which in this patient was near the coronary sinus ostium.

Figure 20.20 shows a fused atrioventricular electrogram near the coronary sinus ostium after termination of the tachycardia.

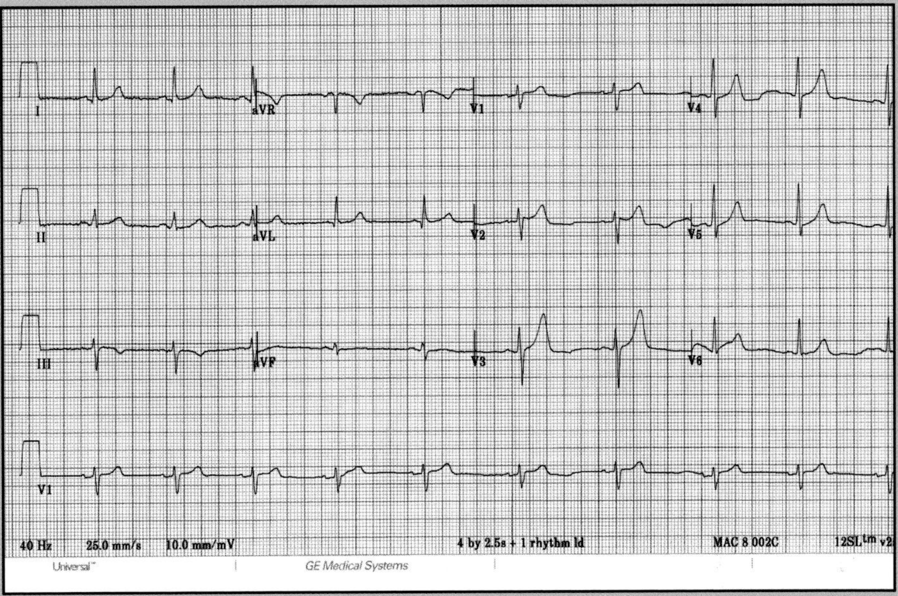

Figure 20.25: The 12-lead ECG obtained post procedure shows no evidence of preexcitation but rather a normal PR interval of 144 msec.

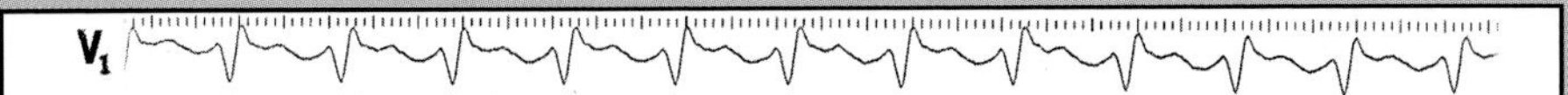

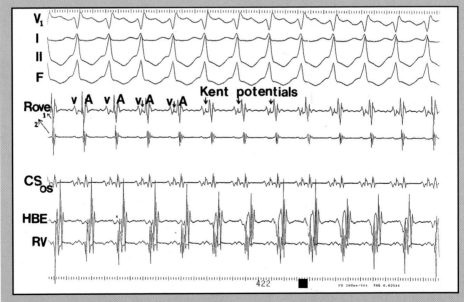

Figure 20.26: An example of electrical potentials recorded directly from an accessory pathway. These are called Kent potentials.

Initial attempts at radiofrequency catheter ablation were unsuccessful from the right side and near the coronary sinus ostium.

Figures 20.21 and 20.22 show right and left anterior oblique fluoroscopic images of the 20-pole catheter and the ablation catheter (placed retrograde across the aortic valve toward the left posterior septum). A fused atrioventricular electrogram was recorded at a left posterior septal location (figure 20.23), and radiofrequency energy resulted in prompt loss of preexcitation (figure 20.24). The 12-lead ECG obtained post procedure (figure 20.25) shows no evidence of preexcitation (normal PR interval of 144 msec).

Also note that occasionally accessory pathway potentials (also called Kent potentials) can be recorded during a tachycardia between the ventricular and atrial recordings (figure 20.26). Radiofrequency catheter energy delivered to the site of these recorded potentials can be very successful.

The overall success rate for patients with WPW syndrome and radiofrequency catheter ablation is on the order of 95 percent. The success rate is highest for left-sided bypass tracts and slightly lower for paraseptal and right-sided bypass tracts. Alternatives to radiofrequency catheter ablation for patients with WPW syndrome include the use of antiarrhythmic drugs such as flecainide. This can help diminish the "all or none" conduction properties of the accessory pathway. There is, however, a significant recurrence rate during follow-up among patients treated medically.

The risks of catheter ablation of accessory pathways include bleeding and/or clot formation (deep venous thrombosis and/or pulmonary embolus), heart block requiring a permanent pacemaker, vascular perforation and/or myocardial perforation (cardiac tamponade), valvular damage, coronary artery dissection, radiation burns due to long fluoroscopy times, cerebrovascular accident, and myocardial infarction. In addition, cardiac arrests and deaths have rarely been reported.

There is a high likelihood of success by radiofrequency catheter ablation in patients with WPW syndrome. Radiofrequency catheter ablation should be considered as first-line therapy for highly symptomatic patients. Pharmacologic therapy should be reserved for those with unsuccessful catheter ablation attempts. In general, asymptomatic patients with the WPW pattern on ECG should not undergo a routine electrophysiology study and/or catheter ablation. High-risk occupations (airplane pilots and bus drivers) and highly competitive athletes (professional ball players) may benefit from curative ablative therapies, thereby permitting safe participation in their respective vocations.

Chapter 21

Ventricular Tachycardia

Ventricular tachycardia, as well as ventricular fibrillation, is a leading cause of sudden cardiac death worldwide. Most people who die suddenly are not experiencing acute myocardial infarction. In fact, only 20 percent of patients who experienced sudden death suffered from acute myocardial infarction. On the contrary, 80 percent of patients who experienced sudden death had coronary artery disease. Sudden death due to ventricular tachycardia and ventricular fibrillation may also occur in any patient with an abnormal cardiac substrate. This includes patients with dilated cardiomyopathy, hypertrophic cardiomyopathy, significant valvular disease (aortic stenosis, mitral stenosis, mitral regurgitation, and pulmonic stenosis), arrhythmogenic right ventricular cardiomyopathy/dysplasia, and primary electrical disorders (such as Brugada syndrome and long QT syndrome).

When a patient presents with ventricular tachycardia, it is important to determine the stability of his or her rhythm and apply basic and advanced cardiac life support. If the patient has an unstable rhythm, advanced cardiac life support including cardiopulmonary resuscitation and early defibrillation needs to be performed immediately. Once you've resuscitated the patient, it is important to rule out a myocardial infarction (by serial cardiac enzymes and ECGs). A ventricular tachycardia or ventricular fibrillation that occurs in the setting of a myocardial infarction is deemed as a transient and potentially reversible problem, and is not necessarily a primary indication for an implantable cardioverter-defibrillator (ICD).

Once the presence or absence of a myocardial infarction has been determined, the workup of a patient's status after ventricular tachycardia includes an ischemia evaluation as well as determination of the precise cardiac substrate. This can be performed with a two-dimensional echocardiogram to assess left ventricular function, valvular disease, and other cardiac pathologies. In addition, the patient may undergo a nuclear and/or echocardiographic stress test. A coronary artery angiogram, including a left ventriculogram to assess left ventricular function, is usually indicated. It is important to document the left ventricular ejection fraction in all patients who may potentially get an ICD, because several primary prevention trials have demonstrated that a low left ventricular ejection fraction may be an indication for an ICD.

Non-Invasive Screening for Ventricular Tachycardia

There are a number of noninvasive techniques that can be used to screen for ventricular tachycardia. A 24-hour Holter monitor is a device that can be worn by the patient. It is connected via electrodes so that the patient's electrocardiogram can be recorded over a 24-hour period. This method is useful for detecting very frequent arrhythmias and giving a baseline analysis of the heart rhythm during that period. In addition, the 24-hour Holter may reveal the variability of the heart rhythm (heart rate variability). The lower the heart rate variability noted over a 24-hour period, the more prone a patient is to ventricular arrhythmia. It is limited, however, by merely recording the rhythm over 24 hours, and may miss less frequent arrhythmias.

Using a 12-lead electrocardiogram, the QT dispersion can be identified. By subtracting the maximum QT interval from the minimum QT interval in all 12 leads, the QT dispersion can be defined. A very prolonged QT dispersion (greater than 70 msec) may indicate that the patient is more prone to a ventricular tachyarrhythmic event.

Loop recorders are devices (usually smaller than the Holter monitor) that can be worn for prolonged periods of time (*i.e.*, over one month). Loop recorders are the size of a beeper, are attached to electrodes, and are connected to the patient. A particularly beneficial feature of the loop recorder is that the patient may experience a fleeting event and press the button afterwards, thereby recording what had occurred prior to the button's deployment. Overall, this method is very useful for infrequent episodes that occur a few times a month. An event recorder may even be smaller than the loop recorder (close to the size of a credit card). They can only record information after activation (no memory loop recording feature).

The signal-averaged electrocardiogram analyzes three orthogonal electrocardiograms. The signal is averaged over a number of beats (200 for example) in order to enhance the signal and diminish the noise. Utilizing special filtering and analysis, late potentials (seen at the end of the QRS complex) can be identified. This signal can indicate a propensity towards ventricular tachycardia and ventricular fibrillation (*i.e.*, the substrate for ventricular tachycardia). At one time, this method was fairly commonplace as a screening technique, but more recently has gone out of favor based on the expanding indications for implantable

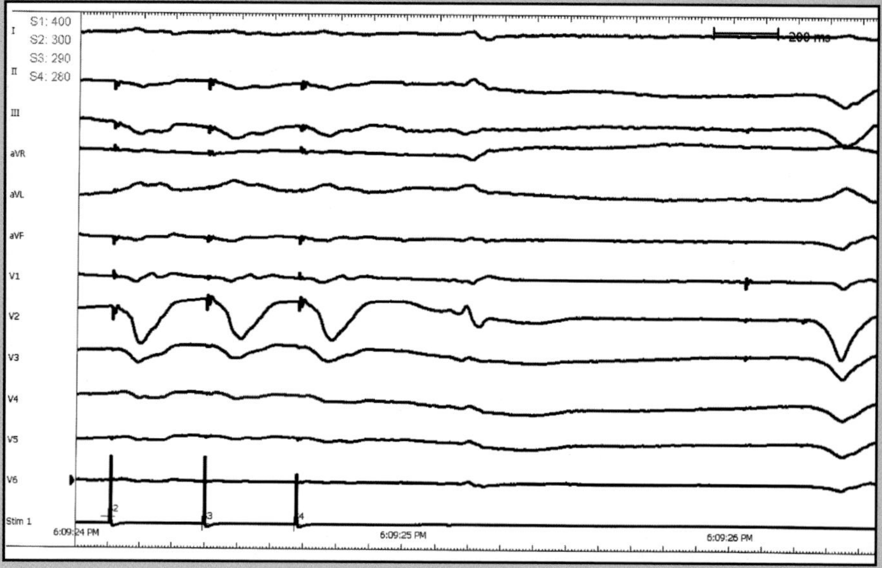

Figure 21.1: Standard programmed electrical stimulation with three extrastimuli performed from the right ventricular apex, resulting in a single extra beat.

cardioverter-defibrillators. It is particularly useful in patients with arrhythmogenic right ventricular cardiomyopathy/dysplasia who often have a very long and prominent late potential at the end of the QRS complex (see Chapter 22, figure 22.5).

Microvolt T wave alternans is another noninvasive diagnostic technique for risk stratifying patients who may be at risk for ventricular tachycardia. By placing the patient on a treadmill, performing a stress test and using a special computerized system, microvolt T wave measurements can look for T wave alternans and risk stratify patients for ventricular arrhythmias. The patient walks on a treadmill until their heart rate is greater than 90 beats per minute; then, computerized signal processing of the electrocardiogram is performed in order to detect microvolt T wave alternans. A positive microvolt T wave alternans test in a high-risk population may be associated with a high risk of clinical ventricular tachycardia or sudden death, whereas a negative study has a low arrhythmic event rate. The results of this test may be similar to invasive programmed electrical stimulation as a risk stratifier (however, the latter can give incremental information related to the site, mechanism, and significance of the induced arrhythmia). In addition, programmed stimulation offers a therapeutic option (*i.e.*, catheter ablation).

All noninvasive methods have limitations for indicating the need for an implantable cardioverter-defibrillator. Invasive testing (programmed electrical stimulation) may be necessary to determine the patient's best potential for ventricular tachycardia and/or fibrillation.

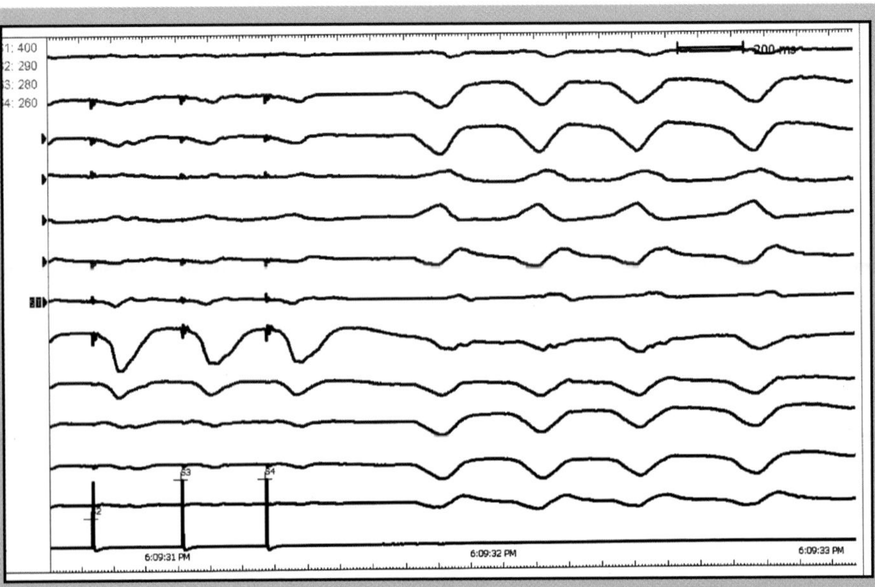

Figure 21.2: By subsequently decreasing the extrastimuli, we see the induction of a four-beat run of nonsustained ventricular tachycardia.

Ventricular Programmed Electrical Stimulation

If a patient has symptoms of palpitations, syncope, or near-syncope, and/or has demonstrated ventricular tachycardia and ventricular fibrillation, it is often useful to perform programmed electrical stimulation. This is a critical component of a standard electrophysiology study (see Chapter 14: Programmed Electrical Stimulation) in order to identify curable tachycardias (*i.e.*, bundle-branch reentrant or fascicular ventricular tachycardia). In addition, programmed electrical stimulation can help determine the utility and possibly help set the antitachycardia algorithm in an implantable cardioverter-defibrillator.

To perform ventricular programmed electrical stimulation, it is necessary to place a catheter into the right ventricle (initially the apex and subsequently the outflow tract, but not necessarily in that order). Pacing with a fixed drive cycle length of 600 msec, 500 msec, and/or 400 msec with progressive placement of additional premature extrastimuli (starting with a single extrastimulus and working up to three extrastimuli), one may be successful at inducing ventricular tachycardia. The method of induction of ventricular tachycardia has been well described elsewhere (again, see Chapter 14).

In general, standard ventricular tachycardia in a patient with a coronary artery disease/myocardial infarction substrate is via the mechanism of reentry. Figure 21.1 refers to an elderly patient with a history of a myocardial infarction and a left ventricular ejection fraction of 40 percent who

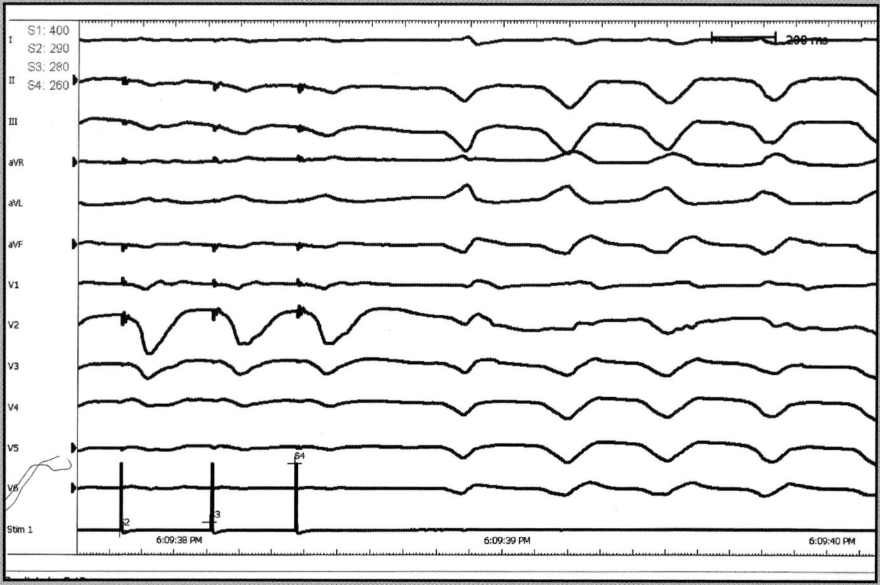

Figure 21.3: The repetition of the same cycle length (as in figure 21.2) with nonsustained ventricular tachycardia, but this time with induced sustained monomorphic ventricular tachycardia.

had a dual-chamber pacemaker present. This patient presented with syncope. The patient was subsequently referred for an electrophysiology study. Figure 21.1 shows standard programmed electrical stimulation with three extrastimuli performed from the right ventricular apex, resulting in a single extra beat (ventricular premature complex). By subsequently decreasing the coupling intervals of the extrastimuli in figure 21.2, one can see the induction of a four-beat run of nonsustained ventricular tachycardia. Figure 21.3 shows the repetition of the same cycle length that previously induced nonsustained ventricular tachycardia, but this time, sustained monomorphic ventricular tachycardia was induced.

Sustained monomorphic ventricular tachycardia is defined as a ventricular tachycardia with the same morphology (shape) in every beat that persists for at least 30 seconds (*i.e.*, sustained). If the ventricular tachycardia is three beats or more but less than 30 seconds, this is defined as nonsustained ventricular tachycardia. However, if the ventricular tachycardia is hemodynamically unstable and the patient is shocked before 30 seconds, it is still called sustained monomorphic ventricular tachycardia. This is a very specific finding, especially in patients with coronary artery disease. Figure 21.4 shows the ventricular tachycardia induced, characterized by a monomorphic morphology. In figure 21.5, you can see the same ventricular tachycardia in a 12-lead ECG form. This patient's ECG demonstrates a wide complex tachycardia with a right bundle-branch block pattern and an extreme right axis, which is very characteristic of ventricular tachycardia.

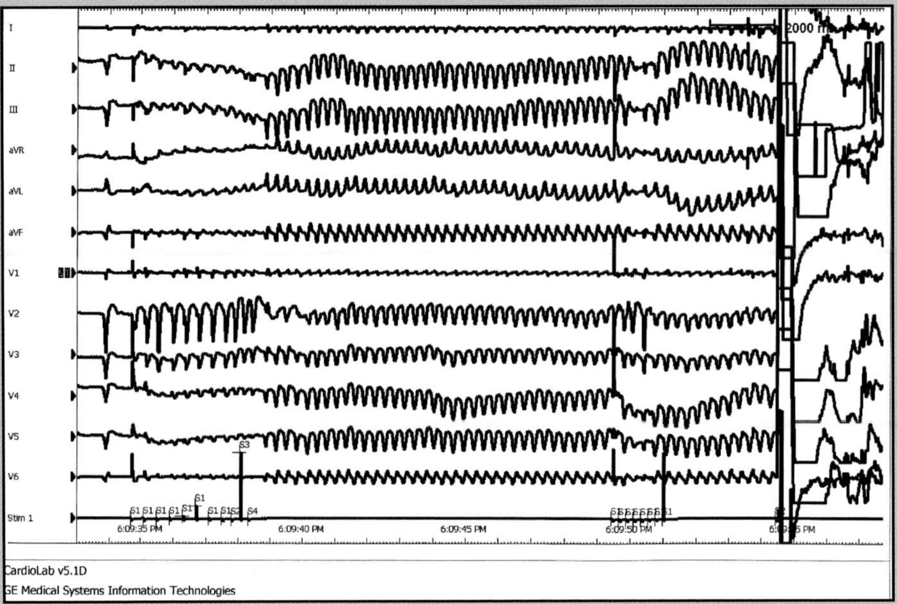

Figure 21.4: Above, the ventricular tachycardia that is induced has a consistent pattern or morphology, resembling that of a specific bundle branch block. This is termed monomorphic ventricular tachcardia.

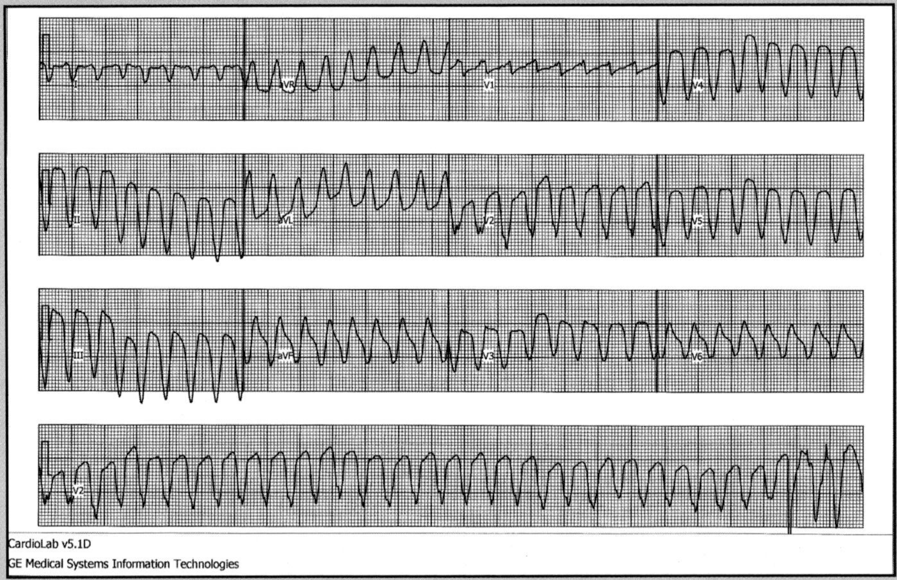

Figure 21.5: The same ventricular tachycardia as in figure 20.4, in 12-lead ECG form. This ECG shows a wide complex tachycardia with a right bundle-branch block pattern and an extreme axis (QRS complex is down in leads I and II), which is very characteristic of ventricular tachycardias.

ICDs Versus Drug Trials

In years past, initial therapy for ventricular tachycardia consisted of antiarrhythmic drug therapy. Subsequent studies have demonstrated the limitations of antiarrhythmic drugs in patients with coronary artery disease. In this population of patients who presented with ventricular tachycardia and/or ventricular fibrillation that are not in the setting of an acute myocardial infarction, studies have demonstrated the benefit of an ICD. The Antiarrhythmic Versus Implantable Defibrillator (AVID) trial, for one, demonstrated the enhanced efficacy of ICDs in patients who presented with hemodynamically significant ventricular tachycardia and/or ventricular fibrillation compared with the best antiarrhythmic drugs (sotalol and amiodarone).

A number of primary prevention trials have also demonstrated the benefit of these devices. The Multicenter Automatic Defibrillator Implantation Trial (MADIT) demonstrated that patients with a prior myocardial infarction who have nonsustained VT, a left ventricular ejection fraction of less than 36 percent, and inducible but not drug-suppressed ventricular tachycardia may benefit from an ICD compared with standard antiarrhythmic drugs. The Multicenter Unsustained Tachycardia Trial (MUSTT) also confirmed that the ICD resulted in the only true benefit in patients who underwent electrophysiology study-guided antiarrhythmic drug therapy and who had nonsustained ventricular tachycardia, left ventricular ejection fraction of 40 percent or less, and prior myocardial infarction.

More recently, the Multicenter Automatic Defibrillation Implantation Trial II (MADIT II) demonstrated that prophylactic implantation of an implantable defibrillator in a patient with no arrhythmia and a prior myocardial infarction with an ejection fraction of 30 percent or less will improve mortality. More importantly, the Sudden Cardiac Death in Heart Failure Trial (SCD-HeFT), the largest primary prevention implantable defibrillator trial in patients with heart failure (2,521 patients), demonstrated that ICDs can improve survival in patients with a left ventricular ejection fraction of less than 36 percent, regardless of the type of cardiac substrate (ischemic or nonischemic cardiomyopathy), and class II or III congestive heart failure. Simple ICD therapy reduced mortality in this population by 23 percent as compared with placebo. Amiodarone therapy, when used for primary prevention, did not improve survival. The results of these and other multicenter trials led Medicare to expand reimbursement of ICDs to include MADIT II and SCD-HeFT indications.

In addition, the Comparison of Medical Therapy, Pacing, and Defibrillation in Heart Failure (COMPANION) trial demonstrated that cardiac resynchronization therapy with the implantable defibrillator in patients who have a wide QRS complex greater than 120 msec, class III or IV congestive heart failure despite optimal medical therapy, and an ejection fraction of less than 36 percent improves survival and quality of life. A biventricular ICD plus optimal medical therapy decreased the risk of all-cause mortality by 36 percent as compared with optimal medical therapy alone.

The role of antiarrhythmic drugs in this population has really been relegated

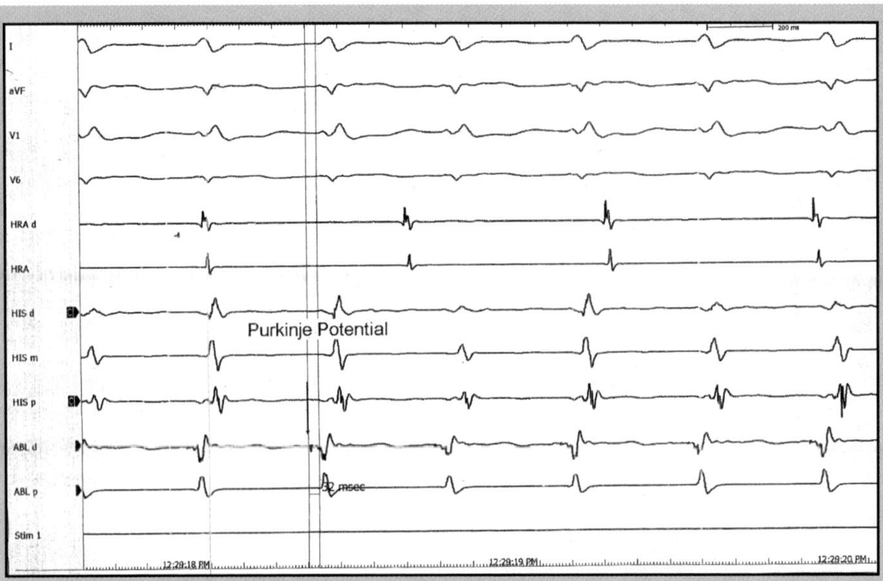

Figure 21.6: A Purkinje potential preceding the left posterior septal ventricular tachycardia in a patient with a structurally normal heart.

to patients who refuse implantation of a cardioverter defibrillator, receive frequent therapies from ICDs, or have a limited longevity due to other comorbid conditions, or as an adjunct to device-based therapy. For example, if a patient has incessant ventricular tachycardia and is receiving frequent shocks with an ICD, the addition of an antiarrhythmic drug such as amiodarone may help suppress the ventricular tachycardia, so that the patient may receive fewer discharges from the device. Chapter 26 reviews the ICD in more detail.

Ventricular Tachycardia Ablation

Depending on the type of cardiac substrate and mechanism, ventricular tachycardia may be successfully treated by radiofrequency catheter ablation. The most approachable types of ventricular tachycardias are idiopathic repetitive monomorphic ventricular tachycardias, which occur in structurally normal hearts. These focal tachycardias are predominantly localized in the right ventricular outflow tract and left ventricular posterior septum.

Traditionally, idiopathic ventricular tachycardias can be mapped in order to identify the earliest point of activation. In addition, a ventricular pace mapping technique can be utilized in order to identify the tachycardia's location. A successful ablation can be performed by pacing from the tip of the ablation catheter and matching the morphology of a 12-lead electrocardiogram during pacing to that during the clinical ventricular tachycardia. Successful pace mapping can be performed by carefully examining all 12 leads and comparing the configuration of the paced bundle-branch block morphology to that of the tachycardia. If the pacing

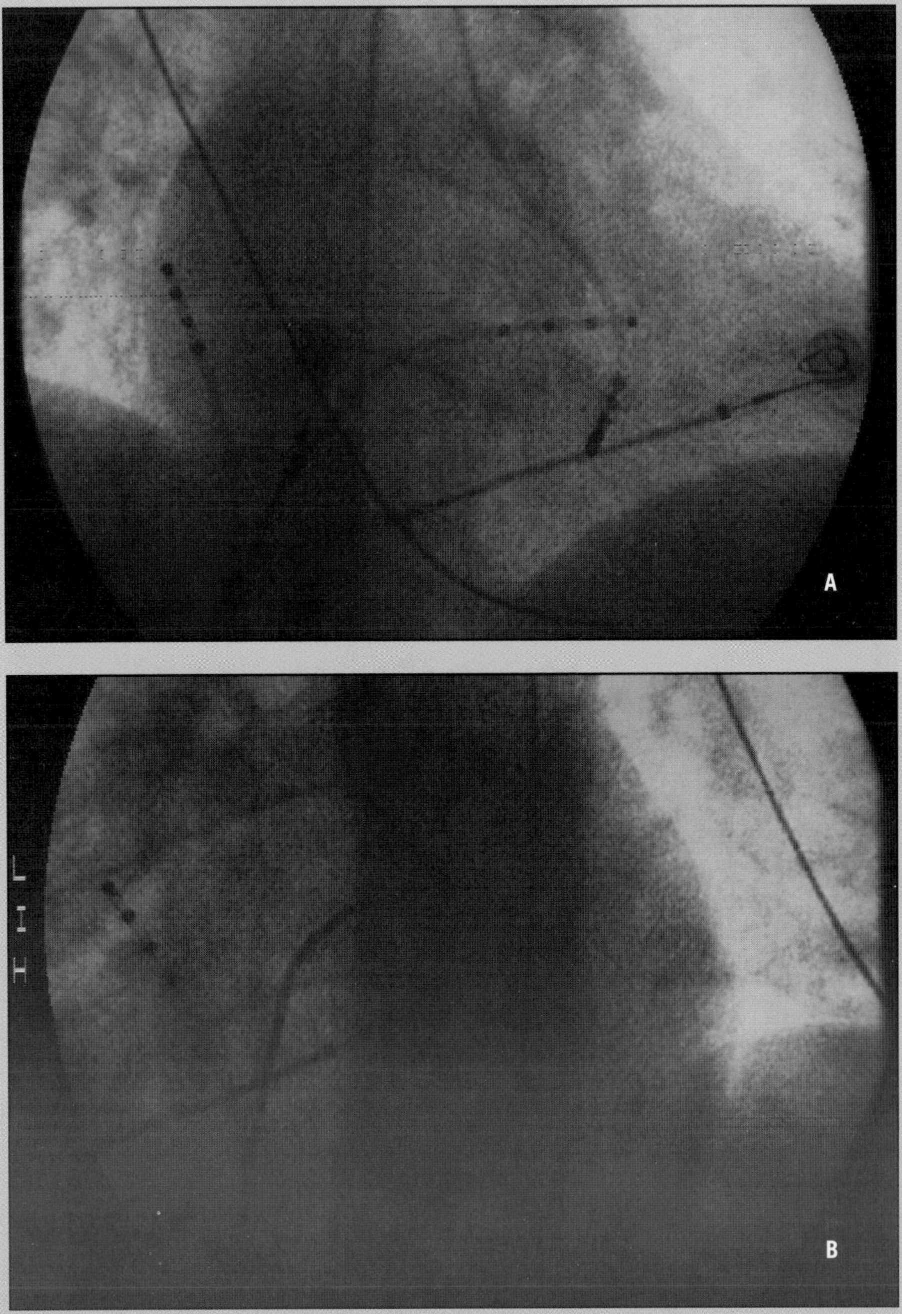

Figures 21.7a and 21.7b: Right and left anterior oblique fluoroscopic projections of a large-tipped ablation catheter in the left posterior septal location.

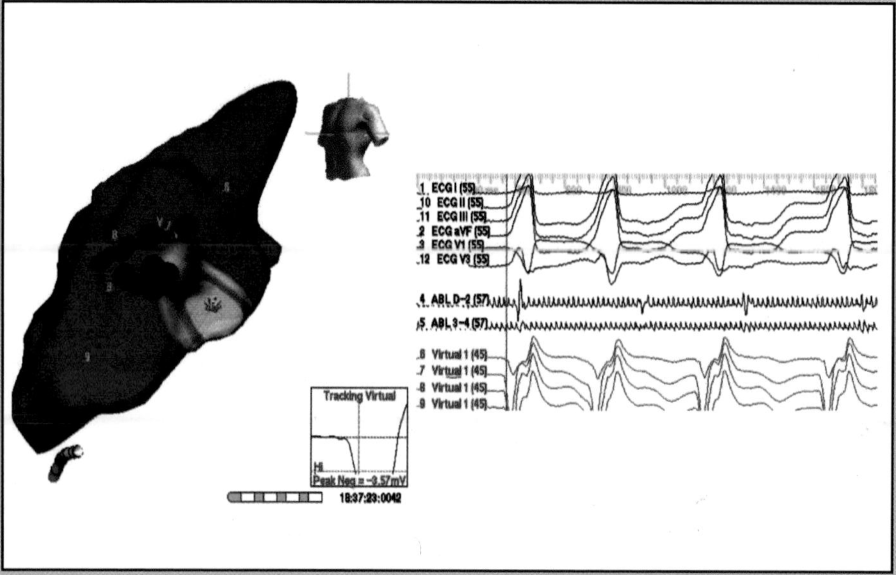

Figure 21.8: A right ventricular outflow tract tachycardia in which the tachycardia origin was modified after radiofrequency energy applications (dark circles).

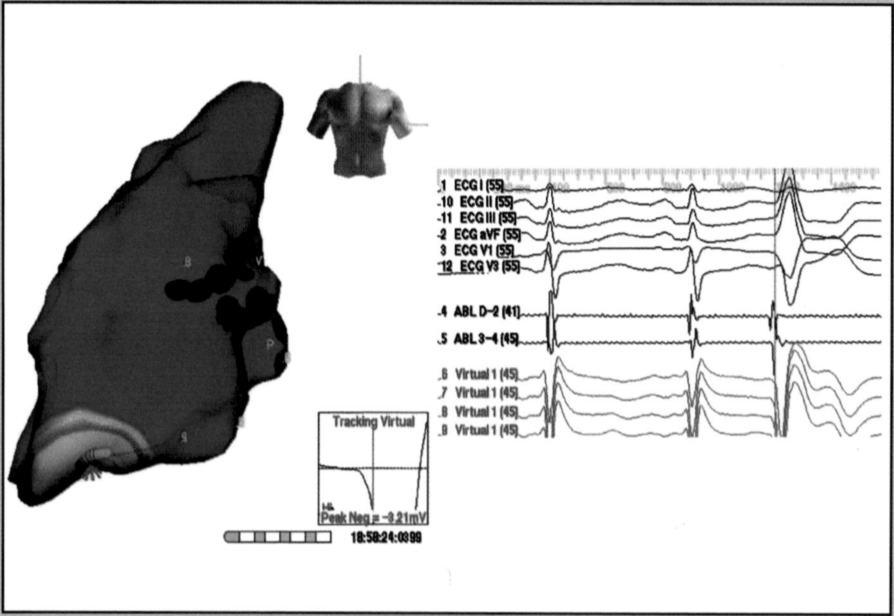

Figure 21.9: A catheter-induced premature ventricular contraction with a different origin as compared to the clinical ventricular tachycardia (figure 21.8).

and clinical tachycardia morphologies are identical, there is a very high likelihood of a successful ventricular tachycardia ablation.

Patients with a left posterior septal ventricular tachycardia often have a Purkinje potential preceding the ventricular tachycardia (figure 21.6). Figures 21.7a and 21.7b show the right and left anterior oblique fluoroscopic images of an ablation catheter that recorded the Purkinje potential. Radiofrequency energy delivered at that location terminated and eliminated the ventricular tachycardia.

More recently, the use of three-dimensional mapping techniques has helped to localize idiopathic and myocardial scar tachycardias. Using a nonfluoroscopic, non-contact three-dimensional mapping modality (the EnSite System, St. Jude Medical, Inc., St. Paul, MN), a rainbow-shape colored target identifies the earliest activation point for the tachycardia. As seen in figure 21.8, radiofrequency catheter ablation of a right ventricular outflow tract focus was performed with the initial activation located at the darkened circular sites. Those initial applications changed the activation to a more inferior septal location. Subsequently, after several lesions at the target site, ventricular tachycardia was no longer inducible.

Figure 21.9 shows a catheter-induced premature ventricular contraction (quite different in location to that of the ventricular tachycardia). At the end of the procedure, there were no premature ventricular contractions and programmed electrical stimulation plus ventricular burst pacing failed to induce ventricular tachycardia (even with isoproterenol).

Figure 21.10 shows the deployment of the EnSite Array™ multielectrode balloon catheter (St. Jude Medical) in the right ventricular outflow tract with the ablation catheter (right anterior oblique projection at 30 degrees). Figure 21.11 shows the same balloon deployment in the right ventricular outflow tract along with the ablation catheter in the 18-degree left anterior oblique projection. The success rate of ventricular tachycardia ablation in patients with idiopathic repetitive monomorphic ventricular tachycardia is approximately 90 percent. The major concern for this ablation is perforation/cardiac tamponade. Valvular damage can also occur.

Patients who have coronary artery disease and a secondary cardiomyopathy may have two types of ventricular tachycardias. The first is micro-reentrant in nature. The tachycardia revolves around a fixed scar related to myocardial infarction or fibrosis. The patient may be mapped using a standard technique known as concealed entrainment. A ventricular tachycardia is induced at a fixed cycle length. If the tachycardia is hemodynamically stable, pacing can be performed near the ablation site at a cycle length faster than that of the tachycardia. If the paced tachycardia is identical in morphology to that of the induced tachycardia, the post-pacing interval is measured and used to determine whether the tip is in the critical slow zone of the tachycardia or outside that region. If the post-pacing interval is approximately the same as the ventricular tachycardia cycle length, the operator should examine the stimulus to QRS duration as a percentage of the ventricular tachycardia cycle length. If the stimulus to QRS interval is less than 30 percent of the tachycardia cycle length, the

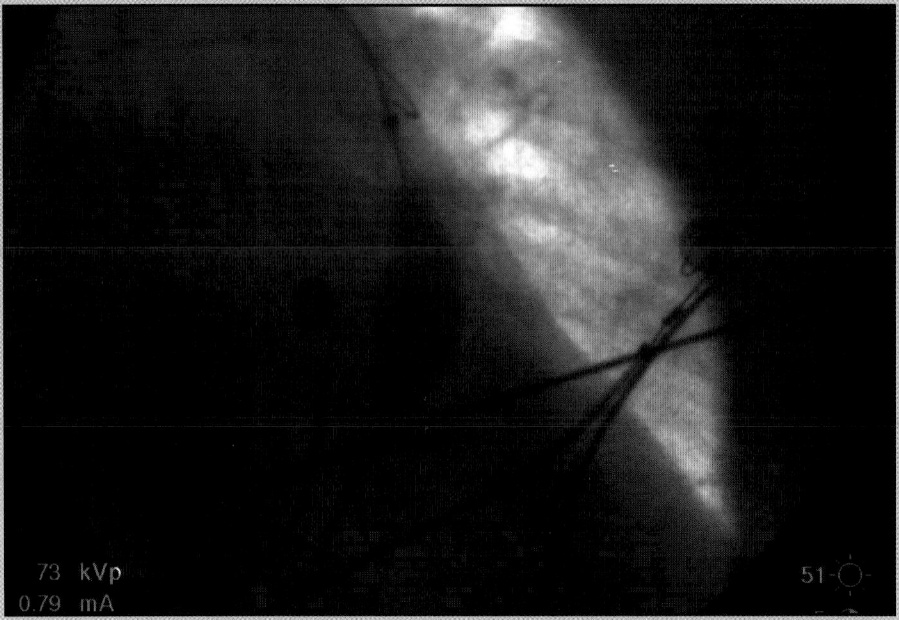

Figure 21.10: The deployment of the EnSite Array™ multielectrode balloon catheter (St. Jude Medical, St. Paul, MN) in the right ventricular outflow tract in the 30-degree right anterior oblique projection.

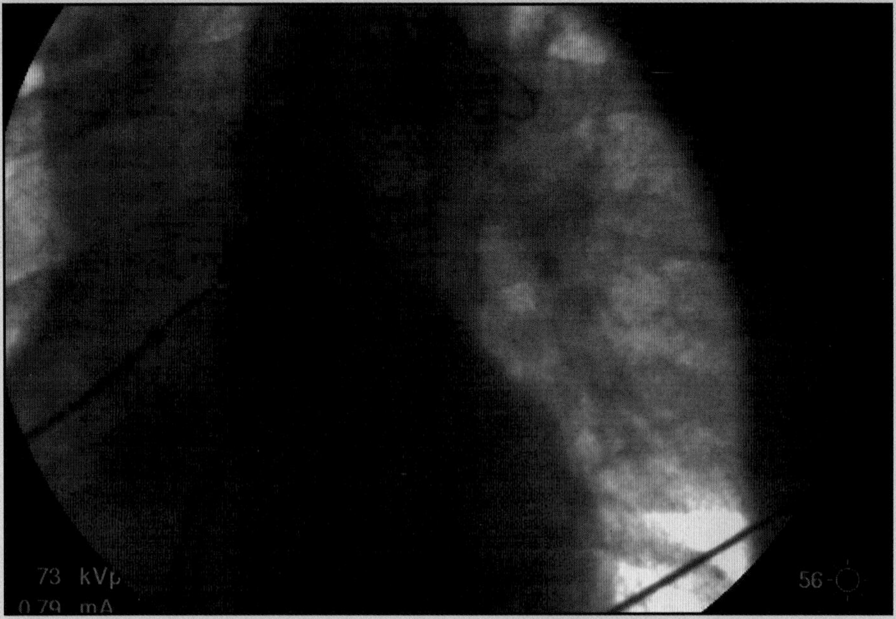

Figure 21.11: The same right ventricular outflow tract balloon deployment seen in figure 21.10, in the 18-degree left anterior oblique projection.

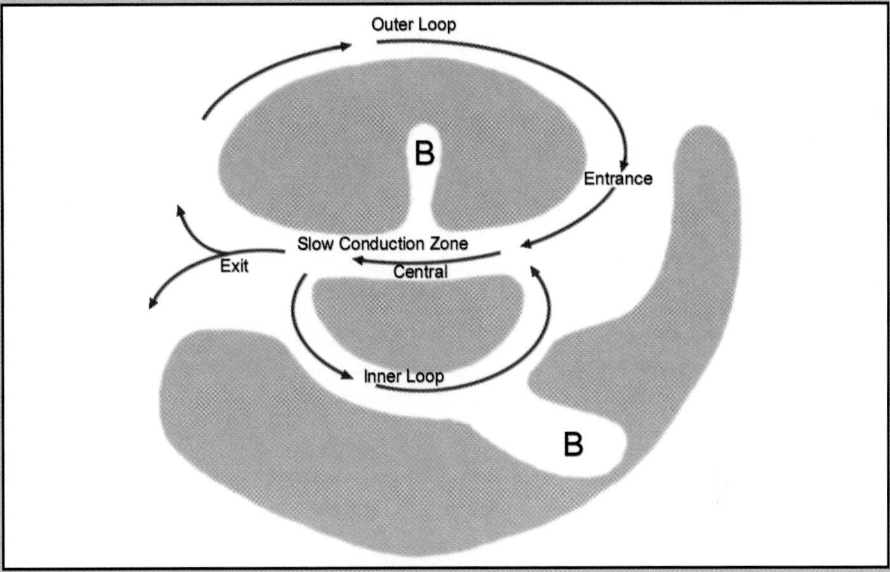

Figure 21.12: Schematic of a myocardial ventricular tachycardia circuit. The slow conduction zone is the critical location to identify, localize, and ablate the tachycardia successfully. Bystander locations are ineffective ablation sites and not critical to the tachycardia circuit. The bystander location is indicated by the letter B.

catheter tip is at the exit site of the slow conduction zone; 30 to 50 percent indicates that it is in a central slow conduction zone; 50 to 70 percent means it is in a proximal slow conduction zone; and greater than 70 percent indicates that it is in an entrance location (figure 21.12).

Case Report: Ventricular Tachycardia Ablation in a Patient with Prior Myocardial Infarction

Figures 21.13a-e show an example of a complicated ventricular tachycardia ablation, from a case originally presented by Tristram Bahnson, MD, in *EP Lab Digest* (2003;3:24–30; reprinted with permission from *EP Lab Digest*). Figure 21.13a shows six different ventricular tachycardia morphologies induced in an EP study. Figure 21.13b shows a CARTO® system voltage map that demonstrates a narrow isthmus (white arrow). Red circles illustrate the location of radiofrequency catheter ablation lesions targeting the central isthmus and tachycardia exit sites, which eliminated all inducible ventricular tachycardia morphologies. Figure 21.13c demonstrates endocardial recordings from the central isthmus during both sinus rhythm and ventricular tachycardia showing fractioned potentials (FP). Pacing from the isthmus induced ventricular tachycardia with a first stimulus to QRS interval equal to the FP to QRS interval during the tachycardia, which demonstrated that this site was critical to the circuit (figure 21.13d). Ablation at this site eliminated VT4, and additional ablations eliminated VT5. Figure 21.13e shows pace mapping that helped to localize VT2. Additional ablation applications described

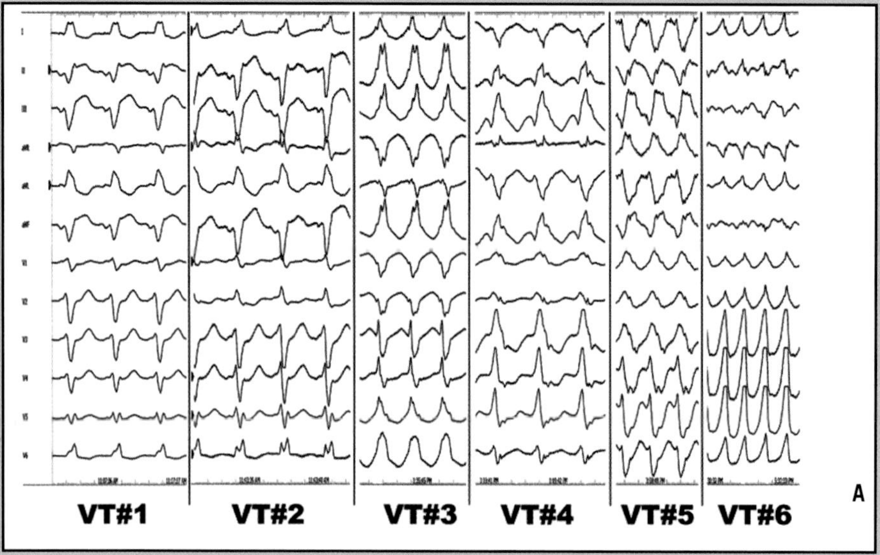

Figure 21.13a: Mapping data from a patient with VT late after myocardial infarction. Six different VT morphologies induced in a patient late after MI. (Reprinted with permission from *EP Lab Digest* 2003;3:24–30.)

in the figure legends eliminated all ventricular tachycardia morphologies.

The success rate for patients with concealed entrainment and myocardial ventricular tachycardia is in the order of 60 to 80 percent. Besides cardiac tamponade and valvular disease, a cerebrovascular accident is a potential left-sided complication. Vigilant anticoagulation should be performed during this procedure.

Bundle-branch reentrant ventricular tachycardia may also have been seen in patients with ischemic or nonischemic cardiomyopathy. These patients typically have a depressed left ventricular ejection fraction (less than 36 percent), a left intraventricular conduction defect (QRS duration greater than 120 msec), and/or left bundle-branch block pattern; they often have severe His-Purkinje disease (HV interval greater than 65 msec) as well. It is common for these patients to have a left bundle-branch morphology ventricular tachycardia similar to a baseline left bundle-branch configuration seen during sinus rhythm.

Bundle-branch reentrant ventricular tachycardia is a macro-reentrant tachycardia that involves the bundle branches (left and right). Typically, the tachycardia travels down the right bundle branch and up the left bundle branch. It can easily be cured via radiofrequency catheter ablation of the right bundle branch.

If the patient has a left bundle-branch block pattern, and complete right bundle-branch block is produced via radiofrequency catheter ablation of the right bundle, one would assume that the patient would develop complete heart block. However, it is uncommon for patients with bundle-branch reentry and left bundle-branch block pattern to

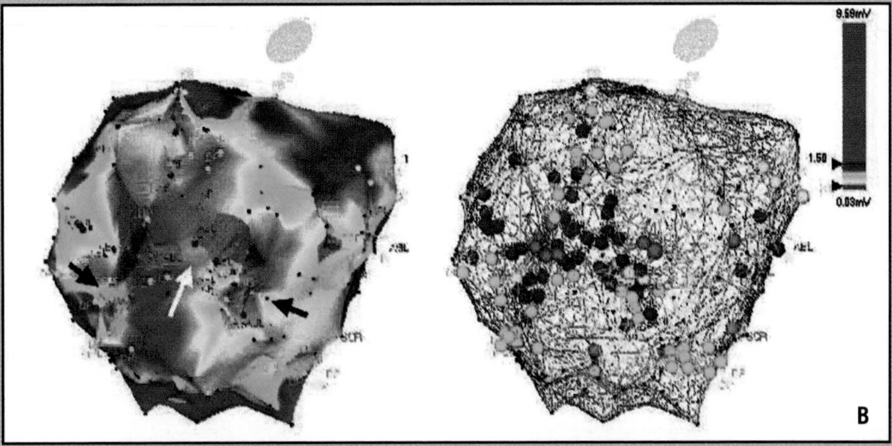

Figure 21.13b (On left) Voltage map of the postero-basal infarct region generated during mapping and ablation using the CARTO® system (Biosense Webster, Inc., a Johnson & Johnson company, Diamond Bar, CA) in a patient exhibiting the multiple VT morphologies depicted in 21.13a. A scale for color coding of endocardial electrogram voltage amplitude appears to the right. Purple areas represent sites with normal (> 1.5 mV) peak to peak bipolar endocardial electrograms. Red areas represent sites with low amplitude (< 0.5 mV). Yellow, green and blue regions correspond to sites with intermediate voltages between 0.5 and 1.5 mV. Areas marked grey represent unexcitable areas where unipolar pacing at 10 mA, pulse width of 2.0 ms, failed to capture. Note that the electrically unexcitable areas produce a narrow isthmus (white arrow). (On right) The "mesh view" on the right allows better visualization of tagged points that were annotated during mapping. Endocardial electrograms demonstrating fragmented potentials and stim-QRS times > 40 ms are tagged as blue circles. Areas consistent with exit sites were also defined by a pace map match to an inducible VT (black arrows). Red circles represent sites where RF lesions were delivered targeting both the central isthmus as well as tachycardia exit sites. All ablation sites were located within the infarct scar. In this case, all inducible VT morphologies were eliminated. (Reprinted with permission from *EP Lab Digest* 2003;3:24–30.)

develop complete heart block. Therefore, the presence of left bundle-branch block pattern in patients with bundle-branch reentrant ventricular tachycardia more commonly is a relative bundle-branch block pattern and not complete blockage of the left bundle branch.

The prevalence of bundle-branch reentry is higher in nonischemic dilated cardiomyopathy patients (up to 30 percent) than in those with ischemic cardiomyopathies (up to 16 percent). It is also not uncommon for patients with coronary artery disease to have both myocardial ventricular tachycardia and bundle-branch reentry. The success rate for catheter ablation of bundle-branch reentry is greater than 90 percent.

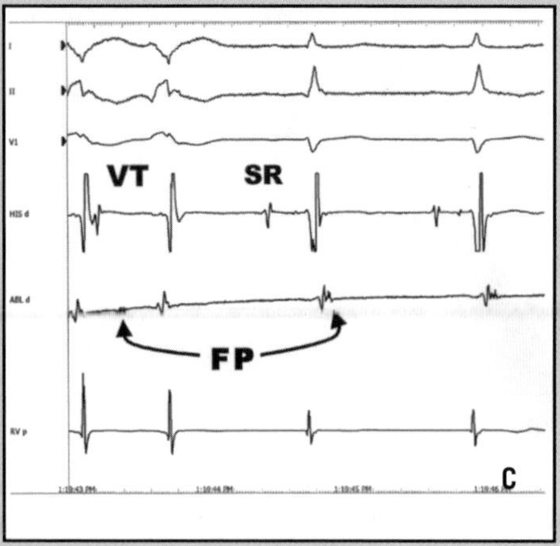

Figure 21.13c: Mapping data from a patient with VT late after myocardial infarction. Endocardial recording from the central isthmus region (figure 21.13b) during VT and during sinus rhythm demonstrated fractionated potentials (FP). During VT, a mid-diastolic low-amplitude potential is recorded, which also appears at the end of the far-field ventricular electrogram during normal rhythm. There is a large difference in timing of the FP relative to the far-field electrogram during VT as opposed to sinus rhythm. (Reprinted with permission from *EP Lab Digest* 2003;3:24–30.)

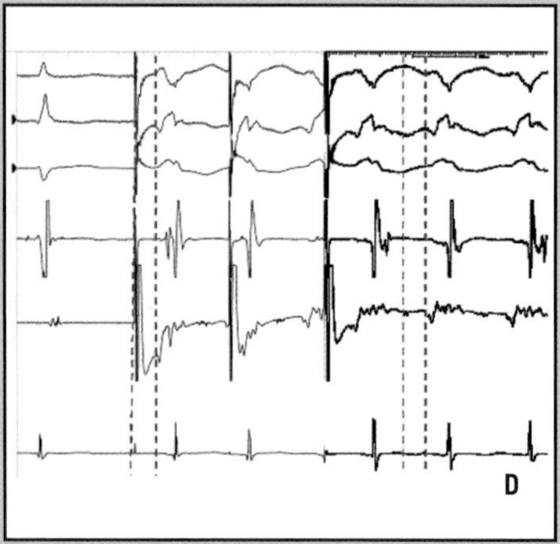

Figure 21.13d: Pacing from the isthmus site induces VT with the first stim-QRS interval equal to the FP-QRS interval during tachycardia, verifying that this site participates in the tachycardia circuit. The first paced beat also matches the QRS morphology of VT. Ablation at this site eliminated VT4. Additional ablation lesions extending toward the infero-septal scar margin eliminated VT5. (Reprinted with permission from *EP Lab Digest* 2003;3:24–30.)

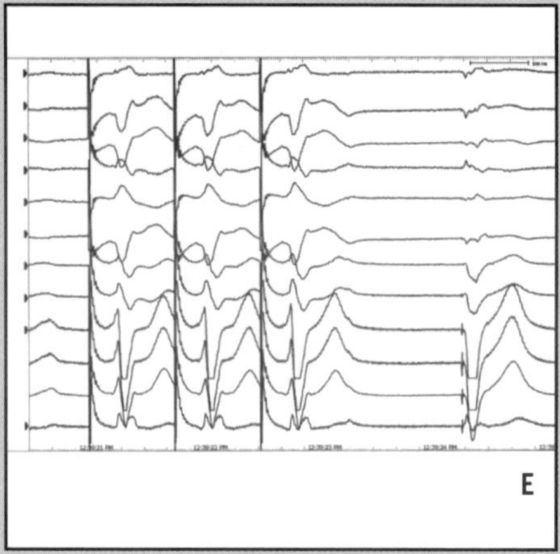

Figure 21.13e: Pace mapping near the basal and septal margin of the infarct scar matched VT2. Note the prolonged stim-QRS interval. Additional ablation lesions toward the septal side of the unexcitable scar areas eliminated VT 1 and 2. Linear ablation guided by pace maps for remaining VT morphologies were made in the lateral region of the infarct scar and eliminated the remainder of the induced VT morphologies. (Reprinted with permission from *EP Lab Digest* 2003;3:24–30.)

Chapter 22

Hereditary Conditions

Hereditary causes of ventricular arrhythmias and aborted sudden death are conditions that are due to genetic mutations. These conditions include congenital long QT syndrome (LQTS), Brugada syndrome, arrhythmogenic right ventricular cardiomyopathy/dysplasia, and hypertrophic cardiomyopathy (HCM).

Long QT Syndrome

In a patient with congenital long QT syndrome, the 12-lead ECG may show prolongation of the corrected QT (QTc) interval. A normal baseline QTc interval of less than or equal to 0.44 seconds does not exclude LQTS; in fact, this may be observed in approximately 12 percent of genetic carriers of this condition. Figure 22.1 shows a 12-lead ECG with a long QT.

Long QT syndrome can be identified in approximately 1 in 2,500 people, placing them at risk for sudden death. These patients often present with near syncope and/or syncope due to polymorphic ventricular tachycardia (torsades de pointes).

The most frequent genetic substrate of LQTS are genes that encode cardiac ion channels. Abnormities in the potassium ion channel genes KCNQ1 (Type I LQTS or LQT1) and KCNH2 (Type 2 LQTS or LQT2) result in the most common types of LQTS. Abnormalities in the sodium channel gene SCN5A (Type 3 LQTS or LQT3) is the third most common cause of LQTS. Commercial genetic testing is available for LQTS and has become an important part of the diagnostic process.

Not all types of LQTS behave in the same manner. For example, LQT1 is adrenergically mediated, in which the QTc interval increases with

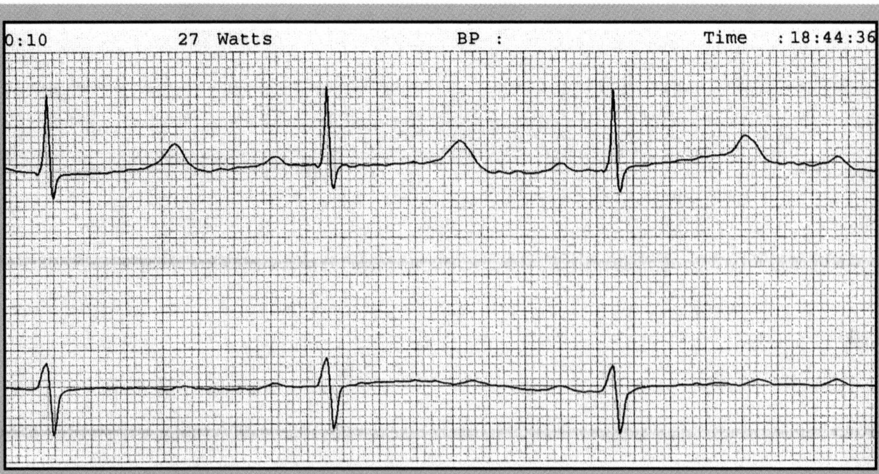

Figure 22.1: Shows a 12-lead ECG with a long QT. This ECG was taken from an 8-year-old girl, whose long QT syndrome was incidentally discovered on a routine ECG. There is no family history of sudden death or cardiac arrest. Leads II (top) and V3 (bottom) are shown at paper speed 10 mm/sec. QTC = 530 ms. She was genotyped as LQT3, the sodium channel subtype. (Reprinted with permission from *EP Lab Digest* 2004;4:1,10.)

exercise. It is one of the classic types of long QT syndrome associated with syncope during exercise or in response to emotions. With this condition, there is a decrease in potassium channel availability. Long QT2 also involves a decrease in potassium channel availability and has a variable response with exercise. Prominent bifid T waves may be seen in the resting electrocardiogram. Long QT3 involves the sodium channel, and is due to impaired inactivation of sodium current. This condition is more malignant (has a higher risk of sudden death) than long QT1 or 2. During exercise, the QTc interval decreases more than normal. Peak T waves may be seen along with the long ST segment. At least four other variants of LQTS have also been described.

Screening for patients with LQTS (blood testing) does not exclude the disorder since not all genes have been identified. Treatment includes beta-blocker therapy and/or mexiletine or cardiac pacing. If recurrent syncope occurs despite these measures, an implantable cardioverter-defibrillator (ICD) is indicated.

Brugada Syndrome

Brugada syndrome is also a lethal disease; however, its incidence is not entirely clear. First described in 1992, the condition presents with a right bundle-branch block pattern on an ECG and persistent ST segment elevation in V1 through V3. These patients typically have normal appearing hearts and present with sudden death. Figure 22.2a and 22.2b show ECGs from a patient with subtle changes to the ST segment elevation in V1 through V3. This patient had a member of the family with Brugada syndrome. He had inducible VT at electrophysiology study,

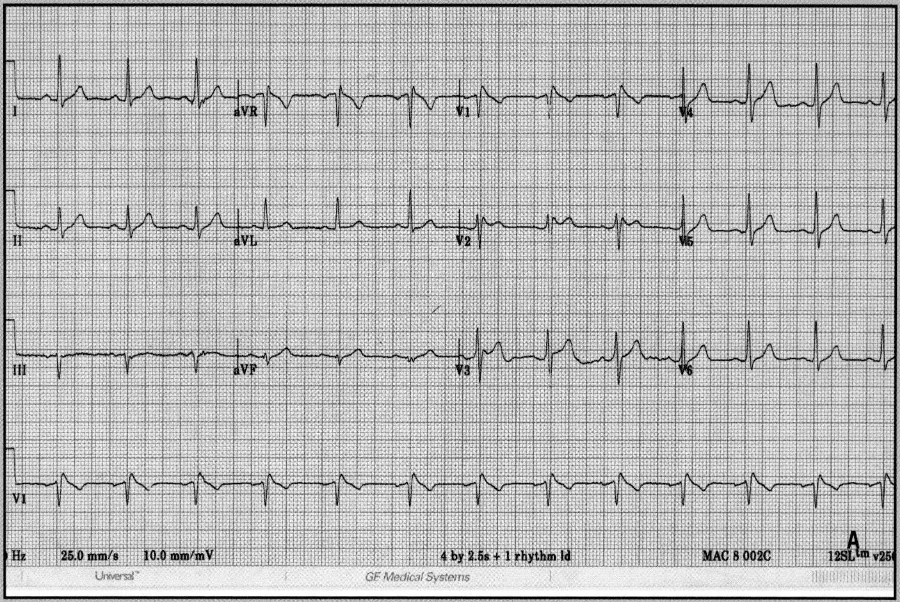

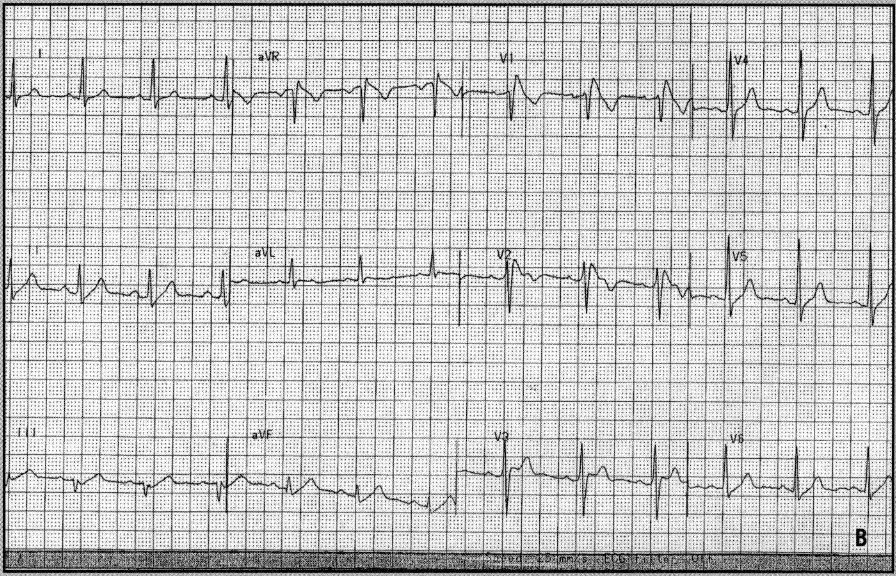

Figures 22.2a and 22.2b: Shows two ECGs from a patient with Brugada syndrome. There are subtle changes to the ST segment elevation in V1 through V3, between the two ECGs.

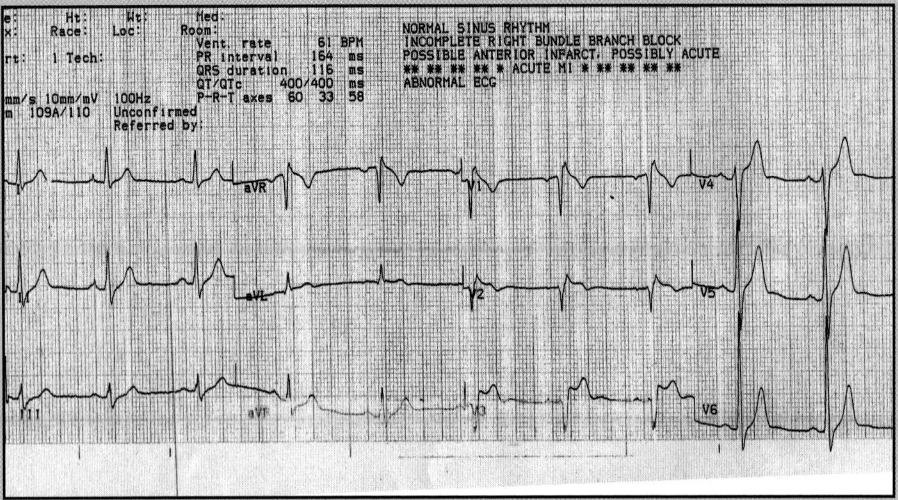

Figure 22.3: Shows an ECG from a patient with ARVC/D with localized widening at the end of the QRS in V1 through V3 (greater than 110 msec).

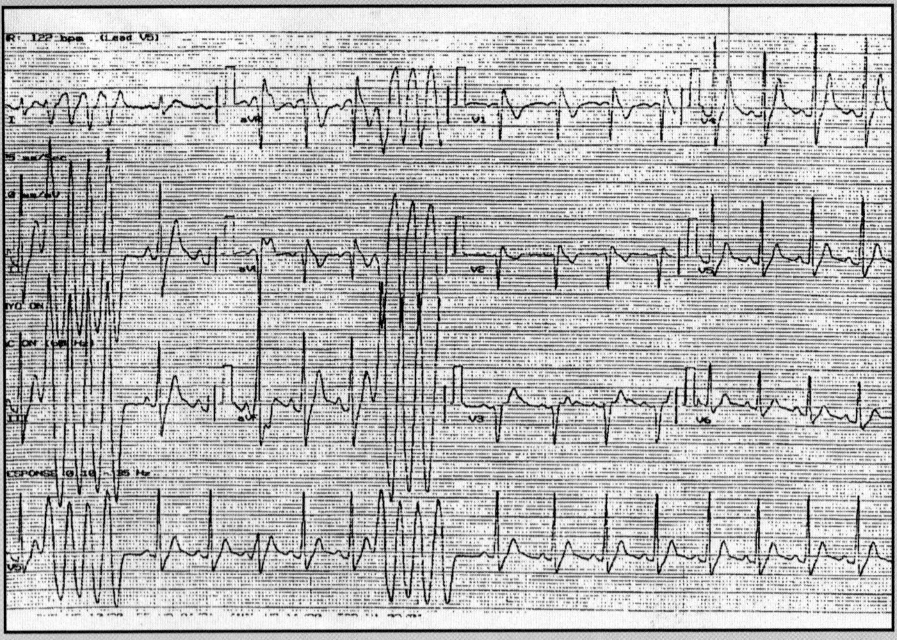

Figure 22.4: Shows rapid bursts of non-sustained ventricular tachycardia in a patient with ARVC/D.

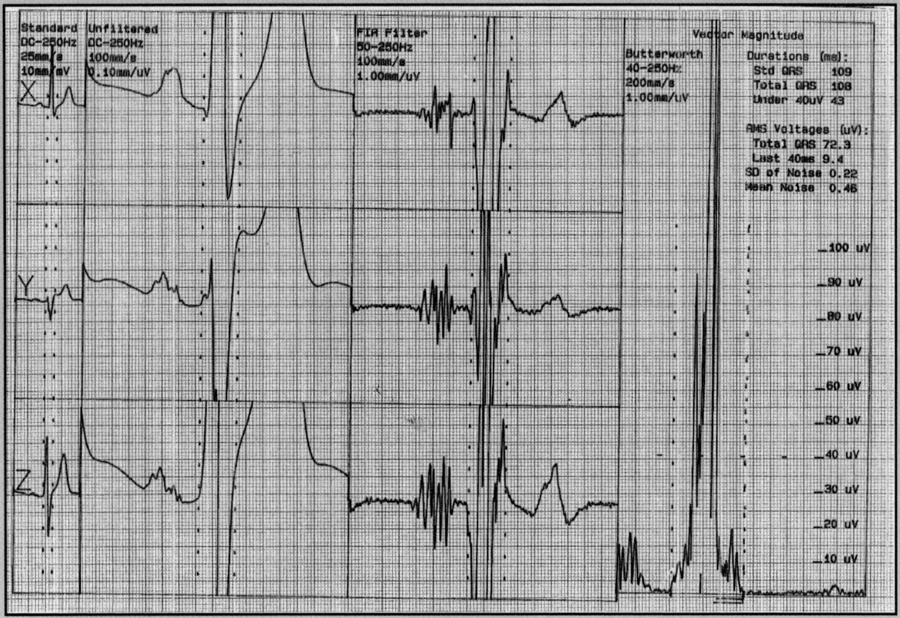

Figure 22.5: Individuals with ARVC/D typically have a very prominent positive signal-averaged ECG with a high frequency, low amplitude late potential. Note that this is the same patient as in figure 22.4.

and subsequently received an implantable cardioverter-defibrillator.

Mutations related to the SCN5A gene have been identified in Brugada syndrome. Genetic transmission is autosomal dominant, with men principally being involved. Occasionally the electrocardiogram may not show a full Brugada pattern, and it is necessary to infuse a Class I antiarrhythmic agent to bring out the classic electrocardiographic findings. Intravenous flecainide or ajmaline may be used to bring out the Brugada pattern; however, in the United States, intravenous procainamide is used, since the former drugs are not available in intravenous form.

Programmed electrical stimulation may be positive in patients with Brugada syndrome. The treatment is an ICD.

Arrhythmogenic Right Ventricular Cardiomyopathy/Dysplasia

Arrhythmogenic right ventricular cardiomyopathy/dysplasia (ARVC/D) is a rare disorder typically involving the right ventricle in which normal muscle is replaced by fat, placing the patient at risk for ventricular tachycardia and sudden death. It occurs in approximately 1 in 5,000 people, and more commonly has an autosomal dominant mode of inheritance (though autosomal recessive inheritance has also been reported). ARVC/D is largely regarded as a disease of the desmosome, in which 40 to 50 percent of ARVC/D patients have mutations identified in genes that encode desmosomal proteins.

In arrhythmogenic right ventricular cardiomyopathy/dysplasia, fat deposition may be identified in the right ventricular wall of

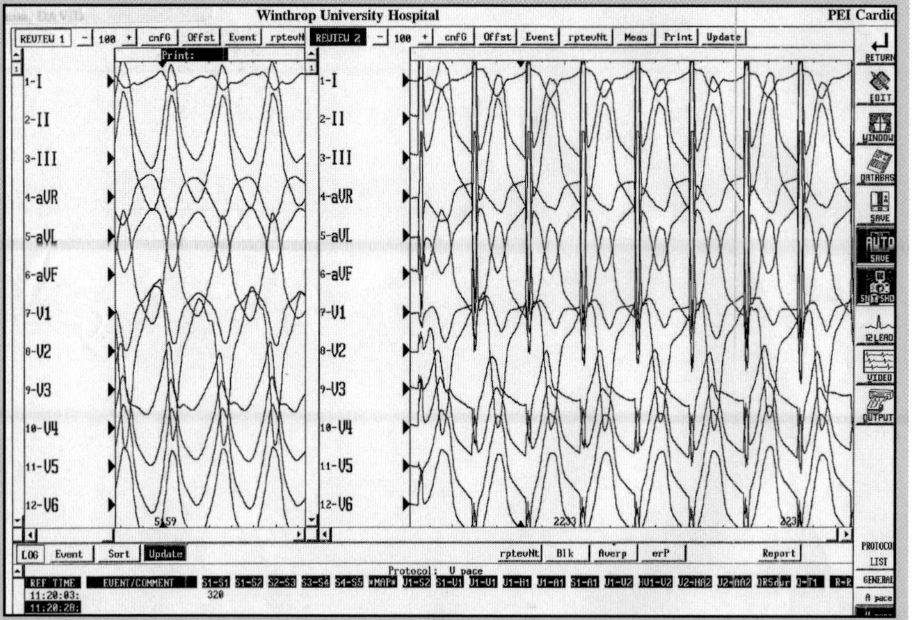

Figure 22.6: This patient had inducible sustained monomorphic ventricular tachycardia; however, pace mapping followed by catheter ablation was unsuccessful in completely eliminating the tachycardia, and an ICD was implanted.

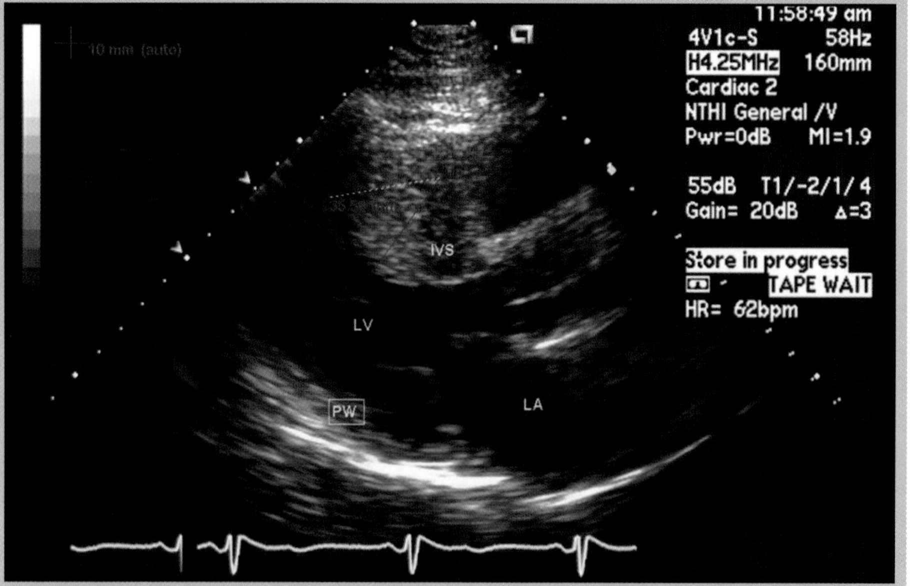

Figure 22.7: Shows a parasternal long-axis view of a two-dimensional echocardiogram showing an extremely large interventricular septum (IVS, greater than 3 cm) as compared to the relatively normal-sized left ventricular posterior wall (PW), placing the patient at risk for ventricular tachycardia/fibrillation.

the myocardium by magnetic resonance imaging, computer tomography scan, or transesophageal echocardiogram. On the electrocardiogram, there is typically a localized widening at the end of the QRS in V1 through V3 (greater than 110 msec) (figure 22.3). This has been termed an epsilon wave. Figure 22.4 shows rapid bursts of non-sustained ventricular tachycardia in a patient with ARVC/D. In addition, individuals with ARVC/D typically have a very prominent positive signal-averaged ECG with a high frequency, low amplitude late potential (figure 22.5). Negative T waves may be seen in V1 through V3, and a left bundle-branch block morphology ventricular tachycardia and/or premature ventricular contraction may be identified. The two-dimensional echocardiogram occasionally shows some right ventricular enlargement; however, thin-slice magnetic resonance imaging can demonstrate the deposition of fat in the myocardium.

ARVC/D patients who have presented with syncope and/or near-syncope and who are inducible via programmed electrical stimulation should receive an ICD. This patient had inducible sustained monomorphic ventricular tachycardia; however, pace mapping followed by catheter ablation was unsuccessful in completely eliminating the tachycardia, and an implantable cardioverter-defibrillator was implanted (figure 22.6). Sotalol may be helpful in preventing frequent and recurrent ventricular arrhythmias (in addition to an ICD).

Hypertrophic Cardiomyopathy

Hypertrophic cardiomyopathy is another hereditary condition in which patients may be prone to ventricular arrhythmias. The molecular genetic basis involves mutations that result in disease of the sarcomere. Genetic mutations have been identified in areas such as the beta-myosin heavy chain gene, troponin T gene, alpha-tropomyosin gene, actin gene, and the myosin binding protein-C gene. The mode of inheritance is autosomal dominant in over 50 percent of cases and sporadic in the remainder. HCM is a relatively common genetic disorder, affecting 1 in 500 individuals. Symptomatic patients with syncope and/or aborted sudden death, nonsustained ventricular tachycardia and/or ventricular tachycardia, or very thickened myocardium (greater than 3 cm) may be at risk for sudden death. Figure 22.7 shows a two-dimensional echocardiographic image of a very thick ventricular septum (3.6 centimeters) in a young man with hypertrophic cardiomyopathy. A prophylactic implantable cardioverter-defibrillator was implanted. Patients who have inducible ventricular tachycardia via programmed electrical stimulation and/or with a significant clinical and/or family history should be considered for an ICD.

Other Conditions

There are other conditions that may predispose to arrhythmias (not necessarily ventricular in origin). Familial Wolff-Parkinson-White syndrome and other forms of supraventricular tachycardia have also been described. Not all the genes for these hereditary conditions have been described here.

Familial clustering of arrhythmias and/or sudden death should suggest a hereditary condition. Genetic testing is of great value to suspected family members only if a specific genetic mutation has been identified. Table 22.1 shows a list of available genetic, testable genes.

Table 22.1: Genes associated with Long QT Syndrome, Brugada Syndrome, Hypertrophic Cardiomyopathy, ARVC/D and other syndromes that are available for genetic testing (courtesy of PGxHealth, New Haven, CT).

Disease	Gene (Subtype)	Protein	% Patients with a Mutation
Long QT Syndrome	KCNQ1 (LQT1)	KvLQT1	30-35%
	KCNH2 (LQT2)	HERG	25-30%
	SCN5A (LQT3)	Cardiac sodium channel	5-10%
	KCNE1 (LQT5)	Beta(MlnK)	~1%
	KCNE2 (LQT6)	Beta(MiRP)	<1%
Brugada Syndrome	SCN5A	Cardiac sodium channel	20-30%
Hypertrophic Cardiomyopathy	MYH7	Beta-Myosin heavy chain	20-30%
	MYBPC3	Myosin-binding protein C	20-30%
	TNNT2	Troponin T	3-5%
	TNNI3	Troponin I	<5%
	TNNC1	Troponin C	Rare
	TPM1	Tropomyosin-1alpha	<5%
	MYL2	Regulatory myosin light chain 2	<5%
	MYL3	Essential myosin light chain 3	Rare
	ACTC	alpha-Cardiac actin 1	Rare
Arrhythmogenic Right Ventricular Cardiomyopathy Dysplasia (ARVC/D)	PKP2	Plakophilin 2	25%
	DSP	Desmoplakin	8%
	DSG2	Desmoglein 2	5%
	DSC2	Desmocollin 2	<1%
	TMEM43	Transmembrane Protein 43	Unknown
Catecholamingeric Polymorphic Ventricular Tachycardia (CPVT)	RYR2	Cardiac ryanodine recepter	50-55%

Part 2: Quiz

Test your knowledge of Part 2:

Question 11. The mnemonic "NAVel" stands for:

A. Next To Artery Valve
B. Knee Anterior Cruciate Ligament And Varicose Veins
C. Nerve, Artery, Vein
D. Near Aorta Vessel

Question 12. An HV interval of 100 msec indicates:

A. Significant AV nodal disease
B. Severe His-Purkinje disease
C. Pre-excitation
D. Intraventricular conduction delay

Question 13. An HV interval of 0 msec indicates:

A. Severe AV nodal disease
B. Severe His-Purkinje disease
C. Pre-excitation
D. Intraventricular conduction delay

Question 14. A patient's baseline sinus cycle length is 1,000 msec. The sinus node recovery time is 1,400 msec. Calculate the corrected sinus node recovery time:

A. 100 msec
B. 200 msec
C. 300 msec
D. 400 msec

Question 15. Which of the following is *not* a mechanism of an arrhythmia?

A. Reentry
B. Facilitated conduction
C. Automaticity
D. Triggered

Question 16. Digitalis toxicity is often associated with:

A. Early afterdepolarizations
B. Delayed afterdepolarizations
C. Reentry
D. Automaticity

Question 17. Which oral antiarrhythmic drug is most consistently associated with a rise in defibrillation thresholds during implantable defibrillator testing?

A. Quinidine
B. Sotalol
C. Mexiletine
D. None of the above

Question 18. Which medication is associated with dose-dependent proarrhythmia and can lower the defibrillation threshold?

A. Quinidine
B. Sotalol
C. Mexiletine
D. Flecainide

Question 19. Which of the following are considered class III antiarrhythmic drugs (Potassium Channel Blockade, Sodium Channel Activation)?

A. Quinidine and procainamide
B. Lidocaine, mexiletine, and tocainide
C. Flecainide and propafenone
D. Sotalol, amiodarone, and dofetilide

Question 20. This antiarrhythmic is considered the most effective but also the most toxic medication, which may adversely affect the thyroid, lung, and liver:

A. Quinidine
B. Flecainide
C. Sotalol
D. Amiodarone

Question 21. The Antiarrhythmic Versus Implantable Defibrillator (AVID) trial demonstrated:

A. Increased survival in patients who received amiodarone or sotalol as compared to an implantable cardioverter-defibrillator.
B. Increased survival in those who received quinidine as compared to an implantable cardioverter-defibrillator.
C. Increased survival in those who received an implantable cardioverter-defibrillator as compared to amiodarone or sotalol.
D. Increased survival in those who received sotalol as compared to amiodarone.

Question 22. The usefulness of class Ic antiarrhythmic drugs in patients with a prior myocardial infarction was questioned by the results of which trial?

A. SCD-HeFT
B. CASS
C. CAST
D. AVID

Question 23. The Sudden Cardiac Death in Heart Failure Trial (SCD-HeFT) demonstrated an improvement in survival in those who received an implantable cardioverter-defibrillator as compared to:

A. Quinidine
B. Sotalol
C. Amiodarone and placebo
D. A pacemaker

Question 24. The delivery of radiofrequency energy as a modality for catheter ablation was first described by:

A. Dr. Melvin Scheinman
B. Dr. Warren Jackman
C. Dr. Morton Mower
D. Dr. Steven Huang

Question 25. The anticipated success rates for persistent atrial fibrillation ablation is greater than 90 percent.

A. True
B. False

Question 26. Which of the following is *not* an indication for an electrophysiology study?

A. Syncope of unknown etiology.
B. Asymptomatic premature atrial contractions.
C. Nonsustained ventricular tachycardia in a patient with a prior myocardial infarction and ejection fraction of 35 percent.
D. Unexplained palpitations with presyncope.

Question 27. What is the most common cause of atrial fibrillation?

A. Thyrotoxicosis
B. Myocardial infarction
C. Hypertension
D. Valvular disease

Question 28. According to the American Heart Association, what is the number of people living in the United States with atrial fibrillation?

A. 1.2 million people
B. 2.2 million people
C. 3.2 million people
D. 4.2 million people

Question 29. Atrial fibrillation that is unable to be successfully cardioverted is called:

A. Paroxysmal atrial fibrillation
B. Persistent atrial fibrillation
C. Chronic atrial fibrillation
D. Permanent atrial fibrillation

Question 30. What did the Atrial Fibrillation Follow-Up Investigation of Rhythm Management (AFFIRM) trial demonstrate?

A. Superiority of antiarrhythmic drug therapy over rate control and anticoagulation.
B. Superiority of rate control and anticoagulation over antiarrhythmic drug therapy.
C. Equivalence of antiarrhythmic drug therapy as compared to rate control and anticoagulation.

Question 31. According to the Canadian Trial of Atrial Fibrillation, what was the best drug for suppression of atrial fibrillation?

A. Amiodarone
B. Propafenone
C. Sotalol
D. None of the above

Question 32. What is the incidence of dual AV nodal pathways in patients referred for EP studies?

A. 10 percent
B. 15 percent
C. 20 percent
D. 25 percent

Question 33. What is the best drug for acute termination of paroxysmal supraventricular tachycardia?

A. Verapamil
B. Adenosine
C. Procainamide
D. Amiodarone

Question 34. Typical AV-node reentrant tachycardia (the most common form) involves an arrhythmia in which conduction occurs:

A. Down a fast pathway and up slow pathway
B. Down a slow pathway and up a fast pathway
C. Down a slow pathway and up a slow pathway
D. Down a fast pathway and up a fast pathway

Question 35. During a successful radiofrequency ablation of the slow AV nodal pathway to treat AV-node reentrant tachycardia, one would most commonly see:

A. A junctional rhythm
B. Complete heart block
C. Ventricular tachycardia

Question 36. Atrial tachycardias often terminate with:

A. Carotid sinus massage
B. Adenosine
C. Quinidine
D. Amiodarone

Question 37. The easiest way to localize a focal atrial tachycardia is by:

A. Point by point intracardiac mapping
B. Body surface mapping
C. Nonfluoroscopic three-dimensional mapping
D. Surface electrocardiogram

Question 38. Patients with atrial flutter have no risk for thromboembolism.

A. True
B. False

Question 39. Patients who undergo atrial flutter ablation using nonfluoroscopic three-dimensional mapping have a better outcome than patients who undergo ablation using a multi-poled catheter across the cavotricuspid isthmus and an ablation catheter.

A. True
B. False

Question 40. When a patient fails external cardioversion and/or defibrillation, which of the following techniques should be considered?

A. Pressure applied over the patches to lower transthoracic impedance
B. Cardiopulmonary resuscitation
C. Infusion of ibutilide
D. Intravenous amiodarone

Question 41. Internal cardioversion should be considered in people who are refractory to standard external defibrillation.

A. True
B. False

Question 42. A switch box utilized to switch between external patches and internal cardioversion/defibrillation is called:

A. The Scheinman box
B. The Griffin box
C. The Cohen box
D. The Booker box

Question 43. The presence of a delta wave on an ECG can be found in:

A. 0.15 percent of the general population
B. 0.5 percent of the general population
C. 1 percent of the general population
D. 5 percent of the general population

Question 44. Most (greater than 50 percent) of accessory pathways are located where?

A. On the right side of the heart
B. On the left side of the heat
C. In the middle of the heart (paraseptal)

Question 45. An ECG that shows delta waves inverted in lead V1 and upright in V2 is consistent with an accessory pathway in which location:

A. A left lateral bypass tract
B. A right free wall bypass tract
C. A right posteroseptal bypass tract
D. A left posterior bypass tract

Question 46. Most patients who experience sudden cardiac arrest are suffering from an acute myocardial infarction.

A. True
B. False

Question 47. What is the best way to treat ventricular tachycardia that is not in the setting of an acute myocardial infarction or due to a reversible cause?

A. Antiarrhythmic drugs
B. Revascularization
C. An implantable defibrillator

Question 48. The following noninvasive markers are useful at predicting the risk of ventricular tachycardia:

A. Ejection fraction
B. The presence of late potentials on a signal-averaged electrocardiogram
C. A positive or indeterminate microvolt T wave alternans test
D. All of the above

Question 49. In patients with myocardial infarction and ventricular tachycardia, the best way to localize and identify a successful VT ablation site is:

A. Concealed entrainment
B. Nonfluoroscopic three-dimensional mapping
C. Point by point mapping
D. Body surface mapping

Question 50. In a patient with dilated cardiomyopathy and a left bundle-branch block pattern, it is important to look for this easily curable form of ventricular tachycardia:

A. Myocardial ventricular tachycardia
B. Bundle-branch reentrant ventricular tachycardia
C. Triggered ventricular tachycardia
D. Epicardial ventricular tachycardia

Question 51. A 43-year-old Asian man presents with ventricular fibrillation and is successfully defibrillated. A 12-lead ECG shows a right bundle-branch block pattern with ST segment elevation in V1 through V3. He has a significant family history of sudden death. The most likely cause of his condition is:

A. Long QT syndrome
B. Brugada syndrome
C. Arrhythmogenic right ventricular cardiomyopathy/dysplasia
D. Hypertrophic cardiomyopathy

Question 52. A 53-year-old man is found to have hypertrophic cardiomyopathy. The intraventricular septum is greater than 3 cm. The best treatment to prevent sudden death is:

A. An implantable defibrillator
B. Amiodarone
C. Verapamil
D. Alcohol septal ablation

Answer key:

11. C.
12. B.
13. C:
14. D.
15. B.
16. B.
17. C.
18. B.
19. D.
20. D.
21. C.
22. C.
23. C.
24. D.
25. B.
26. B
27. C
28. B
29. D
30. C
31. A
32. D
33. B
34. B
35. A
36. B
37. C
38. B
39. B
40. A
41. A
42. D
43. A
44. B
45. C
46. B
47. C
48. D
49. A
50. B
51. B
52. A

Part 3

IMPLANTABLE DEVICES TO DIAGNOSE AND TREAT ARRHYTHMIAS AND HEART FAILURE

Chapter 23

Syncope

Syncope (or loss of consciousness) is one of the most frequent emergency room and hospital diagnoses. Three to six percent of hospital admissions and/or emergency room visits can be attributed to syncope or near-syncope. The workup should follow a simple algorithm. The method of evaluating syncope and determining its etiology should initially consist of a history, physical examination, and 12-lead electrocardiogram. Table 23.1 shows the common causes of syncope. Table 23.2 shows the clinical characteristics of cardiac and noncardiac syncope. Cardiac syncope primarily consists of arrhythmias of all types: tachycardias (rapid heart rhythms) such as ventricular tachycardia/fibrillation and/or supraventricular tachycardia, and bradyarrhythmias such as heart block, sinus bradycardia, and asystole. If the history, physical examination, and/or electrocardiogram point to a cardiac diagnosis, a cardiac workup may be important, followed by an electrophysiology study.

The electrophysiology study is useful at assessing cardiac conduction and presence of arrhythmias. The results of the study can focus the treatment to drugs, catheter ablation (performed at the time of the electrophysiology study), and device-based therapy (pacemaker or implantable defibrillator).

The most common etiologies of syncope are of a noncardiac vascular nature, with neurocardiogenic syncope and orthostatic hypotension accounting for approximately half of all cases. Figure 23.1 shows a schematic of the mechanism of neurocardiogenic syncope. In neurocardiogenic syncope, there is a brain-heart interaction

Table 23.1: Reasons for Syncope

Cardiac Reasons for Syncope	Non-Cardiac Reasons for Syncope
Left-sided heart	Neurocardiogenic
Aortic stenosis	Orthostatic
Hypertrophic cardiomyopathy	Cerebrovascular
Prosthetic valve malfunction	Seizure
Mitral stenosis	Carotid sinus hypersensitivity
Left atrial myxoma	Situational
Right-sided heart	Valsalva
Eisenmenger syndrome	Micturition
Tetralogy of Fallot	Defecation
Pulmonary embolism	Postprandial
Pulmonary stenosis	Vertigo
Primary pulmonary hypertension	Headaches
Cardiac tamponade	Psychiatric
Cardiac arrhythmia	
Sinoatrial disease	
Atrioventricular block	
Supraventricular tachycardia	
Ventricular tachycardia/ventricular fibrillation	
Pacemaker-related	

Table 23.2: Characteristics of Cardiac Syncope

Onset	Onset preceded by tension, dyspnea, diaphoresis, palpitations.
Settings	Any setting.
Posture of patient	Any setting.
Residua	Recovery is immediate or prolonged. There may be signs of seizure or cerebral hypoxia.

such that a catecholamine trigger (adrenaline) causes the heart to beat forcefully (hypercontractile), thereby activating mechanoreceptor C fibers on the posterior left ventricle. Stimulation of these fibers may trigger a hyperactive vagal response with resultant bradycardia and/or hypotension. There are two types of neurocardiogenic syncope responses: a cardioinhibitory response, which is principally bradycardia-driven hypotension, and vasodepressor syncope, in which vasodilatation of the blood vessel is the primary response. In a significant number of patients with neurocardiogenic syncope, a mixed vasodepressor and cardioinhibitory response occurs.

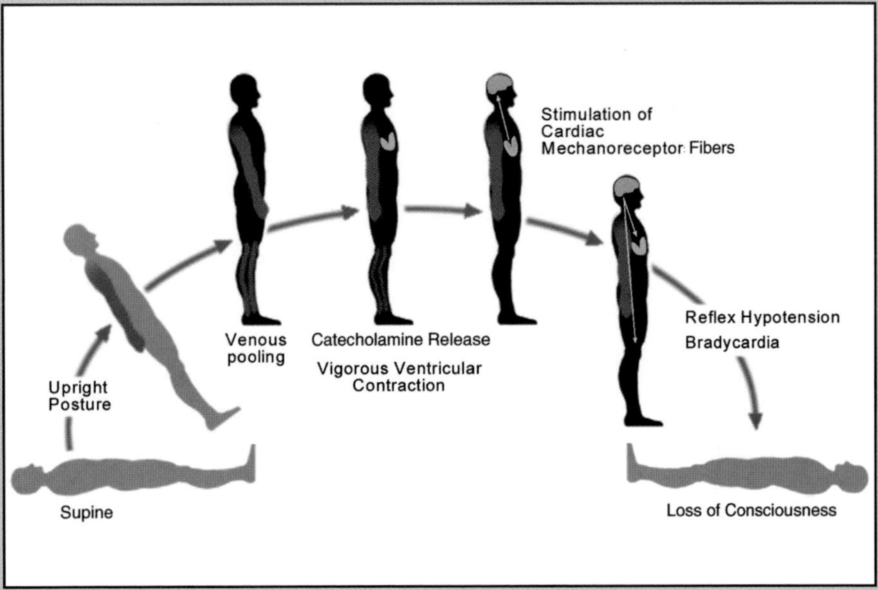

Figure 23.1: Mechanism of neurally-mediated "vasovagal" syncope.

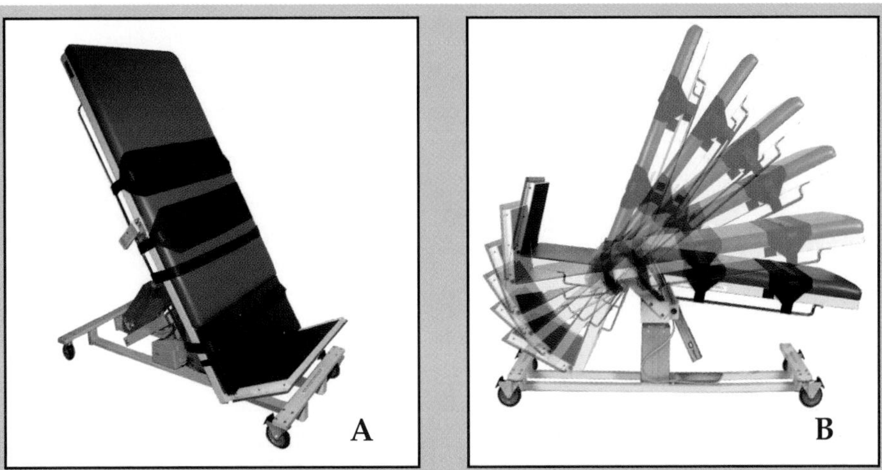

Figures 23.2a and 23.2b: The head-up tilt-table test is a procedure that is used to provoke neurocardiogenic syncope (Rapid Response™ Head Up Tilt™ Table, Medical Positioning, Inc., Kansas City, MO) (courtesy of Medical Positioning, Inc., Kansas City, MO).

The treatment for neurocardiogenic syncope is principally beta-blocker therapy (thereby blocking the catecholamine trigger). Alternatives include fludrocortisone and midodrine. The latter two medications are contraindicated in patients with significant

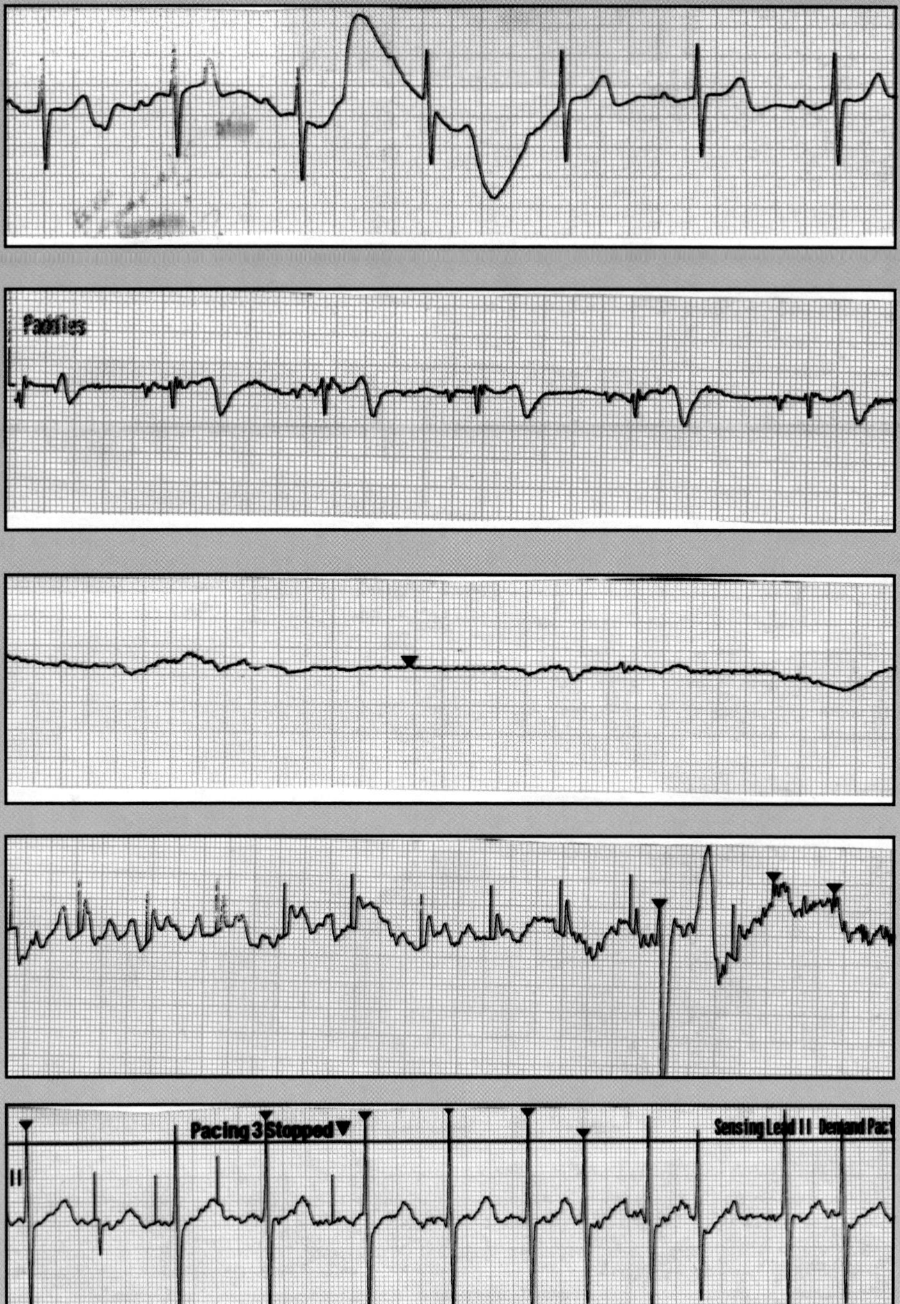

Figure 23.3: Shows asystole occurring as a result of a positive tilt-table test. Beta-blocker therapy is often first-line treatment if not contraindicated.

hypertension. Other causes of syncope include autonomic dysfunction, occasionally seen in patients with diabetes and/or Parkinson's disease (who develop autonomic neuropathy). In addition, patients with dehydration may exhibit orthostatic hypotension in which upon standing, the heart rate increases and blood pressure drops significantly.

An additional 15 percent of patients with syncope may have a primary neurological etiology. In those patients, the history, physical examination, and electrocardiogram often do not reveal any cardiac pathology. A history of an aura, incontinence, and/or focal neurologic problem may point to a neurologic etiology and reveal the necessity of a complete neurologic workup (magnetic resonance imaging, computer tomography scan, and/or electroencephalogram).

The head-up tilt-table test is a procedure that is used to provoke neurocardiogenic syncope (figures 23.2a and 23.2b). It can help in diagnosing autonomic dysfunction as well as orthostatic hypotension. A baseline head-up tilt-table test can be performed by monitoring heart rate and blood pressure while the patient is upright at 60 to 80 degrees for between 30 to 45 minutes. The addition of isoproterenol as a catecholamine trigger (during a 10- to 15-minute tilt test) can increase the sensitivity of the test, but at the expense of its specificity. In Chapter 29, table 29.1 shows a weight-based isoproterenol infusion rate chart. Some centers perform a baseline tilt, and if negative, it is followed by an isoproterenol tilt; whereas others perform a streamlined isoproterenol study only. In patients who have neurocardiogenic syncope, there is concomitant

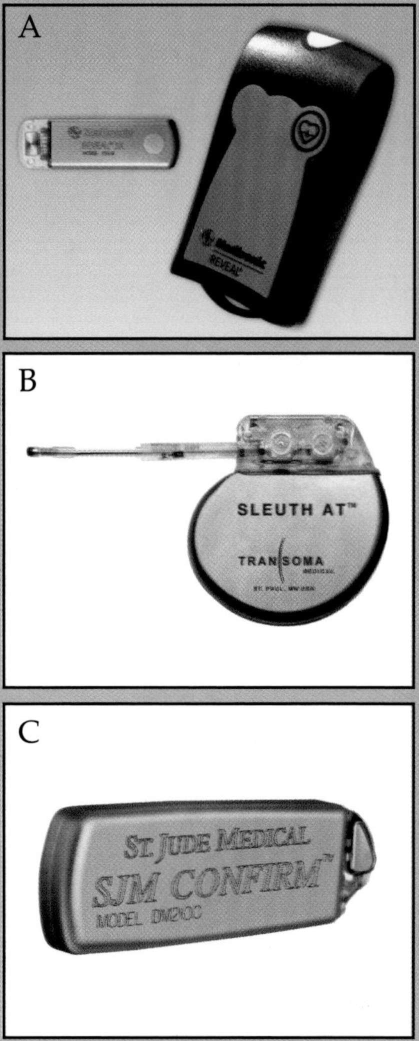

Figure 23.4: In patients with syncope of unknown etiology despite electrophysiological study, tilt-table and neurologic evaluation, an implantable cardiac monitor can be very helpful. (A) Shows the Reveal® DX model 9528 with patient activator, (Reproduced with permission of Medtronic, Inc., Minneapolis, MN). (B) Shows the Sleuth AT™ (Advanced Trending) Implantable Cardiac Monitor (courtesy of Transoma Medical, St. Paul, MN). (C) Shows the Confirm™ Implantable Cardiac Monitor (courtesy of St. Jude Medical, Sylmar, CA).

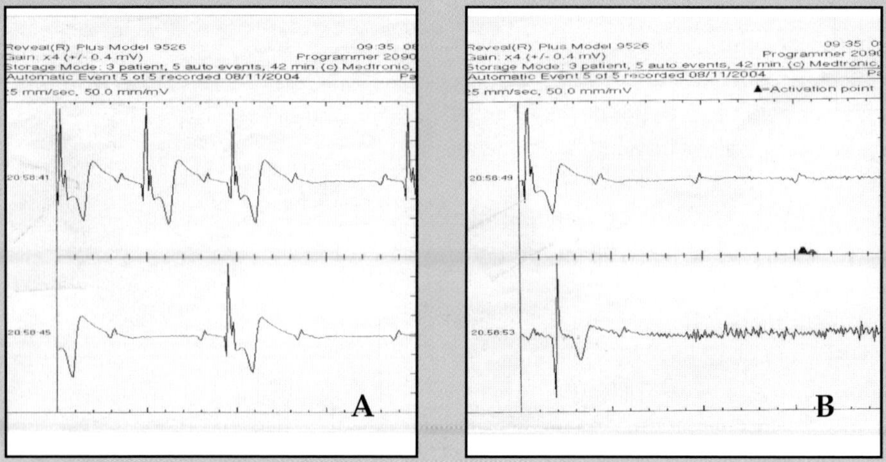

Figure 23.5a and 23.5b: Shows complete heart block detected via implantable loop recorder. Subsequently, a permanent pacemaker was implanted.

hypotension and bradycardia. In patients who have autonomic dysfunction, there is a slow decrease in heart rate and blood pressure over time. In patients who have orthostatic hypotension, there is a drop in blood pressure and an increase in heart rate. In patients who undergo tilt-table testing who have coronary artery disease, the administration of isoproterenol is contraindicated. In those patients, a passive head-up tilt-table test, which consists of up to 45 minutes of upright tilt testing, can be performed. Figure 23.3 shows asystole occurring during a positive tilt-table test. Beta-blocker therapy helped block the catecholamine trigger of this patient's neurocardiogenic syncope.

In patients with syncope of unknown etiology despite electrophysiology study, tilt-table test, and neurologic evaluation, implantable cardiac monitors can be very helpful. This is a small nonvascular device, which is implanted subcutaneously, that can record electrical activity from the heart for up to 36 months. The Winthrop University Hospital experience with this device in over 100 patients demonstrated its utility in diagnosing significant bradycardiac events, supraventricular and ventricular tachycardias that were missed by the electrophysiology study. Figures 23.4a-c show three different implantable cardiac monitoring systems that can record information over a long period of time.

Figures 23.5a and 23.5b show complete heart block recorded by an implantable cardiac monitor that ultimately required implantation of a permanent pacemaker. This type of implantable cardiac monitor can identify an arrhythmogenic etiology in approximately 50 percent of patients with unexplained syncope despite a thorough prior workup.

Chapter 24

Congestive Heart Failure

Congestive heart failure (CHF) has become one of the most common diseases in the United States. Over 5 million people are living with CHF, and approximately 500,000 new cases are diagnosed each year in the United States alone. While this disease is associated with significant morbidity and mortality, with appropriate lifestyle modifications and medical and device-based therapy, quality of life and survival may be improved.

CHF occurs with impaired myocardial filling and/or contraction. This results in either the heart's inability to pump a sufficient amount of oxygenated blood and nutrients to meet the body's needs or the heart's ability to pump blood effectively only by elevating the filling pressures. A manifestation of acute CHF is pulmonary edema, the backup of blood from the left heart into the lungs. Heart failure may be due to myocardial damage (ischemia, long-standing hypertension, the effects of alcohol, etc.). Table 24.1 shows the etiology of congestive heart failure.

CHF is the result of an imbalance in the degree of end-diastolic fiber stretch proportional to the systolic mechanical work achieved. This imbalance can produce a malfunction between mechanisms that keep the interstitium and the alveoli dry and the competing forces that result in fluid transfer to the interstitium. The mechanisms that keep the interstitium and the alveoli dry are the maintenance of plasma oncotic pressure higher than pulmonary capillary pressure, maintenance of connective tissue and cellular barriers relatively impermeable to plasma proteins, and maintenance of a vast lymphatic system.

Table 24.1: The Etiology of Congestive Heart Failure

1. Ischemic Cardiomyopathy.
2. Idiopathic Cardiomyopathy.
3. Valvular Heart Disease (stenotic/regurgitant valvular disease).
4. Hypertensive Heart Disease.
5. Congenital Heart Disease.
6. Hereditary (ARVC/D, Hypertrophic).
7. Toxin-Induced Cardiomyopathy.
   Alcohol/Doxorobicin
8. Infiltrative Cardiomyopathy.
   • Amyloid/Hemochromatosis
9. High Output Failure.
   • Thyrotoxicosis
   • AV Fistulae
   • Pregnancy
   • Chronic Anemia

Opposing forces responsible for fluid transfer to the interstitium include pulmonary capillary pressure and plasma oncotic pressure. When fluid is transferred into the lung interstitium with increased lymphatic flow under normal circumstances, no increase in interstitial volume occurs. When the capacity of the lymphatic drainage is surpassed, however, fluid collects in the interstitial spaces surrounding the bronchioles and lung vasculature, consequently giving rise to pulmonary vascular congestion.

CHF can be classified in one of two groups: 1) forward or backward ventricular failure, or 2) systolic and diastolic dysfunction. Backward failure is secondary to elevated systemic venous pressure, while left ventricular failure is secondary to reduced forward flow into the aorta and systemic circulation. Systolic dysfunction is characterized by a dilated left ventricle with impaired contractility. Conversely, diastolic dysfunction occurs in a normal-sized left ventricle with impaired capacity to relax and accept as well as eject blood.

Table 24.2 shows clinical findings in a patient with congestive heart failure. These include peripheral edema; jugular venous distention; pulmonary congestion; addition of a third or fourth heart sound (S_3 or S_4); and hepatomegaly. Table 24.3 shows clinical symptoms of CHF. These include dyspnea (shortness of breath); decreased exercise tolerance; fatigue; leg swelling (pedal edema); and cerebrovascular symptoms (confusion).

The New York Heart Association Classification of Congestive Heart Failure (NYHA CHF Classification) classifies CHF along therapeutic and function lines for the prescription of physical activity for cardiac patients. This functional classification is in widespread use, and has been adopted by the American Heart Association as well. Table 24.4 shows the NYHA CHF Classification.

CHF is the leading diagnosis-related group of hospitalization for patients over the age of 65, and is associated with a high mortality rate. Men have a mortality rate of 60 percent a year, while women have a mortality rate of 40 percent a year. Furthermore, African Americans have a 150 percent higher

Table 24.2: Clinical Findings of Congestive Heart Failure

1. Peripheral Edema.	4. Pulmonary Congestion/Rales.
2. Jugular Venous Distention.	5. Hepatomegaly.
3. S_3 or S_4 Heart Sounds.	6. Cardiac Cachexia (wasting).

Table 24.3: Symptoms of Congestive Heart Failure

1. Dyspnea.	4. Fatigue.
2. Pedal Edema.	5. Cerebrovascular Symptoms/Confusion.
3. Decreased Exercise Tolerance.	

Table 24.4: The New York Heart Association Classification of Congestive Heart Failure

Class I	Patients with no limitation of activities; they suffer no symptoms from ordinary activities
Class II	Patients with slight, mild limitation of activity; they are comfortable with rest or with mild exertion
Class III	Patients with marked limitation of activity; they are comfortable only at rest
Class IV	Patients who should be at complete rest, confined to bed or chair; any physical activity brings on discomfort, and symptoms occur at rest

mortality rate than white patients, and it is higher in men than women. Though CHF may occur among patients of any age, it is most prevalent in the elderly, occurring in nearly 10 percent of the general population over the age of 75.

Table 24.5 shows standard treatments of CHF. Lifestyle modifications including diet, cessation of smoking, and weight loss as well as environmental changes are prescribed to reduce stress. The more recent guidelines by the American Heart Association, American College of Cardiology, and Heart Rhythm Society have expanded on the above indications and have added room for physician judgment in order to be acceptable as an indication for implantation. An example of this is implantation of a biventricular ICD in a patient with New York Heart Association Class I congestive

Table 24.5: Treatment of Congestive Heart Failure

1. Lifestyle Modifications.

- Exercise
- Diet (Salt Restriction)
- Weight Loss
- Stress Reduction
- Smoking Cessation

2. Optimal Medical Therapy.

- Angiotensin-Converting Enzyme Inhibitor and/or Angiotensin Receptor Blocker
- Aldosterone Inhibitor
- Beta Blocker Therapy
- Digitalis
- Diuretics

3. Device-Based Therapy.

- ICD (EF < 36 percent; NYHA Class II or III)
- Biventricular ICD (EF < 36 percent; NYHA Class III or IV; QRS > 120 ms).
- Current ACC/AHA/HRS guidelines add additional acceptance for less aggressive NYHA heart failure classifications based on physician judgement as well as patient's pacing requirement.

heart failure despite optimal medical therapy and an ejection fraction of less than 36 percent, with the frequent need for ventricular pacing. In addition, the SCD-HeFT indications have been expanded, so it is now permitted (based on physician judgment) to implant a prophylactic defibrillator in a patient with NYHA Class I congestive heart failure despite optimal medical therapy.

Optimal medical therapy includes a beta blocker and an angiotensin-converting enzyme inhibitor and/or an angiotensin receptor blocker. Diuretics, digitalis, and an aldosterone inhibitor can be helpful as well. Prophylactic device-based therapy (ICD or biventricular ICD) can improve mortality and decrease hospitalizations above and beyond medical therapy in patients with left ventricular ejection fractions of less than 36 percent. In particular, these patients with cardiomyopathies of any etiology and NYHA Class II or III congestive heart failure despite optimal medical therapy can benefit from an ICD (for SCD-HeFT indications, see Chapter 26). Patients with NYHA Class III or IV congestive heart failure despite optimal medical therapy and a QRS duration greater than 120 ms can benefit from cardiac resynchronization therapy with a biventricular ICD (for COMPANION trial indications, see Chapter 27). Biventricular ICDs have been shown to reduce both hospitalizations and mortality.

In summary, lifestyle modifications, drug therapy, and device-based therapy can improve the long-term outlook for patients with congestive heart failure.

Chapter 25

Permanent Pacemaker

Permanent pacemakers are implanted in patients who have symptomatic bradycardia. The standard indications for permanent pacemakers include complete heart block, Mobitz type II second-degree AV block, and symptomatic bradycardia. Occasionally, patients may have a condition known as carotid sinus hypersensitivity, characterized by excessive sensitivity to pressure around their neck or by dizziness when they turn their head. This can be diagnosed by pressing gently on the carotid sinus for five seconds (after ruling out any kind of bruits suggesting carotid

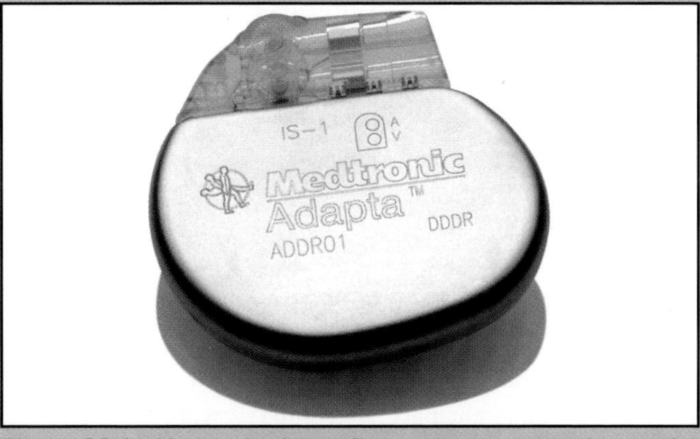

Figure 25.1: Medtronic Adapta™ permanent pacemaker model number ADDR01 (Reproduced with permission of Medtronic, Inc., Minneapolis, MN).

Table 25.1: Indications for Permanent Pacemaker Implantation

1. Complete heart block (not congenital).
2. Mobitz type II second-degree heart block.
3. Symptomatic bradycardia and/or AV block (irreversible).
4. Symptomatic bradycardia and/or AV block requiring essential medications.
5. Symptomatic carotid sinus hypersensitivity.
6. Cardioinhibitory syncope.
7. Syncope with bifascicular block or significant sinus node or His-Purkinje disease.
8. Neuromuscular disease (such as myotonic muscular dystrophy) with any AV block.
9. To prevent or terminate specific tachycardias.

artery obstruction). Table 25.1 shows the more recent indications for permanent pacemaker implantation.

A permanent pacemaker is a mechanical device that consists of a pulse generator (figure 25.1) and pacemaker leads. The most common device implanted is a dual-chamber pacemaker, in which a lead is placed into the right atrium and another pacing lead is positioned into the right ventricle. The tips of these leads may be tined (passive fixation) with little barbs at the end made of polyurethane silicone that hooks into the trabeculae of the myocardium. In addition, active fixation leads have a tiny screw at the end in order to fasten to the heart. Active fixation leads may have an exposed screw coated by a soluble material, or they may be mechanically exposed, extended, and/or retracted. Figure 25.2 shows a variety of devices and leads currently available. Figure 25.3 shows a detachable operation module which is utilized as part of the programmer for implantable devices and may be useful for teaching ancillary personnel, students, and fellows.

Pacing leads may be bipolar (having two poles) or unipolar (a single pole). Modern leads for the right atrium and right ventricle are bipolar. Unipolar leads are more common in pacing systems that are more than 15 years old. It is important to know that bipolar leads and pacemakers may be programmed unipolar. If there is damage to the proximal ring of the pacemaker, it can be reprogrammed to unipolar to function appropriately. In addition, if there is pacemaker pocket stimulation with twitching of the pectoralis muscle, one should suspect conversion to a unipolar type system.

Stimulation: Pacing and Sensing

In order to effectively capture myocardial tissue, an electrical impulse must be delivered from the pulse generator to the pacing lead electrode. Typically, lead impedance is measured and is between 500 to 1,200 ohms, depending on the lead. A low lead impedance suggests an insulation defect, whereas a high lead impedance suggests a lead fracture.

Typically, pacing thresholds are tested at a rate faster than the underlying rhythm, with a pulse duration (pulse width) of 0.5 ms. The pacemaker voltage is sequentially decreased in order to determine where there is loss of capture (a stimulus without

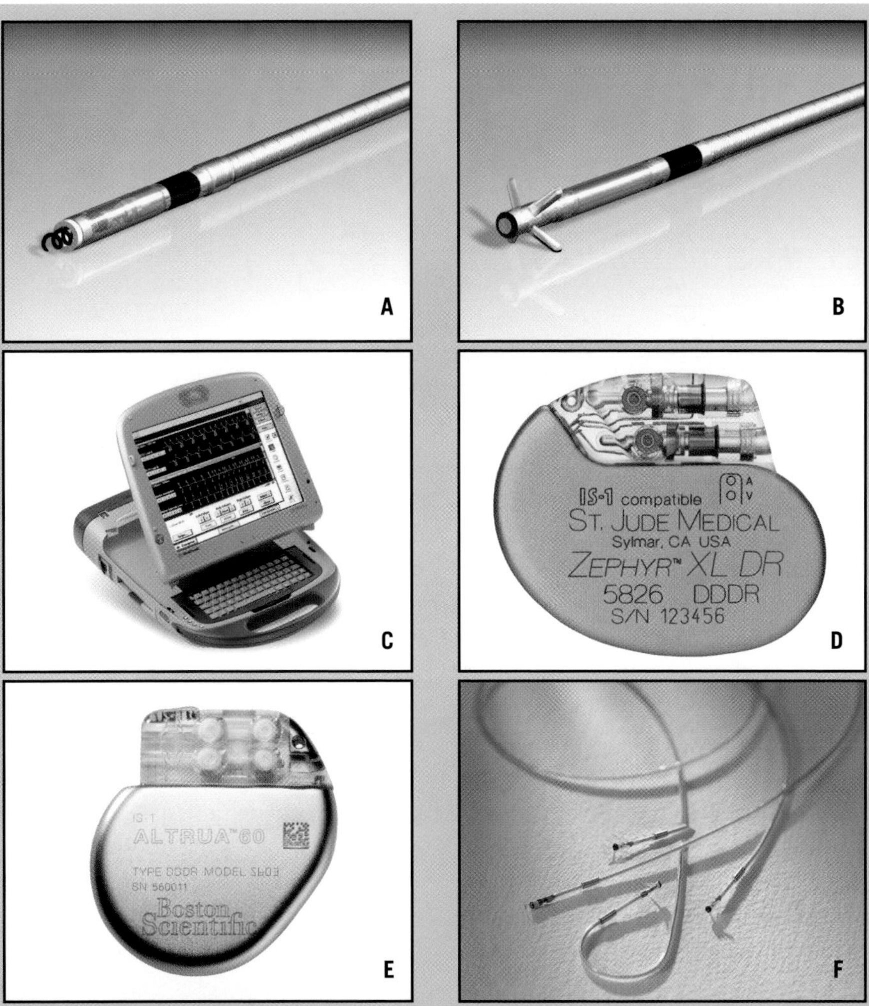

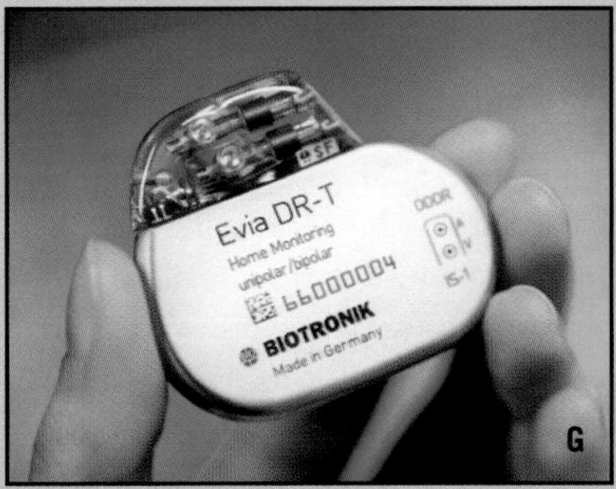

Figure 25.2: (A) CapSureFix® Novus model 5076 (Reproduced with permission of Medtronic, Inc., Minneapolis, MN). (B) CapSure Sense® model 4074 (Reproduced with permission of Medtronic, Inc., Minneapolis, MN). (C) The Medtronic 2090 Programmer used for pacemakers, ICDs, and biventricular ICDs (Reproduced with permission of Medtronic, Inc., Minneapolis, MN). (D) The Zephyr™ XL DR dual-chamber pacemaker (courtesy of St. Jude Medical, Inc., Sylmar, CA). (E) The ALTRUA™ 60 dual-chamber pacemaker (courtesy of Boston Scientific, Natick, MA). (F) The FINELINE® II leads, with active and passive fixation (courtesy of Boston Scientific, Natick, MA). (G) Evia DR-T dual-chamber pacemaker with home monitoring technology (approved in Europe and awaiting FDA approval in the U.S.) (courtesy of BIOTRONIK Inc., Lake Oswego, OR).

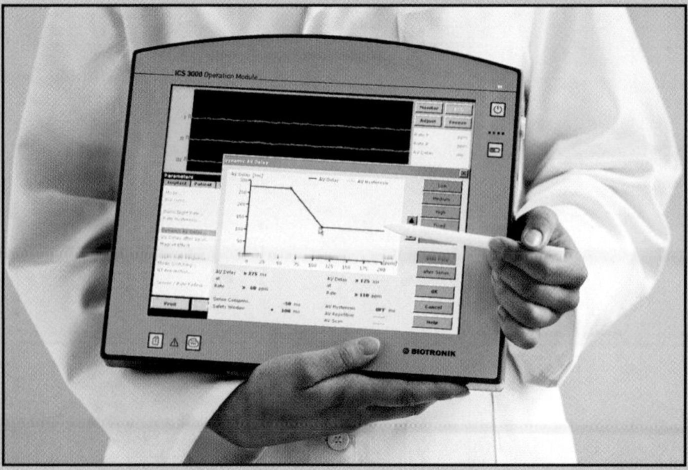

Figure 25.3: ICS 3000 Operation Module Programmer. This Window-based programmer features faster boot up time, 30 GB hard drive, and a detachable Operation Module (courtesy of BIOTRONIK Inc., Lake Oswego, OR).

depolarization) (figure 25.4). The lowest level at which capture occurs is the pacing threshold. In order to assure a 100 percent safety margin, the pacemaker output (voltage) should be doubled from the threshold level. Threshold can also be determined by keeping the voltage fixed and varying pulse width. A strength-duration curve can be generated demonstrating the precise relationship between voltage and pulse width in order to capture the myocardium (figure 25.5). The minimal voltage that provokes a response is called "rheobase." This is the lowest voltage that is approached on the strength-duration curve when the pulse width approaches infinity. The stimulus duration at 2 times "rheobase" is known as "chronaxie." Chronaxie is an energy-efficient point on the strength-duration curve. In general, the chronic pulse width should be less than 0.6 ms, and the chronic voltage should be less than 5 volts.

In order to determine the sensing threshold, the paced rate is programmed below the intrinsic rate in order to sense intrinsic complexes. The sensitivity number is programmed to 5 millivolts (mVs) (the higher the number, the less sensitive it is), and "undersensing" is detected (inappropriate pacer spikes) (figure 25.6). The number is slowly decreased until no undersensing occurs. If the sensitivity number is too low, "oversensing" can occur and appropriate pacing may not occur despite a clinical need.

Typically, the pacing threshold increases over the next month after implantation, but eventually will decrease back towards the implant value by three months (figure 25.7). The addition of a steroid-eluting tip to the lead helps decrease the acute inflammatory response, minimize the initial rise in pacing threshold, and decrease the chronic threshold.

Pacemakers function using complicated timing sequences that sense atrial and ventricular activity. These are well described in standard pacing textbooks. In effect, pacemakers are advanced computers. They are designed to avoid noise and will resort to VOO asynchronous mode.

The pacing mode is determined by a standard four-digit code (table 25.2). The

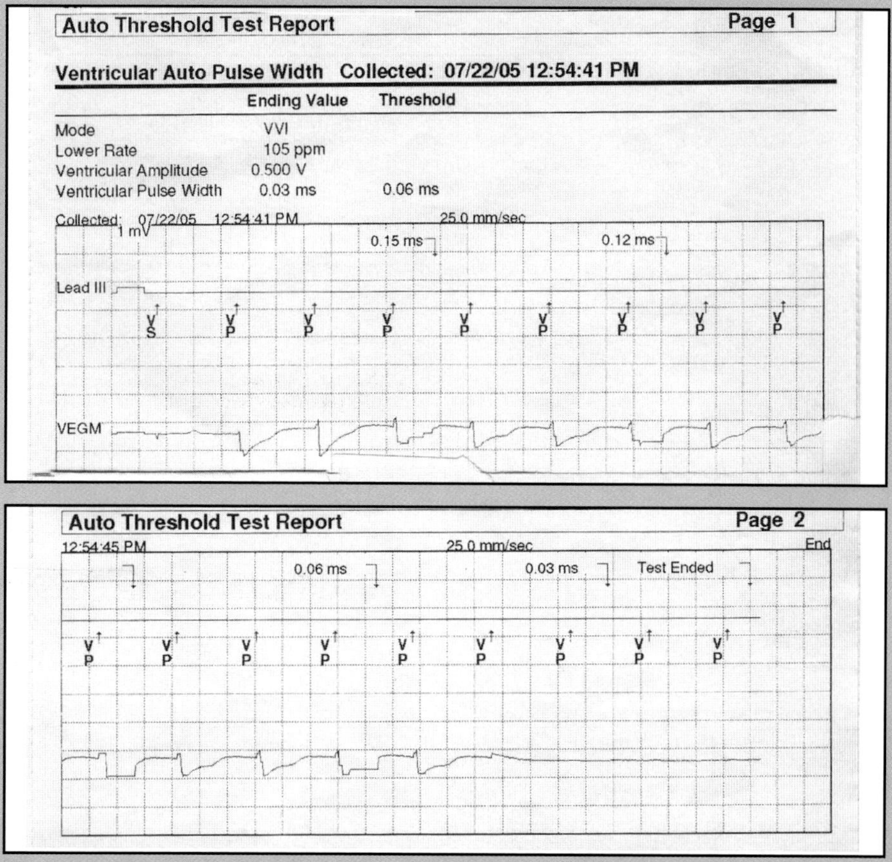

Figure 25.4: Shows threshold testing during right ventricular pacing. Note the loss of pacemaker capture at 0.06 milliseconds.

first letter of the code describes the pacing site, the second letter describes the sensing site, and the third letter describes the sensing modality. The fourth letter is used if rate responsiveness is programmed on. For example, in DDDR pacing, D stands for dual-chamber pacing, sensing, and modality, and R for rate responsiveness.

Modern dual-chamber pacemakers have the ability to switch their modes (*mode-switching*) with the detection of a very rapid onset of atrial fibrillation. Typically, devices mode-switch from DDDR to DDIR (or VDIR) in order not to trace the atrial fibrillation at the upper rate-limit of the device. In addition, these devices have the ability to store intracardiac electrograms from triggered events such as ventricular tachycardia.

Pacemaker Implantation

The pacemaker implantation procedure is associated with several potential complications. First, venous access complications may result in a pneumothorax (collapse of the lung). This complication is seen only in

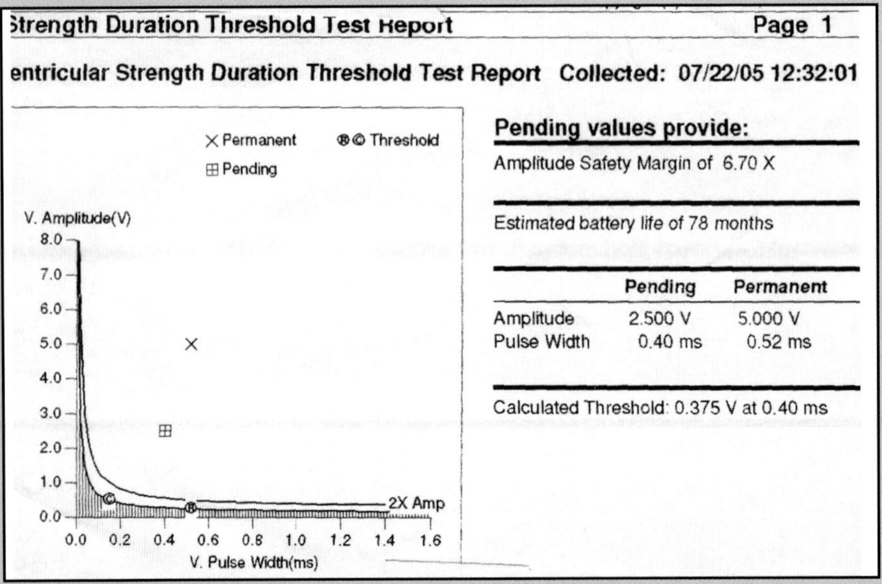

Figure 25.5: Shows a strength-duration curve generated via threshold testing of a pacemaker.

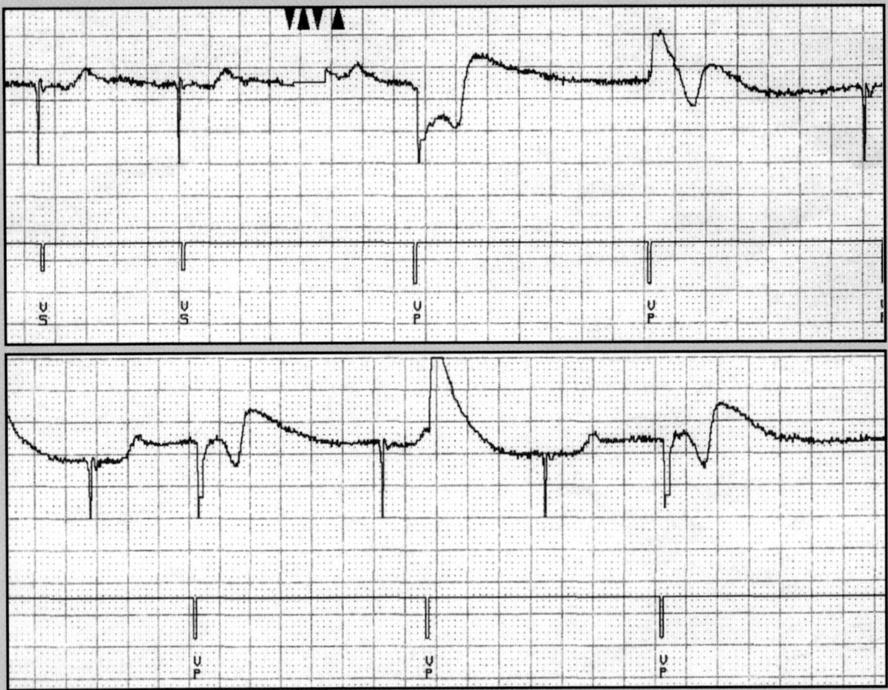

Figure 25.6: Shows sensitivity testing of the right ventricular lead. Note the inappropriate pacemaker spike is indicative of "undersensing."

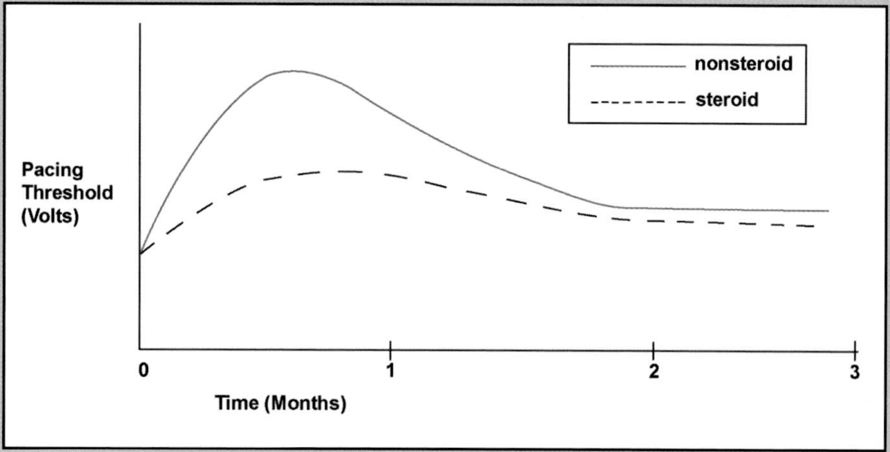

Figure 25.7: Pacing threshold increases after implantation. Steroid-eluting leads help to blunt the acute rise in threshold following implantation and decrease chronic thresholds.

percutaneous subclavian access (sticks), and is not seen with a cephalic vein cut-down approach (in which the actual vessel is exposed and a nick is made in the vessel for lead entry). Pneumothorax requires treatment if more than one-third of the lung has collapsed or if the patient is symptomatic with a drop in oxygen saturation or is complaining of chest discomfort. In that case, the patient may have vascular trauma or perforation resulting in a hemothorax (accumulation of blood in the chest).

Second, the patient may develop a pacemaker pocket hematoma (collection of blood in the pocket). A hematoma requires intervention only if it is unstable (in other words, if it continues to expand) or is extremely large (*e.g.*, the size of a tennis ball). A third possible complication is myocardial perforation (cardiac tamponade). Fourth, the patient may develop an infection and/or a malfunction from the implant. An infected pacemaker (often caused by *Staphylococcus* or *Streptococcus*) will often require explantation and six weeks of antibiotics before the device can be placed on the opposite side. Temporary pacing during this period of time may occasionally be necessary. Malfunctions from pacemakers (dislodgements, isolated component failures, loose-set screws) often require surgical revision.

The implantation of a pacemaker should be performed in a terminally-cleaned room. The cephalic vein cut-down approach is preferred over the subclavian venous approach due to the former's very low incidence of pneumothorax and subclavian crush syndrome (in which trauma occurs due to pressure between the first rib and the clavicle). Most implants are prepectoral. Subpectoral implants are occasionally preferred for cosmetic reasons or to avoid pocket erosion. Pacemaker follow-up should be performed in a facility with skilled personnel with adequate training and proper equipment.

Table 25.2: The NASPE/BPEG Generic (NBG) Pacemaker Code

Position	I	II	III	IV	V
Category	Chamber(s) paced	Chamber(s) sensed	Response to sensing	Programmability, rate modulation	Anti-tachyarrhythmia function(s)
	0 = none A = atrium V = ventricle D = dual (A+V)	0 = none A = atrium V = ventricle D = dual (A+V)	0 = none T = triggered I = inhibited D = dual (T+I)	0 = none P = simple programmable M = multi-programmable C = communicating R = rate modulation	0 = none P = pacing (anti-tachyarrhythmia) S = shock D = dual (P+S)
Manufacturer's designation only	S = single (A or V)	S = single (A or V)			

Table 25.3: Recall Classifications

Class I: Reasonable probability that the use of "product will cause serious adverse health consequences or death."

Class II: Use of a "product may cause temporary or medically reversible adverse health consequences or where the probability of serious adverse health consequences is remote."

Class III: Use of "product is not likely to cause adverse health consequences."

Recalls

Recently, a number of devices (pacemakers as well as implantable cardioverter-defibrillators) have received a recall classification via the United States Food and Drug Administration (FDA). It is important to note that all devices are machines with a small risk of an isolated component malfunction (1 in 9,000 devices). When sequential problems are linked among a series of devices (at a rate greater than the risk of an isolated component malfunction), a specific problem may be identified. The manufacturer, working together with the FDA, has an obligation to notify physicians and their patients so that corrective actions can occur. Table 25.3 shows the three classes of recalls as mandated by the FDA. Not all recalls require device replacement. Careful consideration of a given patient's medical requirements, together with the specific device problem and manufacturer's recommendations, must be considered in order to determine the best mode of management.

Chapter 26

Implantable Cardioverter-Defibrillator

One of the greatest inventions of the modern era has been the implantable cardioverter-defibrillator (ICD). Envisioned by Michel Mirowski and Morton Mower in the late 1970s and early 1980s, this device was initially very large, requiring an open-chest implant and a 10-day hospital stay. The device can now be used to treat life-threatening ventricular tachycardias with a simple transvenous approach.

A single-chamber ICD consists of a pulse generator and lead. Figure 26.1 shows a variety of available ICDs and leads. Dual-chamber and three-chamber (biventricular) devices also exist. In the most simplistic terms, the ICD determines the heart rate of the patient. When the heart rate exceeds a predetermined number (165 beats per minute, for example), the device is programmed to diagnose a ventricular tachycardia and give a correcting impulse (up to 35 joules). ICDs have additional features that can determine the nature of the tachycardia and try to differentiate it from other types of supraventricular tachycardias. These features can be useful in trying to discriminate atrial fibrillation with a rapid ventricular response from ventricular tachycardia. In addition, these devices can be programmed to deliver rapid paced beats in order to terminate ventricular tachycardia and minimize the number of delivered shocks. Finally, bradycardia pacing is also available.

The device was initially indicated for patients who had ventricular tachycardia that was refractory to drug therapy. A myriad of studies, however, have demonstrated the superiority of primary device implantation over antiarrhythmic drug therapy. The AVID (Antiarrhythmic Versus Implantable Defibrillator) trial was the principal study that showed the benefit of the ICD compared with antiarrhythmic drugs. This trial demonstrated that amiodarone and sotalol were inferior to the implantable defibrillator, with respect to mortality in patients who had hemodynamically significant ventricular tachycardia and fibrillation. A number of prophylactic ICD trials have subsequently demonstrated that patients who have significant left ventricular dysfunction (ischemic and nonischemic) may benefit from an implantable defibrillator. Table 26.1 shows the most recent indications for an ICD. Please note that these indications have expanded to permit additional physician judgment, which might warrant an implantable defibrillator. In particular, indications have eased up with respect to implantation indications in inherited conditions such as hypertrophic cardiomyopathy, arrhythmogenic right ventricular cardiomyopathy/dysplasia, cardiac sarcoid, and Chagas disease.

The approach for implanting an ICD is almost entirely similar to that for a permanent pacemaker. The primary approach should be through the cephalic vein in order to eliminate the possibility of a pneumothorax. In addition, this approach (as compared to subclavian venous access) minimizes the risk of subclavian crush syndrome. Placing the lead into the ventricular apex can achieve excellent pacing and sensing, as long as the area in which it is placed does not have a significant scar.

In general, if a patient needs only a defibrillator, implanting a single-chamber defibrillator as a backup is preferred to a dual-chamber device. The Dual Chamber and VVI Implantable Defibrillator (DAVID) Trial demonstrated that dual-chamber pacing (with greater than 40 percent right ventricular pacing) may result in more hemodynamic deterioration, and therefore may be less advantageous to a patient. This is most likely due to pacing of the right ventricle with attendant abnormal depolarization and repolarization properties and worsening cardiac function. When placing an implantable defibrillator in a patient with a history of aborted sudden death from ventricular tachycardia and/or ventricular fibrillation, it should be programmed to minimize ventricular pacing (either by programming down the rate, increasing the atrioventricular delay, and/or employing a specific algorithm to promote intrinsic conduction).

ICD Functions

The following descriptions provide a brief overview of some essential principles related to the function of an ICD.

Detection

The ICD detects electrical signals in the chambers in which leads are implanted. For a single-chamber ICD, right ventricular electrograms are used to determine the rate. In the most simplistic form, *rate detection* is utilized in order to identify a significant tachycardia. In addition, there are a number of detection enhancements used together with rate detection that can help refine detection (table 26.2). *Morphology criteria* can be utilized by the device to compare the configuration of the intracardiac ventricular electrogram during a tachycardia to a sinus rhythm ventricular electrogram. If the electrogram differs significantly, it is more likely to be ventricular

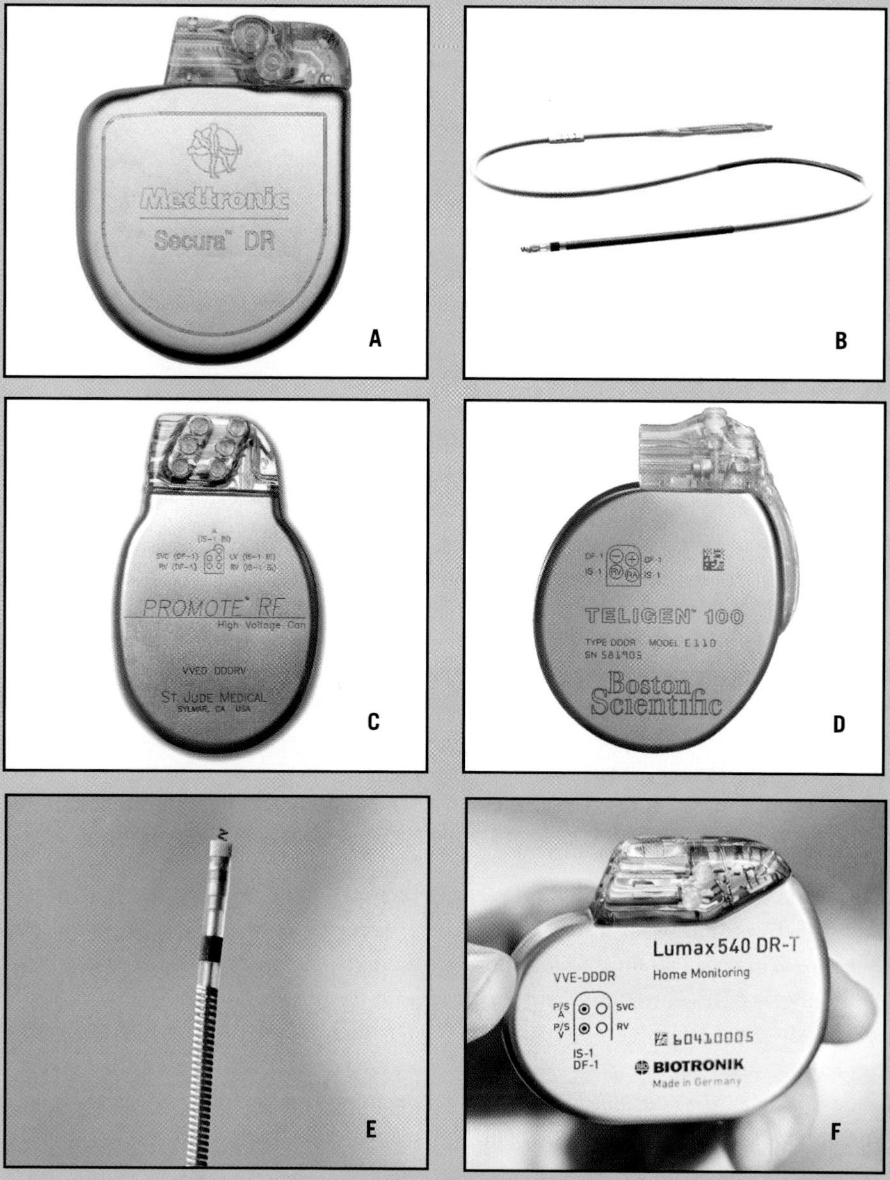

Figure 26.1: (A) Secura™ DR Dual Chamber ICD (Reproduced with permission of Medtronic, Inc., Minneapolis, MN). (B) Sprint Quattro Secure® ICD lead, model number 6947 (Reproduced with permission of Medtronic, Inc., Minneapolis, MN). (C) Promote® RF CRT-D biventricular device (courtesy St. Jude Medical, Sylmar, CA). (D) TELIGEN™ 100 Dual Chamber ICD (courtesy of Boston Scientific, Natick, MA). (E) Linox SD isodiametric, steroid-eluting, active fixation ICD lead (courtesy of BIOTRONIK Inc., Lake Oswego, OR). (F) Lumax 540 DR-T ICD (courtesy of BIOTRONIK Inc., Lake Oswego, OR).

Table 26.1: Indications for Implantable Cardioverter-Defibrillators

1.	Sustained ventricular tachycardia/ventricular fibrillation not in the setting of an acute myocardial infarction (MI) and not due to a reversible cause.
2.	Syncope with LV dysfunction and nonischemic cardiomyopathy; or with inducible sustained ventricular tachycardia at electrophysiology study; or negative electrophysiology study and structural heart disease.
3.	New York Heart Association at least class I heart failure (and preferably II to III) and ejection fraction (EF) of less than 36 percent.
4.	At least 40 days after an MI with an EF of less than or equal to 30 percent.
5.	Nonsustained ventricular tachycardia in a patient having had a prior MI and EF of less than 40 percent with inducible sustained ventricular tachycardia/ventricular fibrillation at electrophysiology study.
6.	Hypertrophic cardiomyopathy or arrhythmogenic right ventricular cardiomyopathy/dysplasia with one or more major risk factors for sudden death.
7.	Symptomatic long QT/Brugada syndrome patients and other familial cardiomyopathies associated with sudden death.
8.	Cardiac sarcoid, Chagas disease, giant cell myocarditis, or LV noncompaction.
9.	Bridge to heart transplant.

Table 26.2: Detection Enhancements

• Morphology Discrimination	• Stability
• Sudden Onset Criteria	• Atrioventricular Timing Sequences

tachycardia or fibrillation than supraventricular tachycardia. In addition, a *sudden onset criteria* makes a reentrant mechanism commonly seen in ventricular tachycardia more likely. This criteria is useful at distinguishing sinus tachycardia from ventricular tachycardia. *Stability criteria,* in which there is little variation in the R-to-R interval, can also be useful in distinguishing ventricular tachycardia from atrial fibrillation. In a dual-chamber ICD, *atrioventricular timing sequences* can be utilized to help enhance detection. Each manufacturer has subtle differences in these timing algorithms, which help to refine arrhythmia discrimination.

Therapy

Devices can administer a variety of therapies to treat ventricular tachycardia (and in more recent devices, supraventricular tachycardia). These include *antitachycardia pacing (ATP),* also called overdrive pacing. This is pacing faster than the tachycardia. *Burst pacing* occurs with rapid pacing, with a fixed coupling interval between each burst stimuli. *Ramp pacing* permits a decrease between each stimuli and is a more aggressive form of ATP. This latter modality is more likely to result in an acceleration of the ventricular tachycardia into ventricular fibrillation. The specific number of stimuli, burst cycle length,

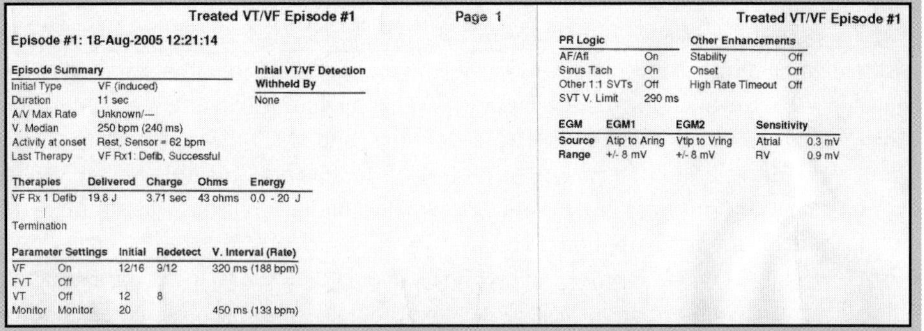

Treated VT/VF Episode #1

Page 1

Episode #1: 18-Aug-2005 12:21:14

Episode Summary	
Initial Type	VF (induced)
Duration	11 sec
A/V Max Rate	Unknown/—
V. Median	250 bpm (240 ms)
Activity at onset	Rest, Sensor = 62 bpm
Last Therapy	VF Rx1: Defib, Successful

Initial VT/VF Detection Withheld By
None

Therapies	Delivered	Charge	Ohms	Energy
VF Rx 1 Defib	19.8 J	3.71 sec	43 ohms	0.0 - 20 J

Termination

Parameter Settings		Initial	Redetect	V. Interval (Rate)
VF	On	12/16	9/12	320 ms (188 bpm)
FVT	Off			
VT	Off	12	8	
Monitor	Monitor	20		450 ms (133 bpm)

Treated VT/VF Episode #1

PR Logic		Other Enhancements	
AF/Afl	On	Stability	Off
Sinus Tach	On	Onset	Off
Other 1:1 SVTs	Off	High Rate Timeout	Off
SVT V. Limit	290 ms		

EGM	EGM1	EGM2	Sensitivity	
Source	Atip to Aring	Vtip to Vring	Atrial	0.3 mV
Range	+/- 8 mV	+/- 8 mV	RV	0.9 mV

Figure 26.2: Shows the ventricular fibrillation induced and detected/treated via the ICD. The detection zones (VT, fast VT [FVT], and VF) are indicated at the bottom of the interrogation. In addition, detection enhancements (PR logic, etc.) are also listed.

coupling interval of the first stimuli to that of the tachycardia, decrement (decrease) between the stimuli cycle lengths, and number of ATP attempts can all be programmed in the device. Low-energy cardioversion as well as ATP therapy may be useful at terminating stable ventricular tachycardia, and is often helpful for treating slower rate ventricular tachycardia. In some instances, ICDs can deliver ATP therapy during capacitor charging in order to attempt to terminate a ventricular tachycardia prior to shock delivery.

Devices have the ability to detect and treat arrhythmias differently, based on the heart rate detected (zone detection). Figure 26.2 shows an interrogation from an ICD showing the induced and detected/treated ventricular fibrillation. The detection zones (VT, fast VT [FVT], and VF) are indicated at the bottom of the interrogation. In a single-zone device, DC energy is delivered after detection of a rapid rate (greater than 188 beats/minute, for example). In a two-zone device, a second zone can provide monitoring or a less aggressive therapy such as low-energy cardioversion or ATP in order to terminate a tachycardia. The use of progressively more aggressive therapies within a zone is termed *tiered therapy*. For example, burst pacing may be utilized first, followed by low-energy cardioversion and then a high-energy shock. A *monitoring zone* is useful at detecting subclinical or slower tachycardias. A three-zone device can permit differential and progressively more aggressive therapies as the heart rates increase. For example, a heart rate from 130 to 160 beats/minute may be programmed as a monitor-only zone, 161 to 195 beats/minute might provide for ATP and then low-energy cardioversion followed by high-energy cardioversion, whereas heart rates greater than 195 beats/minute might provide only for high-energy defibrillation.

Some devices deliver a *committed shock* at times; this means that if a tachycardia is detected and may terminate spontaneously, a shock is still administered by the ICD. Most devices will have a noncommitted shock on the first go around (*i.e.*, be able to divert the shock prior to discharge).

Device-Based Testing

ICDs permit for device-based testing (also called *noninvasive programmed stimulation*, or *NIPS*) in which ventricular tachycardia and/or fibrillation is induced through the device via burst pacing, programmed electrical stimulation, or a shock on the T wave. Figure 26.3 demonstrates a shock on the T wave (arrow), which induced ventricular fibrillation. A 1 joule shock, for example, if delivered in the vulnerable period (approximately 290 msec from the R wave), typically will induce ventricular fibrillation. If unsuccessful, the coupling interval of the delivered shock must be adjusted (lengthened or shortened) in order to induce fibrillation. Testing is performed to assure an adequate defibrillation safety margin (at least 10 joules from the maximum output of the device) and assure the successful termination of the tachycardia. Most devices have maximal outputs of between 27 to 35 joules delivered. With the advent of biphasic shocks, most defibrillators can terminate ventricular fibrillation with an energy output of 8 to 10 joules. Traditionally, a number of shocks were necessary to establish an adequate *defibrillation threshold* (*DFT*); however, with the reliability and success of modern systems, the necessity of extensive testing is not entirely clear. Repeat testing after a *de novo* implant can help identify problems such as a loose setscrew or an unacceptable rise in DFT. In addition, with further programmed stimulation and testing, the ICD programming configuration can be optimized. DFT testing is often recommended following the administration of medications such as amiodarone and mexiletine that have the potential to increase the patient's DFT.

Stored Electrograms

The device has the ability to store the intracardiac electrograms from triggered events including diverted and delivered shocks and ATP therapies. These stored electrograms are useful in identifying whether the tachycardia was supraventricular or ventricular in nature. It is often easy to distinguish the two by comparing the morphology of the ventricular electrogram in sinus rhythm to that of the tachycardia. If it is the same, it is most likely to be a supraventricular tachycardia. In addition, the irregularity of the tachycardia and characteristic atrial arrhythmia might help to identify atrial fibrillation. Figure 26.4 shows atrial and ventricular intracardiac electrograms during ventricular fibrillation (with atrioventricular dissociation). Marker channels indicate appropriate sensing during VF as well as DC energy delivery with termination to a paced rhythm. Figure 26.5 shows a rapid tachycardia in a single-chamber ICD. Following the shock and tachycardia termination (after two premature complexes), the top intracardiac electrograms are identical to that during the tachycardia consistent with a supraventricular etiology.

Life of the Device

All devices have internal clocks and timing sequences for reforming the capacitors, which are necessary to store and deliver DC energy. In addition, these devices track the energy and life cycle of the ICD's battery. Typically, at implant, the device is at beginning of life (BOL); as time progresses, the device reaches middle of life (MOL). Eventually it approaches end of life (EOL) and/or elective replacement indicator (ERI).

A dual-chamber defibrillator may be useful in patients who need the pacing

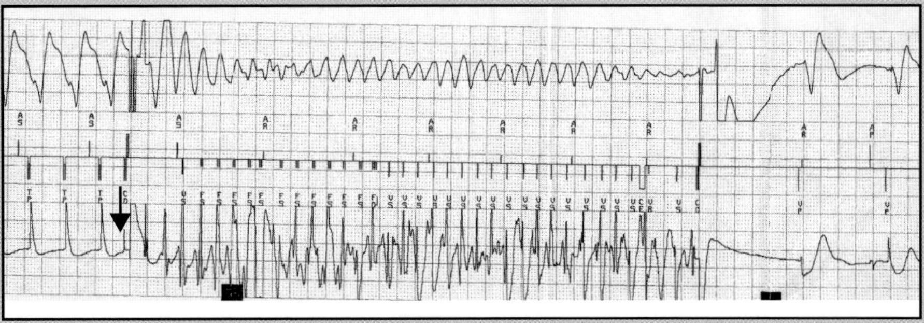

Figure 26.3: Demonstrates a shock on the T wave (arrow) which induced ventricular fibrillation.

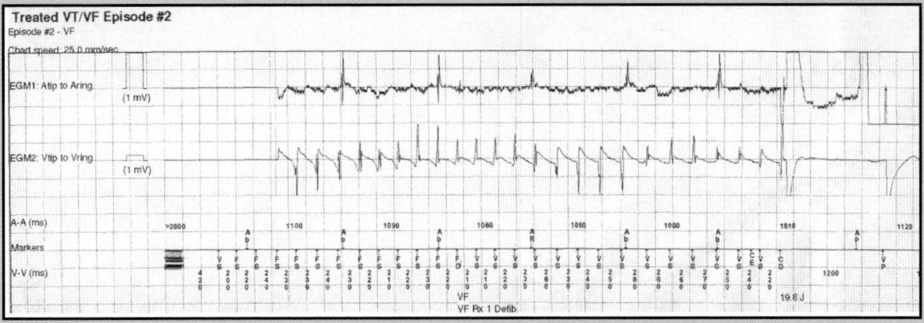

Figure 26.4: Shows atrial and ventricular intracardiac electrograms during ventricular fibrillation (with atrioventricular dissociation). Marker channels indicate appropriate sensing during VF as well as DC energy delivery (19.8J) with termination to a paced rhythm.

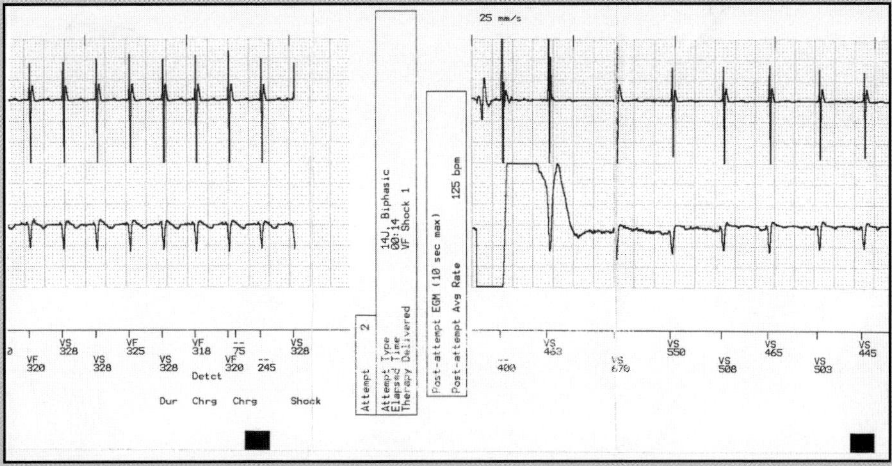

Figure 26.5: Shows a rapid tachycardia in a single-chamber ICD. Following the shock and tachycardia termination (after two premature complexes), the top intracardiac electrograms are identical to those during the tachycardia consistent with a supraventricular etiology.

requirement and hopefully have reasonable AV conduction. Newer implantable cardioverter-defibrillators have algorithms that can maximize intrinsic conduction rather than pace the ventricle. One such algorithm uses atrial pacing, and if two out of four atrial complexes fail to conduct, dual-chamber pacing then occurs. Occasionally, patients who have a continued ventricular pacing requirement may suffer cardiac decompensation as well as congestive heart failure exacerbation. Some patients have received an upgrade to a biventricular device, in which cardiac resynchronization therapy is achieved by simultaneously and/or synchronously pacing the left ventricle and right ventricle. This mode of pacing has helped ameliorate the symptoms of worsening heart failure.

In patients who meet the criteria for cardiac resynchronization therapy (QRS duration greater than 120 msec [however, current Medicare guidelines require a QRS duration greater than 130 msec], a class III or IV congestive heart failure on optimal drug therapy, and an ejection fraction less than 36 percent), a biventricular ICD should be implanted (see Chapter 26, table 26.1).

Chapter 27

Cardiac Resynchronization Therapy

Congestive heart failure affects nearly 5 million people in the United States, with an annual incidence of approximately 500,000 new cases a year. Despite lifestyle modifications (diet plus sodium restriction) and optimal medical therapy (angiotensin-converting enzyme inhibitors, beta blockers, diuretics, digitalis, aldosterone inhibitors), a significant percentage of these patients find their way back into the hospital for more intensive therapy. It is for this population in which optimal medical therapy has reached its limits that cardiac resynchronization therapy (CRT) has been shown to be beneficial.

CRT, or biventricular pacing, is a form of device-based therapy for congestive heart failure caused by dilated cardiomyopathy (ischemic or nonischemic). Using a specialized pacemaker, CRT recoordinates the action of the right and left ventricles in these patients in an attempt to improve heart function.

In approximately 15 to 30 percent of all patients with heart failure, an abnormality in the heart's electrical conduction system known as bundle-branch block causes the two ventricles to beat in an asynchronous manner. Rather than the two ventricles beating nearly simultaneously, they beat slightly out of phase due to regional delays in the electrical activation of the chamber. This asynchrony greatly reduces the efficiency of the ventricles in patients with heart failure by reducing systolic function and increasing systolic volume. Cardiac

Bi-Ventricular Pacing to Improve Cardiac Hemodynamics

J.J. Lattuca, T.J. Cohen, and M.M. Mower
Sinai Hospital, Baltimore, Maryland, and CPI, St. Paul, Minnesota

Incoordinate contraction pattern might be partly responsible for hemodynamic impairment in heart failure. To determine if narrowing the QRS width by simultaneously pacing several sites on the heart would improve hemodynamics, pacing was done on three dogs comparing pacing right and left ventricles alone with both sides simultaneously using a Seamed external pacer device. Artificial AV interval was set shorter than intrinsic, and animals were paced at 150, 175, and 190 BPM. Three replicate measurements were made at each setting. Results (simple means of all measurements) were as follows:

	Cardiac Output (L/min)	Aortic Pressure (mmHg)	Rt. Atr. Pressure (mmHg)	QRS Width (sec)
RV pacing	2.44	60	13.3	.100875
LV pacing	2.61	60	12.7	.10943
Both pacing	2.83	73.3	7.7	.0761

While increased cardiac output and aortic pressure with narrowed QRS complex indicate improved systolic function, the marked right atrial pressure reduction in even more impressive and suggests a favorable effect on diastolic relaxation as well. The clear implication is that some patients in congestive heart failure with conduction defects could be dramatically helped by reducing elevated right atrial pressure through such means.

Figure 27.1: The first abstract on biventricular pacing, published in The American Federation of Clinical Records in 1988.

resynchronization therapy recoordinates the beating of the two ventricles concurrently, whereas typical pacemakers pace only the right ventricle.

In 1987, Jack Lattuca, Todd Cohen, and Morton Mower performed a series of animal studies demonstrating that simultaneous pacing of the right and left ventricles resulted in lower right heart pressures and greater cardiac output than pacing each chamber individually. They coined the term "biventricular pacing" in a 1988 abstract (figure 27.1). Subsequent human trials in the postoperative open-heart population confirmed these findings using epicardial pacing wires. A long-term practical transvenous solution was eventually developed using the coronary sinus vein as a conduit to the left ventricle.

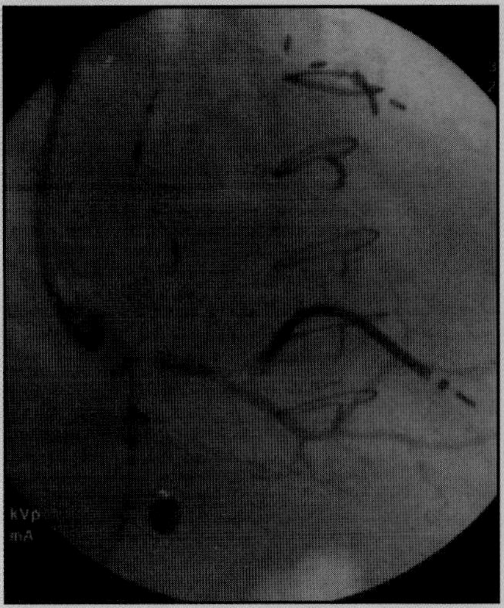

Figure 27.2: A subselected coronary sinus venograph, which is helpful in identifying a lateral left ventricular branch.

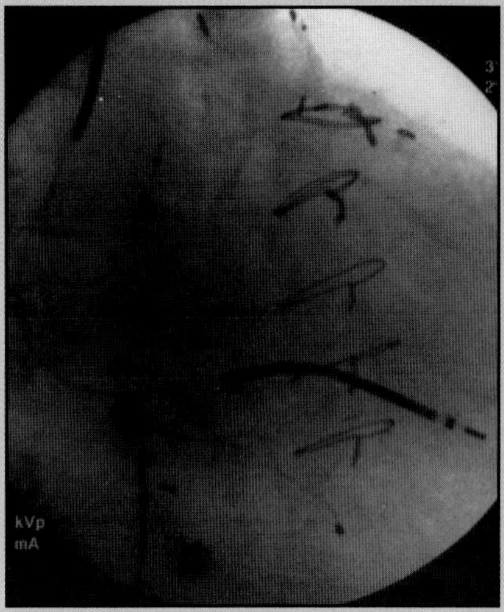

Figure 27.3: Subsequent lead placement in the patient from figure 27.2.

The MIRACLE/MIRACLE ICD trial demonstrated the clinical utility of transvenous CRT, and led to the approval of these systems by the United States Food and Drug Administration. Figure 27.2 shows a venogram of the coronary sinus vein. Figure 27.3 shows the placement of a specially designed left ventricular pacing lead in a lateral branch of the coronary sinus vein. Figure 27.4 shows another example of a coronary sinus venogram. Figure 27.5 shows the left ventricular pacing lead placed in the central coronary sinus branch.

In the MIRACLE studies, CRT in the form of biventricular pacing improved symptoms and the quality of life, increased exercise tolerance, and partially reversed maladaptive remodeling by reducing the size of the dilated left ventricle and improved the energy usage of the heart. These beneficial effects support the hypothesis that long-term CRT decreases the risk of death and complications related to heart failure in patients with intraventricular conduction delays. In addition, Abraham and colleagues demonstrated in a small study a 77 percent reduction in days hospitalized after receiving CRT (published in the *New England Journal of Medicine* 2002;346:1845–1853).

Subsequently, the COMPANION trial, completed in fall 2003, showed that CRT with a backup defibrillator can reduce both hospitalizations and all-cause mortality. In particular, there was a nearly 40 percent reduction in mortality with CRT-ICDs, as compared with optimal drug therapy (statistically significant).

The decision as to whether a CRT defibrillator is appropriate for a particular patient is best determined on an individual basis by the patient and his or her physician. The COMPANION study, however, makes a compelling argument that every appropriate Class III or IV New York Heart Association CHF patient with a projected survival greater than one year and meeting

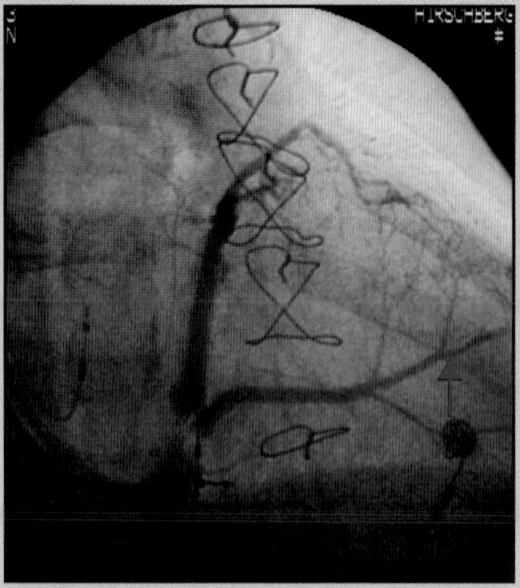

Figure 27.4: Shows a coronary sinus venograph with three large branches seen (image obtained in right anterior oblique projection). Arrow indicates target branch for left ventricular lead (figure 27.5).

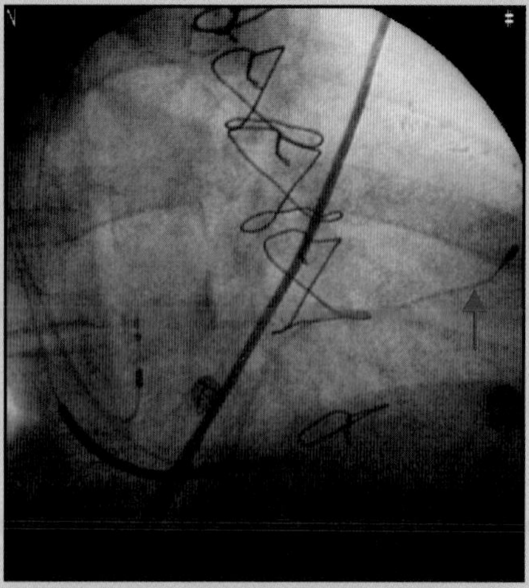

Figure 27.5: Shows left ventricular lead placement (indicated by arrow) in the central vessel observed in figure 27.4 in order to effectively pace the left ventricle (right anterior oblique projection).

the standard biventricular device criteria should receive an ICD as backup (and not just a biventricular pacemaker). The latter has been relegated to patients in which only quality, not quantity, of life is desirable.

The most recent indications for implantation of a CRT defibrillator have been broadened. Table 27.1 lists the most recent indications for a biventricular device. The general indications include patients who have moderate to severe heart failure (New York Heart Association Class III or IV) despite optimal medical therapy, left ventricular dysfunction (with a left ventricular ejection fraction of less than 36 percent), and a QRS duration of more than 120 msec.

Table 27.1: Indications for a Biventricular Device

1a. New York Heart Association Class III or IV congestive heart failure on optimal medical treatment.

And

1b. Ejection fraction of less than 36 percent.

And

1c. Wide QRS complex greater than 120 milliseconds or frequent ventricular pacing.

Or

2. Ejection fraction of less than 36 percent plus New York Heart Association Class I or II patients on optimal medical treatment who are receiving a pacemaker and/or ICD and frequent pacing is anticipated.

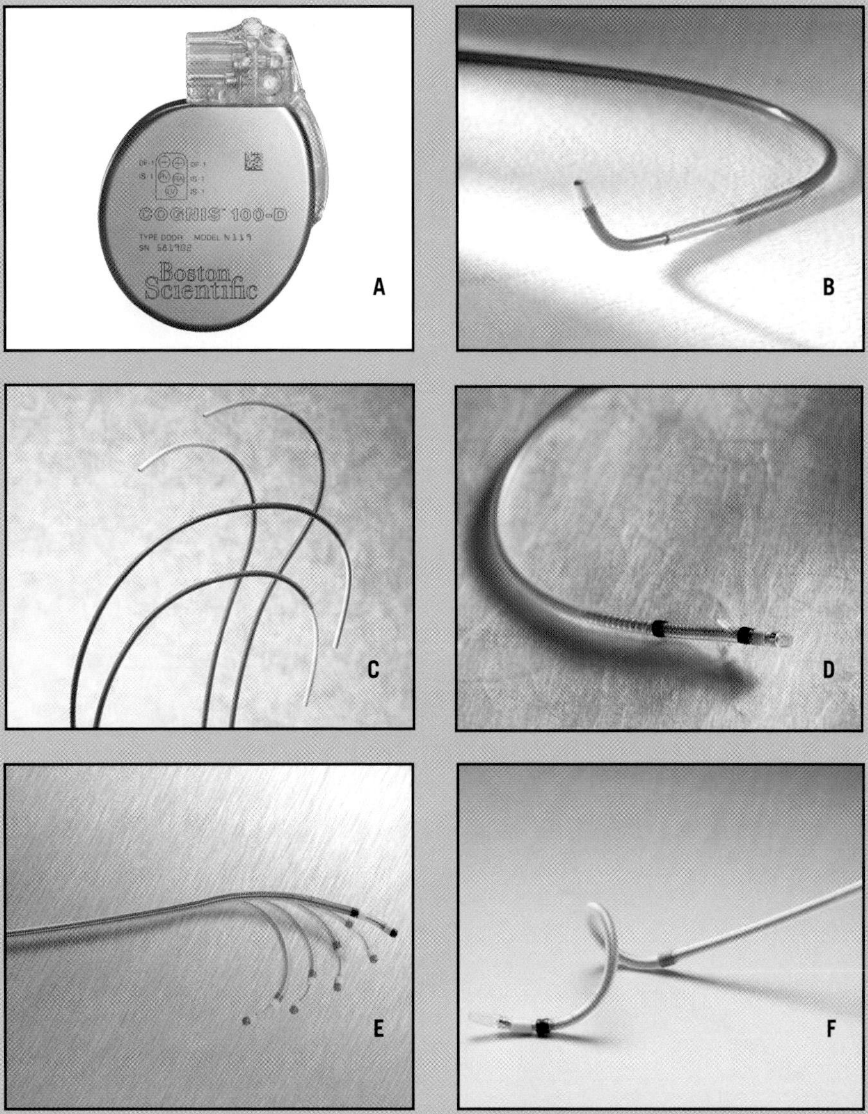

Figure 27.6: (A) COGNIS™ 100-D dual-chamber biventricular ICD (courtesy of Boston Scientific, Natick, MA). (B) RAPIDO® Dual Guide Catheter System (courtesy of Boston Scientific, Natick, MA). (C) RAPIDO ADVANCE® guide catheter (courtesy of Boston Scientific, Natick, MA). (D) EASYTRAK® 2 bipolar LV lead (courtesy of Boston Scientific, Natick, MA) (E) ACUITY™ STEERABLE LV lead (courtesy of Boston Scientific, Natick, MA). (F) ACUITY™ SPIRAL LV lead (courtesy of Boston Scientific, Natick, MA).

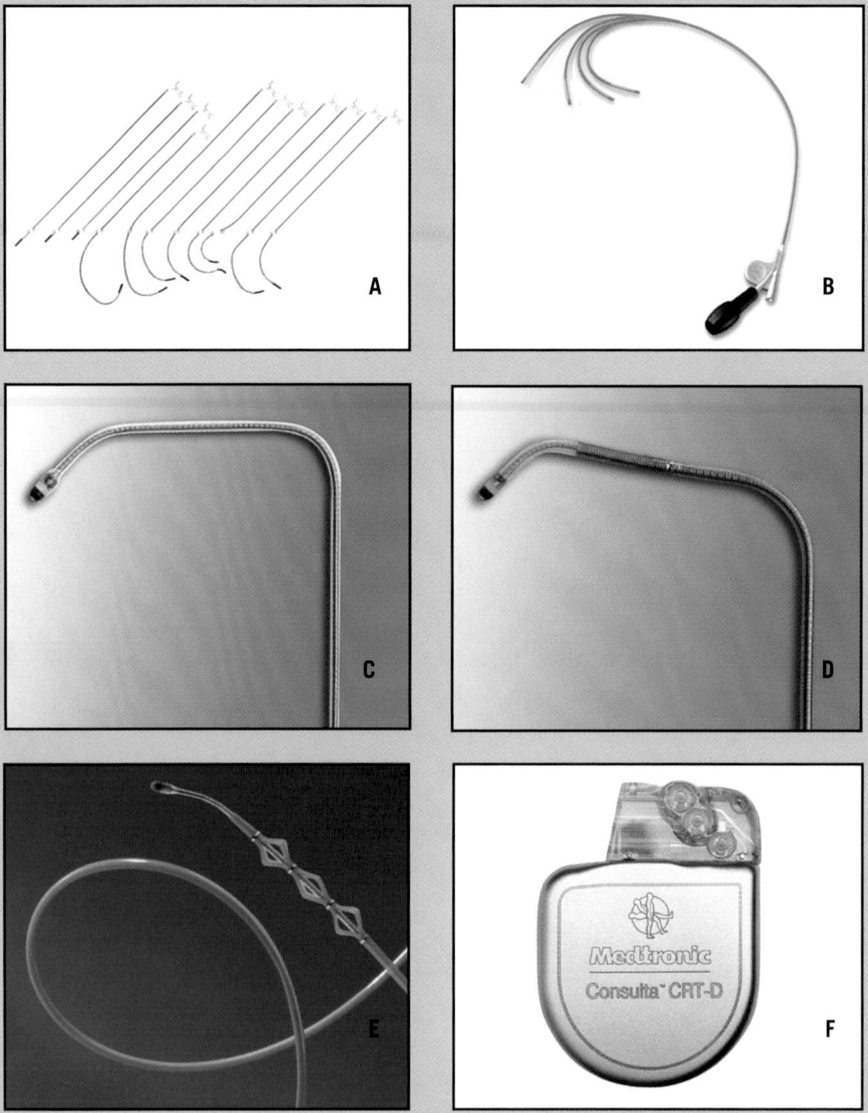

Figure 27.7: More examples of biventricular devices and left ventricular leads currently available. (A) Attain Command™ Coronary Sinus Cannulation Catheters (Reproduced with permission of Medtronic, Inc., Minneapolis, MN). (B) Attain Deflectable steerable introducer sheath, model number 6226DEF (Reproduced with permission of Medtronic, Inc., Minneapolis, MN). (C) Attain OTW left ventricular unipolar pacing lead, model number 4193 (Reproduced with permission of Medtronic, Inc., Minneapolis, MN). (D) Attain OTW left ventricular bipolar pacing lead, model number 4194 (Reproduced with permission of Medtronic, Inc., Minneapolis, MN). (E) Medtronic Attain StarFix® OTW (over-the-wire) model #4195 (Reproduced with permission of Medtronic, Inc., Minneapolis, MN). (F) Consulta™ CRT-D biventricular ICD (Reproduced with permission of Medtronic, Inc., Minneapolis, MN).

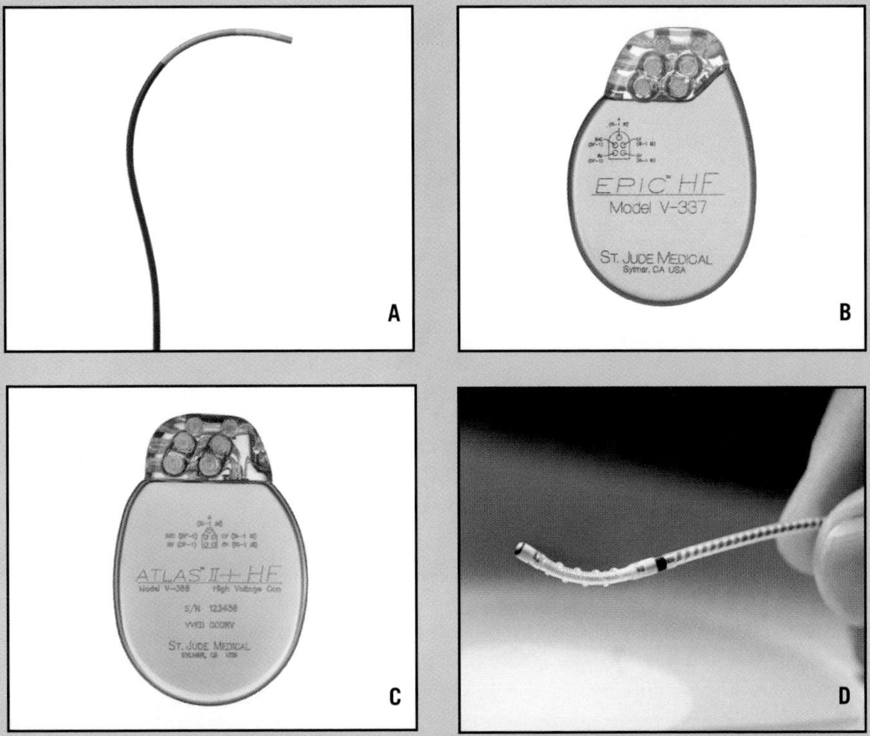

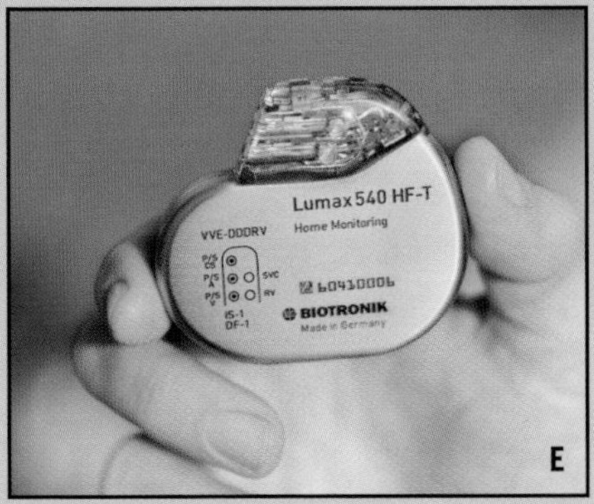

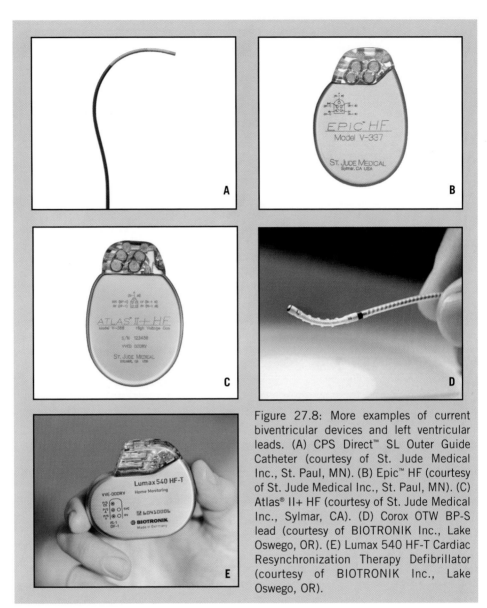

Figure 27.8: More examples of current biventricular devices and left ventricular leads. (A) CPS Direct™ SL Outer Guide Catheter (courtesy of St. Jude Medical Inc., St. Paul, MN). (B) Epic™ HF (courtesy of St. Jude Medical Inc., St. Paul, MN). (C) Atlas® II+ HF (courtesy of St. Jude Medical Inc., Sylmar, CA). (D) Corox OTW BP-S lead (courtesy of BIOTRONIK Inc., Lake Oswego, OR). (E) Lumax 540 HF-T Cardiac Resynchronization Therapy Defibrillator (courtesy of BIOTRONIK Inc., Lake Oswego, OR).

The current guidelines permit physician judgment to include lesser degrees of congestive heart failure in patients who will receive frequent right ventricular pacing.

Overall, cardiac resynchronization reduced the degree of ventricular dyssynchrony (as evidenced by a shortened duration of the QRS interval). This effect was accompanied by both an increase in the left ventricular ejection fraction and a decrease in the left ventricular end-diastolic dimension and in the magnitude of mitral regurgitation. Additionally, CRT improved quality of life, decreased hospitalization, increased exercise capacity, and decreased mortality.

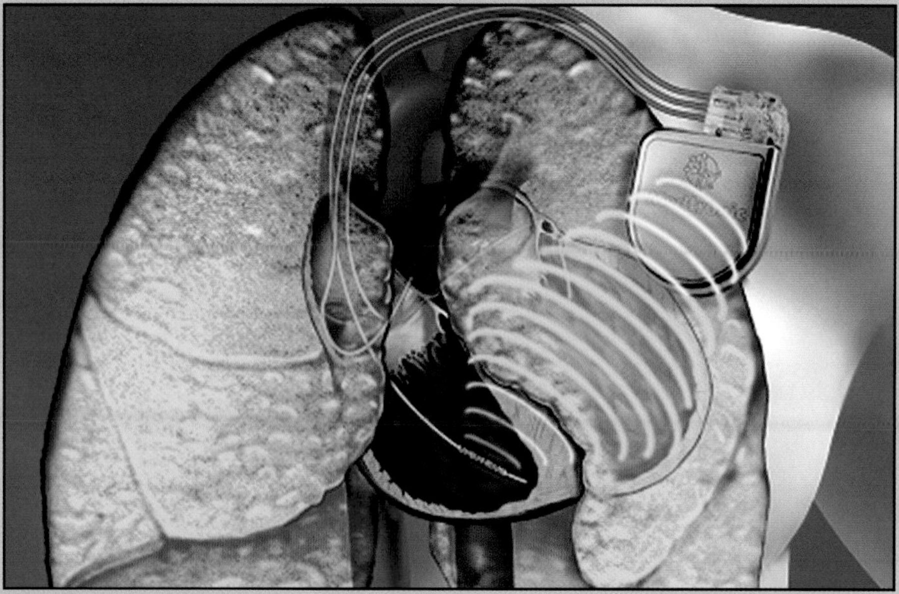

Figure 27.9: Manufacturers are beginning to add physiological signals for monitoring and treating heart failure in devices. Measurement of intrathoracic impedance (between the right ventricular lead and pulse generator) indicating the degree of fluid accumulation in the lungs (Reproduced with permission of Medtronic, Inc., Minneapolis, MN).

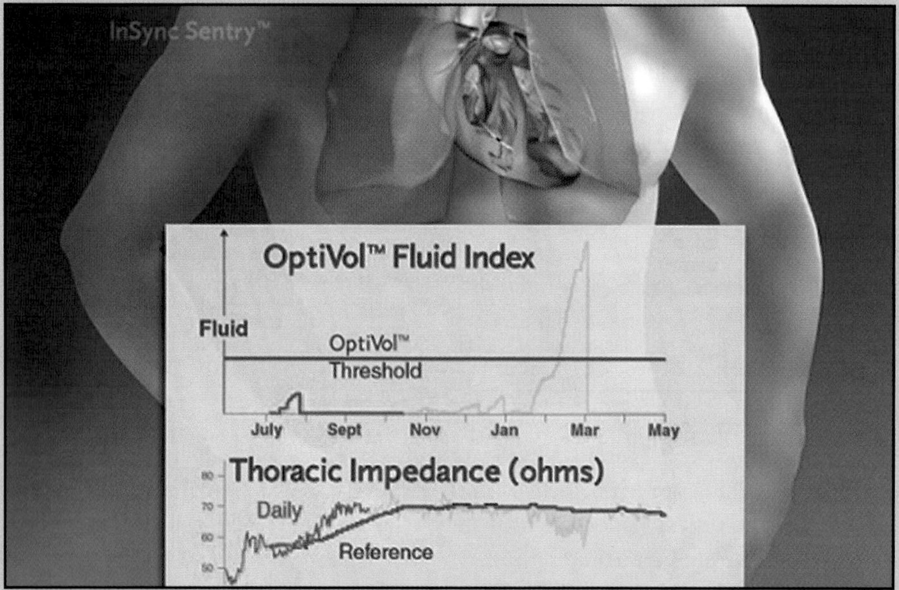

Figure 27.10: Thoracic impedance can be trended to gauge the degree of congestive heart failure and determine the need for additional therapy. This photo shows the OptiVol™ Fluid Index (Reproduced with permission of Medtronic, Inc., Minneapolis, MN).

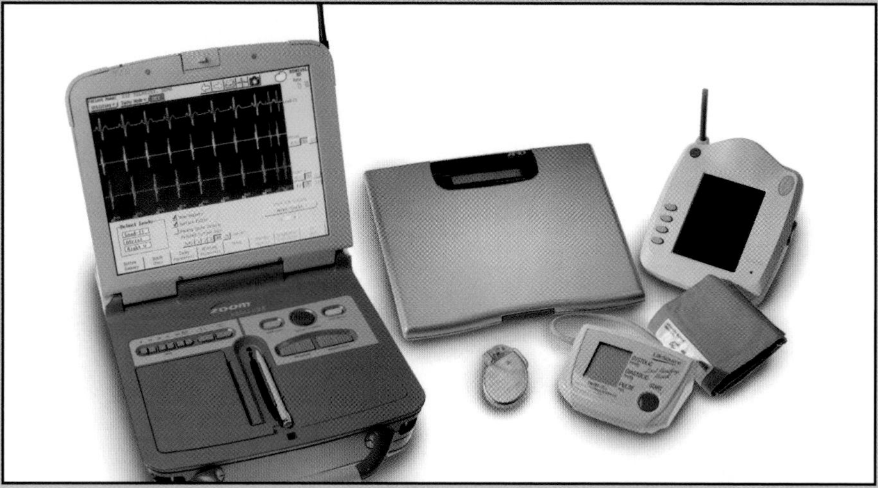

Figure 27.11: Shows the Contak Renewal® 3 RF CRT-D device, surrounded by the LATITUDE® Patient Management weight scale, LATITUDE Patient Management blood pressure monitor, LATITUDE Communicator, and Zoom LATITUDE® programmer, which integrate with an Internet-based patient management system to treat arrhythmias and congestive heart failure (courtesy of Boston Scientific, Natick, MA).

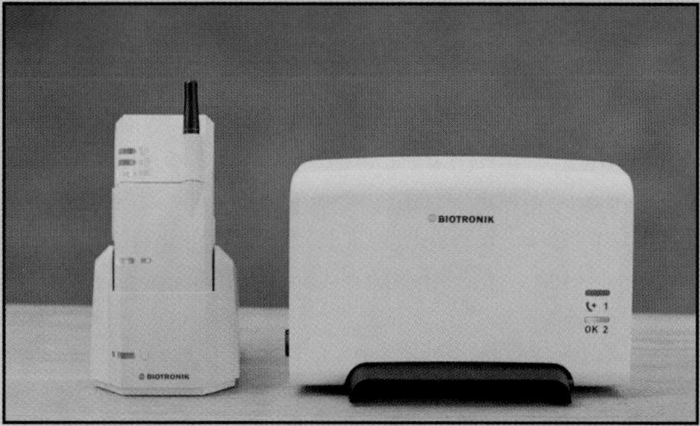

Figure 27.12: BIOTRONIK Home Monitoring® includes CardioMessenger, a GSM-based wireless communication solution with a bedside unit that uses traditional landline telephone technology (courtesy of BIOTRONIK Inc., Lake Oswego, OR).

At Winthrop University Hospital, in approximately 400 biventricular implants, approximately 98 percent were successful using a transvenous approach. Specifically designed steerable catheters and delivery sheaths may help access the coronary sinus vein (the guide vessel to a left ventricular branch). Two of our four electrophysiologists place all three leads through a single cephalic vein using diaphragm-occlusive sheaths. This approach eliminates subclavian crush syndrome and long- and short-term complication risks. In rare instances of difficult access, an epicardial left ventricular lead can be used. Inconsistent benefits have been derived in a small number of failed cases with biventricular right-sided pacing (right ventricular apex and outflow tract pacing). Figures 27.6, 27.7, and 27.8 show a variety of biventricular devices, left ventricular leads, and lead delivery systems. Manufacturers have added physiological signals such as intrathoracic impedance for monitoring and treating heart failure into devices (figure 27.9). Figure 27.10 shows monitoring fluid accumulation in a given patient. This type of monitoring can be performed in person or via remote monitoring over the Internet. Remote monitoring systems can also integrate heart rhythm analysis with changes in body weight and blood pressure—features that are useful in managing CHF (figure 27.11). Figure 27.12 shows a wireless home monitoring system.

In the long term, with skilled implanters, approximately two-thirds of patients can expect a single New York Heart Association classification improvement in clinical symptoms, a six-point increase in ejection fraction, and a shortened QRS complex. Factors that may limit the clinical outcome include the presence of chronic obstructive pulmonary disease (these patients usually remain short of breath from lung disease post implant), and less than ideal initial left ventricular vein lead locations (the best is a lateral location). Phrenic nerve pacing should be avoided during implantation, and if present, post procedure may require reprogramming and/or lead repositioning. In addition, biventricular pacing may be useful after AV junction ablation, especially in patients with worsening left ventricular function and mitral regurgitation. It has the potential to improve severe mitral regurgitation (on top of medical therapy). Newer devices permit programming of not only the paced rate and AV delay, but also allow for varying the timing of RV-LV pacing (V-to-V timing sequence). It should be emphasized that patients with severe comorbid conditions may not be candidates. In addition, for reasons that are not entirely clear, approximately 25 to 30 percent of seemingly appropriate candidates for cardiac resynchronization therapy fail to respond to this treatment. Investigation into two-dimensional echocardiographic parameters that would be useful in selecting patients who may be candidates for biventricular ICD failed to identify any preferred parameters for this purpose.

Chapter 28

Lead Extraction

Implanted pacemaker and defibrillator leads may occasionally require explantation in order to remove infected hardware or make room for newer leads. The techniques used in accomplishing this task include tools for stabilizing the inner lumen of the lead, cutting sheaths that might also include the use of laser and/or radiofrequency energy, and additional monitoring and the availability of a cardiovascular surgical team (in case immediate thoractomy for a vascular/cardiac repair is required).

Dr. Michael Glikson and colleagues most recently reported on this in the January 2009 issue of the Heart*Rhythm* Journal, the official journal of the Heart Rhythm Society. In their article, the investigators analyzed data from the Mayo Clinic ICD database between August 1993 and May 2002, and found 78 ICD patients with 101 abandoned leads. However, there were no signs of lead-related deep venous thrombosis or sensing malfunction. They concluded that abandoning leads is not harmful to patients, and a lead extraction to prevent inappropriate sensing or deep venous thrombosis may be unnecessary.

It is important to note that lead extraction may result in significant mortality (related to operator experience), vascular and/or cardiac perforation/damage, and retained and/or fragmented/dislodged foreign bodies related to the extraction technique. Lead extraction is not a benign procedure; it requires patience, experience, and the immediate backup of a cardiovascular surgical team. Laser lead extractions are performed at our hospital in the operating room with the immediate availability of a cardiac surgeon.

Table 28.1 shows the historically, generally accepted indications for lead extraction. These include lead and/or device infection. If the patient

Table 28.1: Commonly Accepted Indications for Lead Extraction

1. Lead and/or device infection, possibly including endocarditis.
2. Venous thrombosis as a result of lead(s) obstructing the vein.
3. Lead migration, erosion, and/or dislodgment of a damaged and/or malfunctioning lead.

remains septic despite antibiotics, all device hardware should be removed. This includes patients with antibiotic refractory endocarditis. Rarely, venous thrombosis and/or superior vena cava obstruction can occur as a result of lead or leads obstructing venous return to the myocardium. Lead removal can be useful in this circumstance. Occasionally, venous obstruction can prevent lead access. The removal of a malfunctioning lead or leads with extraction sheaths can provide a conduit in order to place a new, fully functional lead or leads. Lead erosion, migration, and dislodgment might require removal and/or repositioning, depending on the particular clinical circumstance.

An important tool for any facility performing lead extraction procedures is the laser sheath (figures 28.1 and 28.2; Spectranetics SLS® II, Spectranetics Corporation, Colorado Springs, CO). The laser sheath employs ultraviolet Excimer laser light at a 308 nanometer wavelength to break down scar tissue holding leads in place, thereby permitting their removal. The laser is delivered by a ring of glass fibers sandwiched between two layers of polymer tubing. The laser sheath is connected via a cable to a generator, which produces the laser energy.

Because of the powered action of the laser sheath, leads can be removed from the scar tissue with gentle sheath advancement. This approach is clinically demonstrated to be safe as well as more effective and more time efficient than manual mechanical dissection methods. The laser energy penetrates only about 50 microns ahead of the sheath tip, and the pulsed delivery results in low temperatures around 50 degrees Celsius.

The laser sheath is particularly helpful when there is substantial fibrosis, when leads are fragile or stretchy, when one or more functional leads are being retained, and when lead removal is being performed to create implant access through a venous occlusion.

The laser sheath is usually used in conjunction with a lead locking device, such as the Spectranetics LLD® (Spectranetics Corporation, Colorado Springs, CO). The lead locking device is inserted in the hollow inner lumen of the lead and locked to secure it for application of traction. The LLD design employs an expanding braided mesh to deliver traction along the entire lead length.

Figure 28.3 shows a locking stylet that can secure the inner lumen and lead so that it is more stable at the tip and body during the extraction procedure (Liberator® locking stylet, Cook Medical, Bloomington, IN). It can often be difficult to cut through hardened calcified scars with the laser lead extraction system; however, the Evolution system (figure 28.4; Evolution® Mechanical Dilator System, Cook Medical) can spin the tip with cutting teeth, and if used carefully, can cut through calcified fibrotic scar in order to free up the lead.

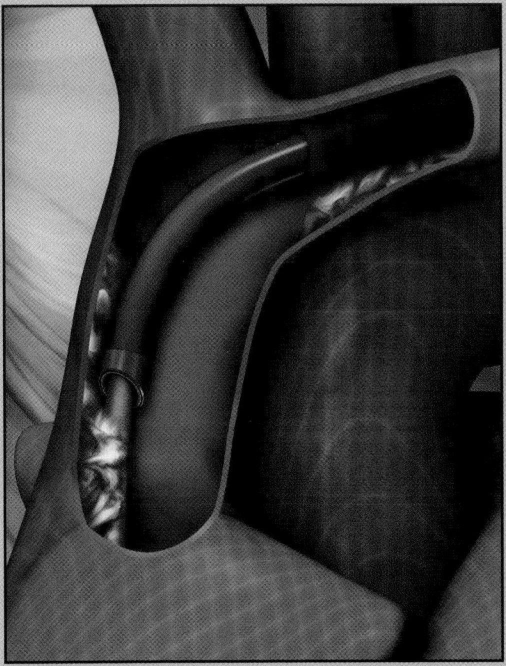

Figure 28.1: The SLS® II Laser Sheath (courtesy of Spectranetics Corporation, Colorado Springs, CO).

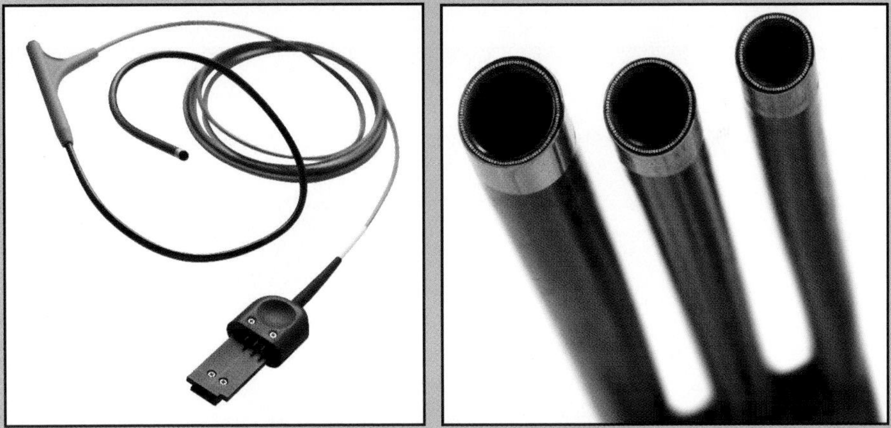

Figure 28.2: The SLS® II Laser Sheath (courtesy of Spectranetics Corporation, Colorado Springs, CO).

Each of these systems has their pros and cons, and an experienced operator should be familiar with a variety of tools to accomplish a high degree of successful lead extraction procedures with a low complication rate. Lastly, familiarity with tools for a femoral lead extraction approach can be useful when the thoracic approach is unsuccessful.

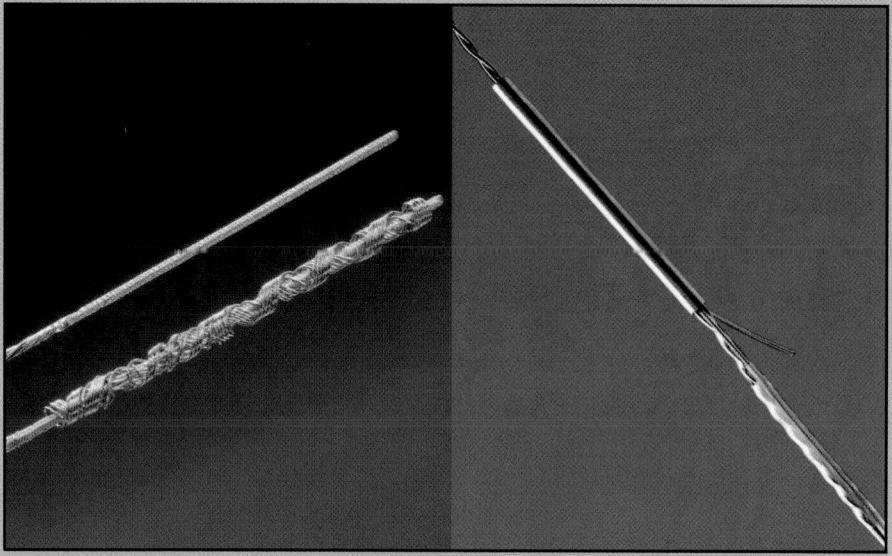

Figure 28.3: (At left) The Liberator® locking stylet (courtesy of Cook Medical, Bloomington, IN). (At right): The Bulldog™ lead extender (courtesy of Cook Medical, Bloomington, IN).

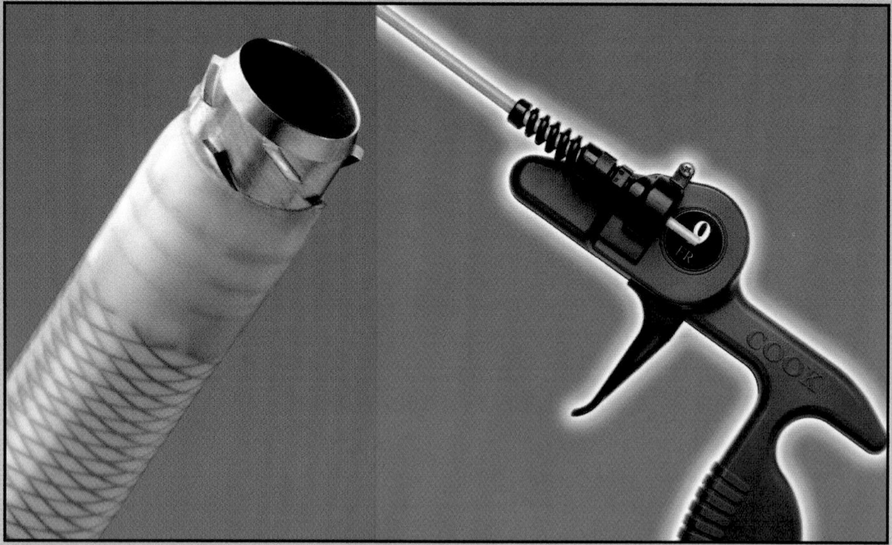

Figure 28.4: The Evolution® Mechanical Dilator System (courtesy of Cook Medical, Bloomington, IN).

Part 3: Quiz

Test your knowledge of Part 3:

Question 53. A 73-year-old woman is in church praying after the death of her husband. She feels sweaty, lightheaded, and dizzy and passes out. This patient should:

A. Undergo an electrophysiology study
B. Undergo a tilt table test
C. Be treated conservatively with hydration (such as for a common faint)
D. Receive a permanent pacemaker

Question 54. A 17-year-old girl has significant lightheadedness and dizziness every time she stands up. Her baseline blood pressure is 80/50 mmHg. She is markedly orthostatic. She is very dizzy any time she arises from bed and walks. The best treatment for her is:

A. A permanent pacemaker
B. Support stockings and fludrocortisone
C. Quinidine
D. Beta blockers

Question 55. Initial treatment from the patient in question 54 fails. The next treatment would be:

A. An implantable defibrillator
B. Sertraline
C. Midodrine
D. Psychiatric counseling

Question 56. A 57-year-old man with recurrent syncope and a mild bradycardia on Holter monitor underwent invasive electrophysiology testing, which was negative. A tilt-table test was also negative. The next recommended study would be to:

A. Implant a loop recorder
B. Implant a pacemaker
C. Implant a defibrillator
D. Treat with beta-blocker therapy

Question 57. A patient who receives an implantable cardiac monitor for recurrent syncope of unknown etiology often requires:

A. Catheter ablation
B. An implantable defibrillator
C. A permanent pacemaker
D. Amiodarone

Question 58. Which is more common in the United States?

A. Atrial fibrillation
B. Congestive heart failure

Question 59. The patients who have shortness of breath present with marked limitations of activity and are comfortable only at rest have:

A. Class I New York Heart Association congestive heart failure
B. Class II New York Heart Association congestive heart failure
C. Class III New York Heart Association congestive heart failure
D. Class IV New York Heart Association congestive heart failure

Question 60. The major medical treatment for congestive heart failure includes:

A. Digitalis
B. Diuretics
C. Angiotensin-converting enzyme inhibitor and/or angiotensin receptor blocker
D. Beta blockers
E. c and d

Question 61. A 57-year-old man with a prior myocardial infarction and ejection fraction of 25 percent has persistent symptoms of shortness of breath with minimal exertion despite optimal medical therapy with an ACE inhibitor and a beta blocker. His QRS duration is 150 milliseconds with a left bundle-branch block. The next best therapy is:

A. An implantable defibrillator
B. An implantable defibrillator with cardiac resynchronization therapy (biventricular implantable defibrillator)
C. A cardiac resynchronization therapy pacemaker
D. Biofeedback

Question 62. Which of the following is *not* an indication for a permanent pacemaker?

A. Asymptomatic bradycardia
B. Complete heart block
C. Mobitz type II second-degree heart block
D. Myotonic muscular dystrophy with high grade AV block

Question 63. The most common cause of pacemaker infections is:

A. E. coli
B. Pseudomonas
C. Staphylococcus or streptococcus

Question 64. A recall issued by the U.S. Food and Drug Administration (FDA) for implantable devices means that the device should be explanted and/or replaced.

A. True
B. False

Question 65. Which of the following conditions should *not* receive an implantable defibrillator?

A. Cardiac sarcoid
B. Chagas disease
C. LV noncompaction
D. Mitral valve prolapse

Question 66. A 62-year-old man has a nonischemic cardiomyopathy and class II congestive heart failure despite optimal medical therapy. His left ventricular ejection fraction is 30 percent. This patient should receive:

A. A permanent pacemaker
B. An implantable cardiac monitor
C. An implantable defibrillator
D. A biventricular implantable defibrillator

Question 67. A patient who had a myocardial infarction and has a documented ejection fraction less than 30 percent should wait at least how many days before receiving an implantable defibrillator?

A. 30 days
B. 40 days
C. 50 days
D. 60 days

Question 68. A patient presents with ventricular fibrillation in the setting of a markedly elevated and abnormal potassium level. This patient should:

A. Receive an implantable defibrillator
B. Receive a permanent pacemaker
C. Undergo treatment for hyperkalemia
D. Be treated with a beta blocker

Question 69. The use of progressively more aggressive therapies within a defibrillator zone is termed:

A. Tiered therapy
B. Zoned therapy
C. Ramp therapy
D. Burst therapy

Question 70. Which of the following is *not* a primary prevention indication for an implantable defibrillator?

A. A patient with prior myocardial infarction and ejection fraction of less than 30 percent
B. A patient with class II New York Heart Association congestive heart failure and ejection fraction of less than 36 percent
C. A patient with sustained ventricular tachycardia not in the setting of an acute myocardial infarction

Question 71. A 50-year-old man with prior myocardial infarction and an ejection fraction of 30 percent but without any symptoms of congestive heart failure can benefit from cardiac resynchronization therapy.

A. True
B. False

Question 72. Remote monitoring of implantable devices can be accomplished through all the following systems except:

A. CareLink®
B. LATITUDE®
C. Facebook

Question 73. What percent of patients who receive appropriate cardiac resynchronization therapy fail to respond?

A. 10 percent
B. 20 percent
C. 30 percent
D. 40 percent

Answer key:

53. C
54. B
55. C
56. A
57. C
58. B
59. C
60. E
61. B
62. A
63. C
64. B
65. D
66. C
67. B
68. C
69. A
70. C
71. B
72. C
73. C

Part 4

ADMINISTRATION

Chapter 29

Intravenous Drug Administration/ Preoperative Checklist

Intravenous Drug Administration

The responsibility for the administration of intravenous (IV) drugs in the EP lab lies with the nurse, under the direction of the physician. Because IV medications are delivered directly into the bloodstream, their dispensation requires more knowledge and greater precautions than do other methods of drug administration. Drug serum levels reach higher concentrations, and adverse reactions occur more rapidly and are usually more severe with the use of IV medications. Therefore, it is important to recognize the problems associated with IV drug administration and to impose caution when dispensing drugs by IV push.

IV administration ensures prompt onset of action and reduces ambiguity allied with the incompleteness of drug absorption by other routes. IV administration requires regular monitoring by a nurse, because this route increases the risk of side effects or toxicity.

It is important for the EP nurse to display an understanding of the drug to be administered by exhibiting knowledge regarding the rationale for the use of a specific drug in a particular patient, the rate of the drug administration, the drug's possible side effects, the drug's normal dosage range, and the compatibilities and incompatibilities of the drug with other IV drugs and fluids.

Table 29.1: Isoproterenol Infusion Rate (micrograms/kilogram/min) for Single-Stage HUT

WEIGHT Pounds (lb)	Kilograms (kg)	INFUSION RATE
80	36.3	1.8
85	38.6	1.9
90	40.9	2.0
95	43.1	2.2
100	45.4	2.3
105	47.7	2.4
110	49.9	2.5
115	52.2	2.6
120	54.5	2.7
125	56.8	2.8
130	59.0	3.0
135	61.3	3.1
140	66.6	3.2
145	65.8	3.3
150	68.1	3.4
155	70.4	3.5
160	72.6	3.6
165	74.9	3.7
170	77.2	3.9
175	79.5	4.0
180	81.7	4.1
185	84.0	4.2
190	86.3	4.3
195	88.5	4.4
200	90.8	4.5
205	93.1	4.7
210	95.3	4.8
215	97.6	4.9
220	99.9	5.0
Greater than 220		5.0

The rate of drug administration is very important because it is directly linked with the rate of absorption. The rate of absorption of a drug is of chief significance, because it is reflected in the concentration of the drug in the serum and at the target site. It determines the drug's time of onset of action and the time of peak effect. If absorption is too slow compared with elimination, the drug might never reach the minimum effectual therapeutic serum concentration. The rate of absorption, while relying on the rate of administration, is subsequently reliant on the characteristics of the patient (weight, age, individual health factors) as well as the characteristics of the drug itself (solubility, acidic vs. basic). Tables 29.1 and 29.2 show infusion rate tables for the drug isoproterenol, an IV drug used most regularly as a bronchodilator and a heart stimulant, and commonly administered in the EP laboratory (table 29.1 demonstrates infusion administered as micrograms/kilogram/minute [weight based], whereas in table 29.2, infusion is given in micrograms/minute).

Prior to any invasive EP procedure, it is important to discontinue any drugs that may interfere with the procedure, such as anticoagulants. Warfarin must be discontinued no fewer than five days prior to surgery. To prevent clotting, heparin can be administered intravenously up to six hours prior to surgery.

The IV administration of sedatives, hypotics, and analgesics is an important part of the nurse's role (see Chapter 30). Specific training is necessary in conscious sedation, including having an understanding of: 1) these medications; 2) their effects and side effects; and 3) the treatment of oversedation (*i.e.*, administration of reversal agents and airway management).

A similar, and equally important, consideration is drug interactions. Many patients receive more than one pharmaceutical agent, and the interactions among multiple drugs can cause serious complications. It is possible that two concurrently-administered agents influence some of the same pathways, and the effects of both agents can decrease each other's effects. For example, when isoproterenol is administered along with a beta-adrenergic blocking agent, the effects of isoproterenol are attenuated.

It is possible to administer two interacting drugs in tandem, provided that precautions such as dosage adjustments are taken. It is important to remember, though, that interactions between pharmaceutical agents apply not only to their intended therapeutic action, but also to their inherent side effects.

Preoperative Checklist

The vast majority of EP procedures are elective. It is critical that every patient who undergoes an EP procedure has a thorough evaluation. The evaluation should consist of a history and physical examination as well as an electrocardiogram. It is also important to have a thorough assessment of the cardiac substrate (the patient's left ventricular function and ejection fraction). An ischemia evaluation, which may consist of a radionuclear study, a stress echocardiogram, and/or a cardiac catheterization procedure, may be appropriate as well. In addition, for these elective procedures, the patient should be hemodynamically stable; not suffering from an electrolyte abnormality,

Table 29.2: Isoproterenol Infusion Rate Based on micrograms/minutes

MICROGRAM/MINUTE	ML/HR
Concentration of 0.2mg/100ml of D5W	
1	30ml/hr
2	60ml/hr
3	90ml/hr
4	120ml/hr
5	150ml/hr
6	180ml/hr
7	210ml/hr
8	240ml/hr
9	270ml/hr
10	300ml/hr

drug toxicity, or ischemic event; not actively bleeding; or infected. Additional preprocedural testing should include electrolytes, BUN and creatinine, glucose, complete blood count (including platelets and white blood cell count), coagulation profile including INR, type and screen, urinalysis, and chest x-ray.

It is important for the electrophysiology operator to directly see and examine the patient and review all pertinent data prior to the procedure. It is not acceptable for the operator to meet the patient on the table without having previously seen him or her, except in the case of an emergency. Electrophysiology emergencies are few and far between. These include placement of a temporary pacemaker in a patient with complete heart block or treatment of incessant ventricular arrhythmias requiring pace termination or ventricular tachycardia catheter ablation. The term "electrical storm" refers to incessant ventricular tachycardia or fibrillation that result in numerous ICD shocks. Aggressive treatment with anti-ischemic medications, intraaortic balloon counterpulsation, antiarrhythmic medications (lidocaine and/or amiodarone), and/or urgent revascularization can be helpful. When all else fails, emergent catheter ablation can be helpful.

To ensure that the basic standards are met during electrophysiology procedures including implants, a preoperative checklist is necessary. The Joint Commission also demands that a "time-out" be performed prior to the procedure. This is where, after the patient has been prepped and draped, the entire team pauses immediately prior to the start of the procedure to perform a final check that it is the right patient, right procedure, and right site.

In addition, informed consent should be performed prior to the patient being placed on the procedural table. The informed consent process is not the signing of the consent form. It is the discussion between the patient (and/or his or her healthcare proxy) and the physician regarding the risks and benefits of the procedure and any alternatives to the procedure. Questions are often asked and answered during this period.

Appendix A shows the checklist developed with the input of our electrophysiology team. This checklist is not a part of our medical records and is intended to be performed prior to any EP procedure. Occasionally, findings at the time of the checklist may result in a procedural delay. In addition, the values established in our checklist are for our hospital and may not be universally applicable. For example, if a patient has chronic renal insufficiency and has a stable hematocrit of 27, it may be unnecessary to transfuse that patient to a hematocrit of 28 just to meet the criteria. More importantly, the operator should document in the medical records that the blood count has been stable, that there are no active signs of bleeding, and that the patient has chronic renal insufficiency. The operator may also document that the risks of transfusion outweigh the benefits.

Anticoagulation is an area that deserves an important amount of attention. Preoperatively, all anticoagulants are held for the necessary amount of time. In addition, the use of a preoperative checklist assures a review of these anticoagulants, thereby reinforcing the appropriate timing of reinitiation postoperatively (depending on the pressing need for immediate anticoagulation). If a patient is cardioverted from chronic atrial fibrillation during the procedure, postoperative heparin and warfarin must be initiated in order to avoid complications (*i.e.*, transient ischemic attack or cerebrovascular accident).

Chapter 30

Members of the EP Team

The electrophysiology team is made up of a diverse group of individuals who work together to perform a single service: arrhythmia management. This group consists of administrators, transporters/orderlies, nurses, practitioners (physician assistants/nurse practitioners), vendors (selling catheters and other devices), technicians (Ph.D.s, radiologic technologists, EP technicians), secretaries, physicians, and physicians-in-training. All these individuals must integrate into the facility in which they operate, regardless of whether the facility is an in-hospital institution (as most EP centers are) or a freestanding facility.

A hierarchy among the EP team is important to ensure continuity of care. Figure 30.1 shows a possible hierarchy in which there is a director as well as a coordinator who helps supervise and organize a large fleet of staff and their activities on a day-by-day basis.

Besides the team members, many other individuals contribute to the success of the EP center. The hospital administration must believe in and be committed to the service in order to provide the adequate space, facility, and equipment. Substantial capital is necessary to equip and maintain such an EP laboratory, which continuously requires disposable and implantable equipment. A commitment to the overall success of the program means that the facility, the staff, and the volume of equipment must grow commensurate with the growth of the program.

Electrophysiology has been growing at an exponential rate due to an expansion of the types of implantable devices and the indications

Hierarchy of the Electrophysiology Team

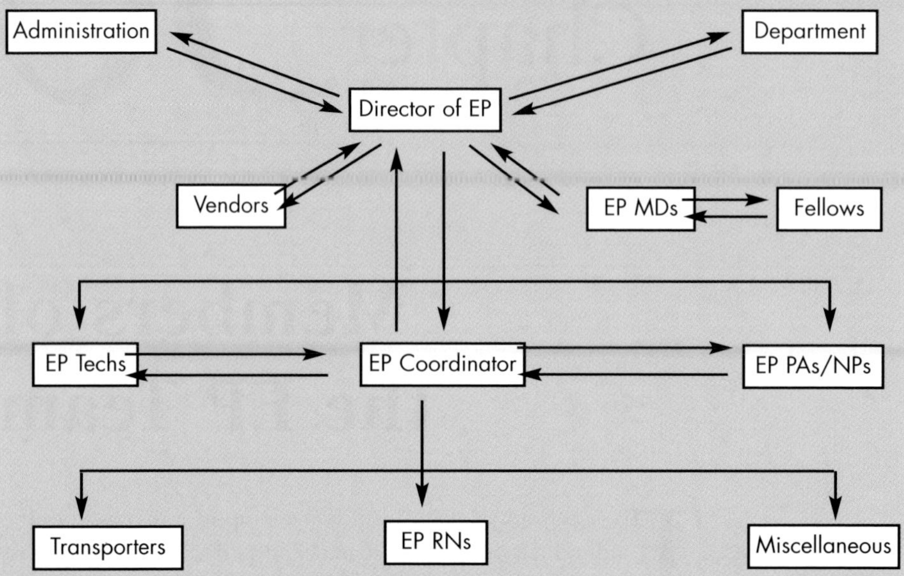

Figure 30.1: A possible hierarchy in which there is a director as well as a coordinator who help to direct a large fleet of staff and coordinate their activities by a day-by-day basis.

for use of implantable devices (based on the results of prophylactic implantable cardioverter-defibrillator trials). Many facilities have found it difficult to keep up with the growth of their EP program. The application of radiofrequency catheter ablation and other ablation modalities has also expanded both the number and types of EP procedures. For a facility to tackle atrial fibrillation, there must be a commitment to time, space, and staffing specifically for the procedure. Performing high-volume atrial fibrillation ablation procedures requires additional resources that may not be available at every institution.

The optimal setting for complex EP procedures is an institution with an open-heart program. This is because these electrophysiologic procedures, device implants, and ablative procedures have the risk for cardiac and vascular perforation. Immediate access to a cardiac surgical team can help prevent mortality associated with such an event.

EP team members include physicians, practitioners, nurses, and EP technicians—specially trained radiologic technologists who assist the nursing staff with sterile fields, patient preparation, and operation of the fluoroscopy. All lab team members are certified in advanced cardiac life support. The nurses ideally should have experience in intensive care and go through formal training in the department. Such training minimizes the need for micromanagement within the lab, allowing the trained professionals to do their job.

The following outlines the different roles of some of the personnel who are critical to electrophysiology lab functions.

The EP Clinical Coordinator

The role of the EP clinical coordinator is multifaceted and requires organization, foresight, and problem-solving skills (figure 30.2). In a way, the lab is like a store in that it should be ready to serve its customers (EP operators and patients) to their satisfaction (within the constraints of the facility, staff, and equipment). A myriad of functions and staff members are coordinated by the EP clinical coordinator in concert with the lab director.

Procedural labs should be terminally cleaned after the last case and prior to any implant. Supplies need to be adequately stored in a well thought-out manner so that the staff can access them easily. Emergency medications and crash carts also need to be easily accessible. Appropriately-trained personnel must be ready to work and able to staff any procedure, whether it is a catheter ablation, an implant, or a simple diagnostic study.

Cases are determined the day before for each lab, and calls are made to determine that appropriate preoperative preparation is conducted, ensuring that the most recent lab and test results will be available. If there is potential for delay, such as pending results (*i.e.*, a stress test, an angiogram, or an INR), then another patient and/or physician will be slotted in that spot. Once the patient is determined fit for testing or implantation, the accessory personnel are coordinated—device representatives, specialized technicians, and anesthesia are notified if necessary.

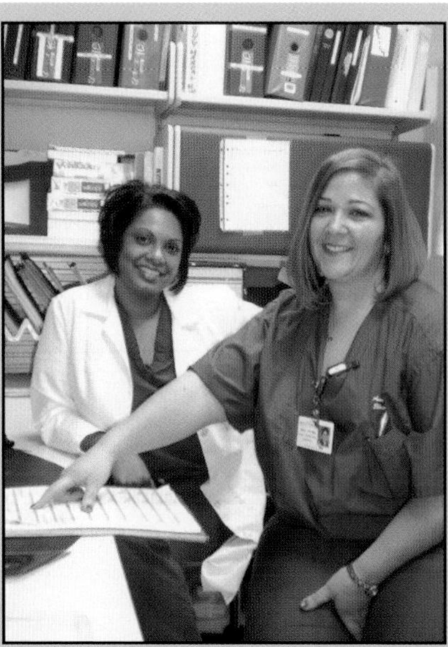

Figure 30.2: The EP coordinator and assistant nurse manager facilitating turnover.

The clinical coordinator determines the patient flow for the remaining cases. Flow decisions are based on patient status, case complexity, and physician availability. One system that has worked well is the assignment of block time (half or a full day) to specific operators based on clinical volume. The physician with the block time for that day takes priority in an invasive lab and a smaller procedure room (for tilt-table testing, cardioversions and ICD checks).

Patients are transported and brought into the room once it is determined that they have met the preoperative checklist criteria (Appendix A). If there are any deviations from the checklist or concerns about patient status, the physician is informed prior to placing the patient on the table. Once the physician makes the decision to move forward with the case,

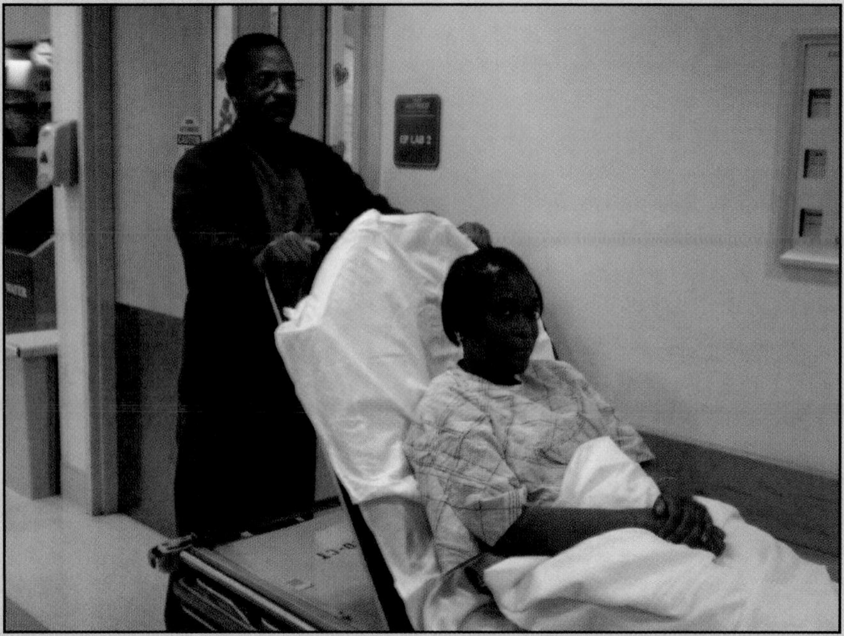

Figure 30.3: An EP lab transporter in action.

he or she should document that a "time-out" was performed in the progress notes before proceeding. Major deviations from the checklist usually result in cancellation of the case.

Transporters are helpful in moving patients and equipment quickly and safely and help to provide a smooth flow in and out of the rooms. There may be as many as two transporters working on a single room—one cleaning, the other bringing patients to and from the lab (figure 30.3). The coordinator assists in the timing of transport by checking in with the teams, determining which cases are wrapping up, and then initiating prep or paperwork on the next case. Ideally, the turnover is kept to 20 minutes between cases in the invasive labs, and five to seven minutes in the tilt/noninvasive procedural rooms.

The schedule for the day may unexpectedly change, requiring shifting of time slots and personnel. Judgments are made with respect to realistic goals for case completion, and the coordinator often reviews the schedule with the director several times throughout the day as issues arise, resulting in cancellations and other modifications.

The Practitioner

The physician assistant and/or nurse practitioner plays an important role in the electrophysiology laboratory (figure 30.4). These practitioners are versatile and able to perform many of the tasks that help extend the physician's practice. These include assisting with consultations, conducting clinical follow-ups (rounding), handling a pacemaker clinic, and being

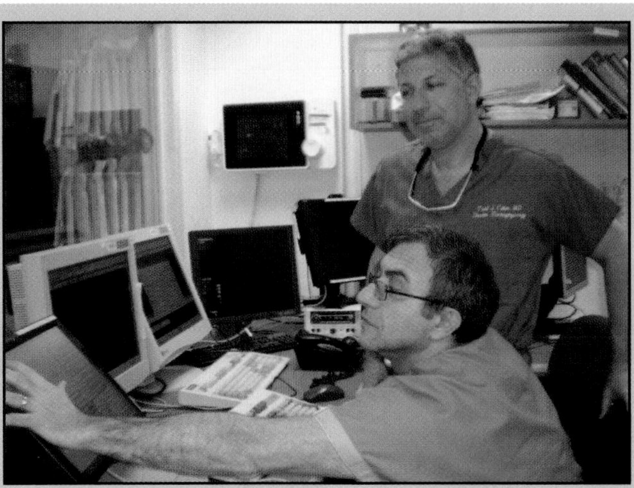

Figure 30.4: The author teaching a PA in the EP lab.

involved in preoperative, operative, and postoperative management.

In addition to helping with clinical follow-up, practitioners can be credentialed to perform a myriad of services under the physician's direction in the electrophysiology laboratory. Among these services are line placement, assistance with device implants and tilt-table testing, operating the computerized EP laboratory, and device interrogations. Working very closely with the electrophysiologist, they are taught specific techniques such as how to insert sheaths and catheters in the femoral veins and arteries, how to make the device pockets, and how to close the pockets at the end of the cases.

An important task for the practitioners is helping with consultations and physical examinations, conducting pre-admission testing, identifying postoperative complications, and assisting with critical situations in the EP lab. Before every one of our procedures, a preoperative order must be placed in the chart by the practitioner. The practitioners can be very helpful in educating the patients, explaining the procedures, and helping with paperwork, although the ultimate responsibility for the consenting process falls on the physician.

In summary, the practitioners serve an important role on the arrhythmia service. Physician supervision and practitioner inclusion as a critical member in the service are pivotal in ensuring the success of their role.

The Director of the EP Laboratory

Being a director of electrophysiology is a challenging task. The director must integrate all EP members (radiology technicians, nurses, transporters, vendors, and physicians) into a clinically productive team with the ultimate goal of delivering uncompromised care.

In order to ensure that a high level of clinical standards is met, the director must implement a detailed preoperative checklist. This ensures that the patients are appropriately consented and "pre-oped" for the procedure. They must also be free of infection and be hemodynamically stable.

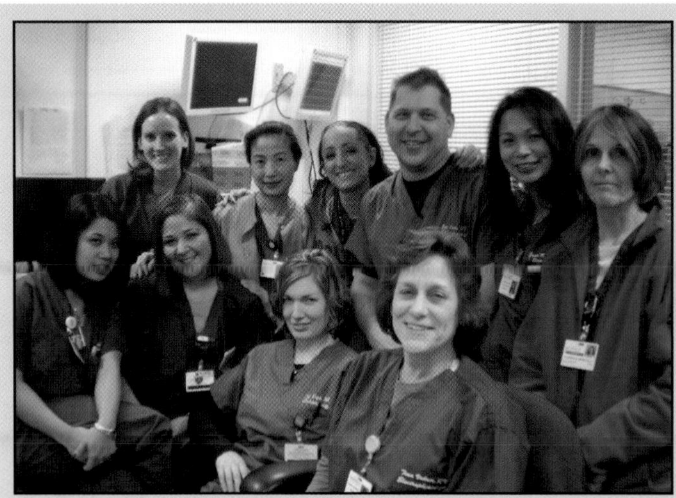

Figure 30.5: Nurses in the EP lab.

The nurses help the director in assuring that these standards are met for every single case. In addition, the nurse coordinator helps the director with the flow of patients in the electrophysiology laboratory. When the facilities are limited due to equipment breakdown, fair and adequate alternative access is sought.

The director must ensure professional behavior via all staff and vendors in the laboratory. It is important to minimize laboratory access only to essential personnel necessary for each specific procedure. In addition, all personnel should be familiar with each institution's policies and procedures, including code of conduct, professionalism, and privacy, in order to deliver care without compromise to the patients, in a safe environment. In addition, the director is responsible (together with administration and EP coordinator) for assuring that all personnel are appropriately trained and credentialed in each of their particular areas of expertise.

It is also the director's responsibility to help the hospital or the facility control laboratory costs. This includes costs related to disposable items and implantable devices. Adequate justification must be demonstrated in order for administration to approve additional resources (equipment, laboratory space, and staffing).

In summary, the director has a key role in making sure that the entire electrophysiology team functions as a whole. All the cogs in the wheel and all the gears of the motor must be oiled, and an occasional tune-up is necessary.

The Electrophysiology Nurse

If electrophysiology is the heart of cardiology, then the electrophysiology nurse is its backbone (figure 30.5). The EP nurse should possess a basic understanding of electrocardiograms including interpretation. Training should include a minimum of two years of recent critical care experience, advanced cardiac life support (and where appropriate, pediatric advanced life support certification), operating room certification in surgical scrub technique, infection control training and certification, and a solid pharmacology foundation (including cardiac medications, their effects and dosages, conscious sedation, etc.). All laboratory nurses performing conscious sedation should be registered nurses (RNs).

The nurse's role in the electrophysiology laboratory is multifaceted. He or she is a caregiver, advocate, surgical assist, teacher and equipment troubleshooter. A preoperative checklist ensures that current labs and chest x-rays are available and that any abnormalities are addressed by the physician prior to placing the patient on the table. The basic physical assessment determines if a patient is fit for this elective procedure. A patient's status may change overnight, and the EP nurse is responsible for identifying potential problems prior to the procedure. The subtleties like comfort and ability to lie flat, changes in respiratory status or vital signs, a slight drop in hemoglobin or an increase in white blood cell count can be identified prior to the procedure. The RN is ever aware of potential procedural risks for infection, injury, knowledge deficits, anxiety, etc., and a patient-specific plan of care is developed, goals are set and the plan is carried out.

The electrophysiology laboratory, although it may not always meet the technical specifications of a true operating room, should be treated like an operating room regardless of the procedure to ensure the highest degree of sterility. Hospital scrubs and appropriate personal protective equipment are worn by all the staff. The patient is brought into the lab wearing only a hospital gown. The set up includes remote access defibrillators (two per room: one connected to the patient via large external patches and one as a backup). The defibrillator is checked daily prior to initiating any procedure. A crash cart with intubation and emergency equipment including a pericardiocentesis needle (in case of cardiac tamponade) and pharmaceutical box with advanced cardiac life support medications is present and checked each day. A patent intravenous line is inserted prior to the procedure, preferably on the side of any contemplated device implant in case a venogram is required. Oxygen is administered via nasal cannula routinely at 2–3 liters per minute. Normal saline is infused at a low rate, a 12-lead electrocardiogram is recorded continuously as part of the electrophysiology computerized recording system, automated blood pressure is measured, and pulse oximetry is recorded. Medications are tailored to the procedure and are readily available.

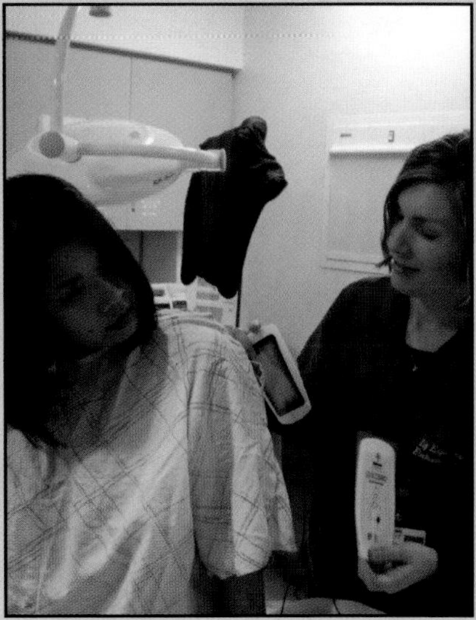

Figure 30.6: RN prepping a patient.

Continuous monitoring of the patient and documentation of their status is performed every 10 minutes, or more often

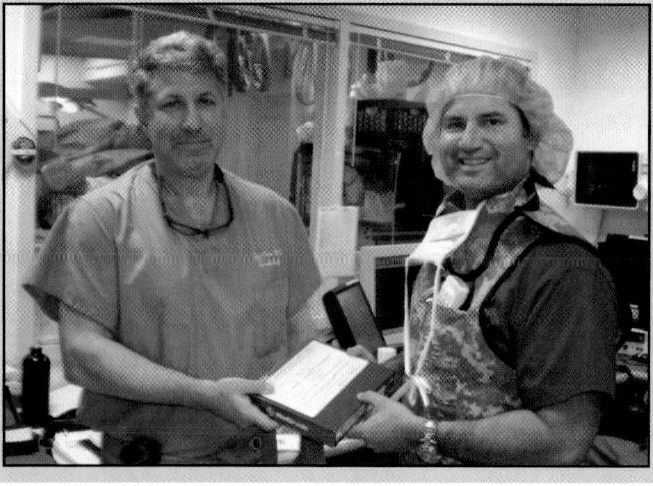

Figure 30.7:
A radiologic technologist with the author preparing equipment for a pacemaker implant.

depending on the clinical circumstance. The EP nurse can work with either another RN or an electrophysiology technician to facilitate timely preparation of the room, sterile tables, and the patient (figure 30.6). The patient is able to address all EP staff by name, and their comfort and safety is the RN's primary concern. Emotional support and ongoing teaching is provided throughout the procedure.

During the procedure, the nurse continues to monitor the patient's vital signs as well as their status and response to conscious sedation. One RN is dedicated to the administration and monitoring of conscious sedation, and the other RN is responsible for circulation duties during the procedure (*e.g.*, adding catheters and sterile supplies, administration of medications ordered by the physician, assisting with stimulation, and updating the physician on patient status as needed throughout the procedure). The radiologic technologists assist the RN with retrieving supplies, etc.

If the procedure is an ablation, the EP nurse is responsible for assisting with the operation of the radiofrequency generator or other ablation equipment (intracardiac echo machine, nonfluoroscopic three-dimensional mapping, laser lead extraction equipment, transseptal equipment). He or she utilizes progress reports and flow sheets to document the catheters that are inserted, conscious sedation administered, and anticoagulation given during the procedure with accompanying activated clotting times (ACT) levels. An ACT record sheet is utilized in which a baseline ACT level is measured and routine ACT levels are recorded every 20 minutes with the doctor's anticoagulation course of action (*i.e.*, amount of heparin administered; see Appendix D). In addition, ablation applications are documented and emotional support is provided (in addition to conscious sedation) in order to optimize patient comfort.

If the procedure is a surgery, the RN is responsible—together with the electrophysiologist—for conscious sedation unless an anesthesiologist is present. Another RN or technician will act as a sterile scrub assistant and help with prepping and draping the patient. The RN prepares the surgical tables and post procedure accounts for all gauze, sharps, and instruments used.

The EP nurse is the physician's eyes and ears in the laboratory, and must rely on the nursing process and judgment to identify, interpret and escalate if there are necessary changes in the patient's condition. There is no role for complacency; SVT can deteriorate into VF in a moment, and one needs to be ready with adenosine as well as the defibrillator. At the end of the procedure, the nurse is responsible for removing venous and arterial sheaths and obtaining hemostasis. Additional emotional support during such time allows the patient to verbalize concerns and questions regarding the study findings, directing the patient to the physician when necessary. A thorough report (including procedure, access site, how the patient tolerated the procedure, medications administered and their effect, review of systems post procedure) is provided to the recovery room receiving RN, and the patient's vital signs should be at or near baseline. If sedation has been administered, then the Aldretti score (assessment of patient's sedation level) should be at or above 8 (10 being fully awake and alert and not sedated) before transport to a recovery area.

Post procedure, the EP nurse ensures that all documentation is complete, that orders are on the chart, that a bed has been secured and that the physician has spoken to the family. As the staff works together turning over the room, they are preparing for the next case. Any surgical device implants require terminal cleaning of the room. Procedure-specific supplies are brought in, and a new checklist is initiated prior to the next patient being placed on the table. The team in the room works closely with the electrophysiology coordinator in ensuring safe, rapid turnover to meet the volume demand as well as the standards of care for their patients.

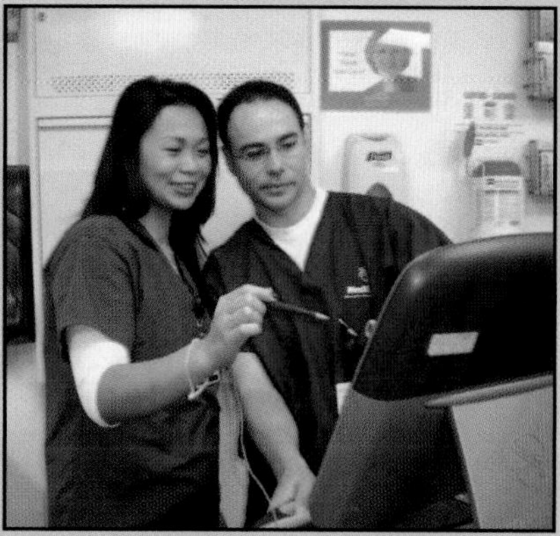

Figure 30.8: Vendor and RN interrogating a device.

The Radiologic Technologist

Trained to perform more tasks than standard technologists, radiologic technologists (figure 30.7) can become a critical element of the EP laboratory, performing many of the tasks of the practitioners and nurses. These tasks include helping to set up the procedural room, monitoring the patient, overseeing inventory management (including stocking each laboratory with catheters and sheaths), breaking down the rooms, transporting patients and helping with the electrophysiological computer laboratory (the stimulation/monitoring equipment), including equipment maintenance and service. All of these tasks are performed in addition to the movement of fluoroscopy

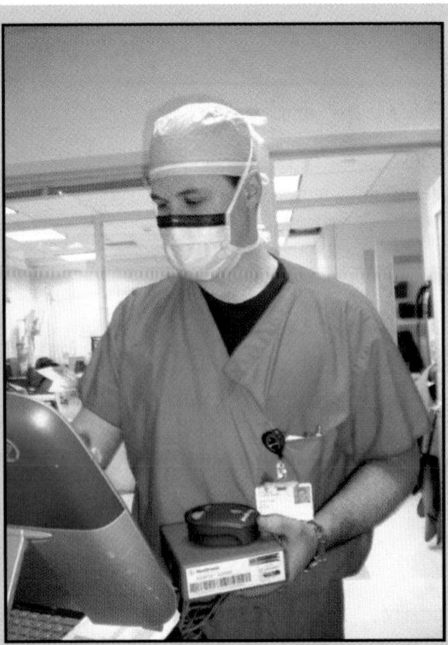
Figure 30.9: Vendor preparing for a device implant.

equipment. These technologists also help coordinate cases and keep a log of patient flow through the laboratories.

In addition, the technologists help minimize the staffs' exposure to radiation. Not only do they help set up shielding in our laboratory, but they also help educate the staff and make sure that noncritical personnel are at least six feet from the image intensifier during a procedure in order to minimize radiation exposure. Working closely with the radiation safety officer in the hospital, they monitor all electrophysiology staff and inspect our leadlike aprons twice a year. In our lab, in addition to lead shielding and leadlike aprons, we have used radiation-protective shields to provide additional protection (RADPAD®, Worldwide Innovations and Technologies Inc., Overland Park, KS). Placing this shield between the operator and the image intensifier can reduce radiation exposure to the operator by an additional 50 percent.

Other technologists [*i.e.*, Registered Cardiovascular Invasive Specialists (RCIS) and/or certified electrophysiology technologists] may also serve important roles in the EP lab; however, the radiologic technology license is necessary for their ability to move, position, and utilize radiation equipment (*i.e.*, fluoroscopy).

The Vendor

Pacemaker, defibrillator, and catheter sales representatives can play a key role in the EP laboratory (figure 30.8). They are responsible for providing the appropriate materials for both implant and disposable use in addition to providing additional expertise regarding the use of their particular products.

The vendor sales force can be divided into two categories: the device-based sales reps and the catheter-based sales reps. Most of the implantable materials for the device-based products are brought in by the vendors. A small number of products (leads and stylets) may be left by the vendors for use during cases in which another vendor is primary. For example, for the implant of a device by Boston Scientific, a defibrillator lead from Medtronic, Inc. or St. Jude Medical, Inc. may be used because of its true bipolar nature. A hospital might purchase these leads or have them left on consignment for this purpose. The pulse generators themselves may be purchased in advance or brought from outside via the vendor.

Catheter-based sales representatives supply a variety of diagnostic and therapeutic catheters. For the most part, these catheters are sold to the hospital and kept for their intended purpose with par values set as a function of their usage. The catheter-based sales reps are responsible for providing appropriate products and addressing any performance needs as they occur.

Both the device-based and the catheter-based sales representatives are expected to provide value-added service to the EP program. The device representatives will assist with pacemaker/defibrillator clinics, hospital interrogations, and reprogramming, as well as helping with devices during surgical procedures (obviously not touching the patient) and providing educational support to the staff (figure 30.9). They also assist with recording important data for implant reports as well as recording device-tracking and performance information that must go to the manufacturer. In addition, sales reps will on occasion bring engineers to further educate the staff.

Should any technical questions occur during the procedure, the lab can contact a vendor's 24-hour service via its toll-free phone number (table 30.1).

Table 30.1: Vendor Contact Information

Boston Scientific:	1-800-Cardiac
Medtronic, Inc.:	1-800-Medtron
St. Jude Medical, Inc.:	1-800-Paceicd

All sales representatives must go through privacy and infection-control training, similar to that of all hospital employees. They must go through hospital security and be seen by employee health to ensure adequate safety to our area. In addition, a certain level of expertise is expected before a sales representative is allowed to function in an EP lab or operating room. A list of skilled individuals who are allowed to enter the area should be maintained. Any new sales individuals must be cleared by the director or the coordinator of the electrophysiology laboratory.

Chapter 31

The Future of Electrophysiology

The future of electrophysiology is extremely exciting. With all the advances in technology over the past two decades and the results of prophylactic implantable defibrillator trials, tremendous growth is projected. Within the field of electrophysiology, novel catheter designs and alternative energy sources for ablation (ultrasound, microwave, and cryothermia) will improve the safety and efficiency of complex catheter ablation procedures. In addition, novel electrode designs and catheter configurations may simplify the ability to create circumferential and linear lesions (*e.g.*, pulmonary vein isolation). Additional technological developments may minimize the operator's direct exposure to radiation. These methods include the application of robotics to the field of electrophysiology. For example, the operator can manipulate catheters remotely from a control room and deliver electrodes precisely using a system that is magnetically driven (Stereotaxis, St. Louis, Missouri) (figure 31.1). With this method, a magnetic responsive guidewire may be manipulated, which can remotely feed a catheter up through the vasculature of the human body in order to facilitate catheter mapping and ablation. In addition, robotic remote navigation systems have been developed and implemented. These systems are mechanically driven (figures 31.2-31.4) (Hansen Medical Inc., Mountain View, California). Hansen Medical's Sensei® system uses computer-based technology to help in manipulation of a catheter. Their disposable Artisan™

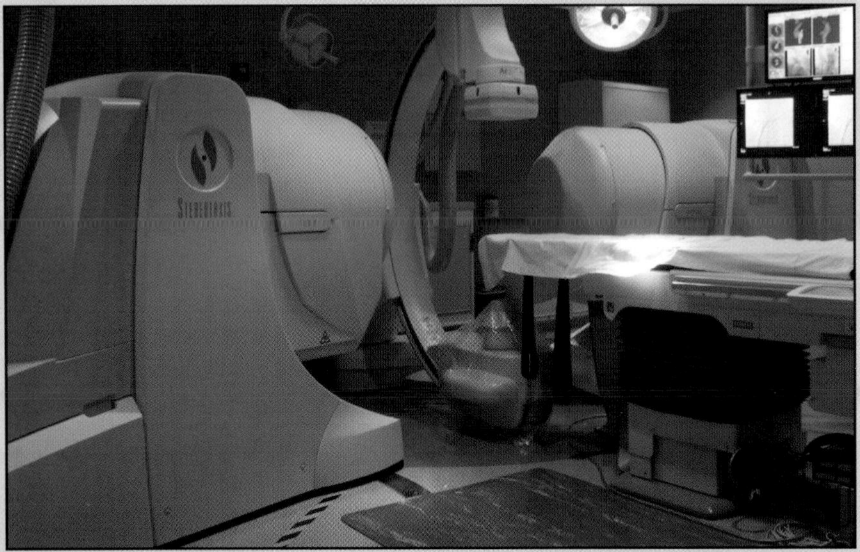

Figure 31.1: Stereotaxis lab. (Reprinted with permission from *EP Lab Digest* 2009;4:16) (Photo courtesy of Gary L. Hansen).

Control Catheter is comprised of inner and outer steerable guide catheters that accommodate indicated percutaneous catheters. A newer system, manufactured by Catheter Robotics Inc., in Budd Lake, New Jersey, utilizes a simpler approach in which the only invasive equipment used is that of standard catheters and sheaths. The latter system does not require a large catheter control system, but only a small remote controller similar in size, shape, and feel to that of a standard catheter handle. The Hansen Medical and Stereotaxis systems have been used to perform atrial fibrillation ablation. Clinical investigation of the Catheter Robotics system is necessary prior to approval by the United States Food and Drug Administration (FDA).

Figure 31.5 shows the Catheter Robotics system. This remote catheter manipulation system attaches to a standard fluoroscopic table. The remote controller does not take up any significant space, and immediately integrates with current electrophysiology laboratory computerized work stations. Additionally, this system allows the operator to immediately access the mapping catheter, remove it and manually manipulate it, and then replace it back in the robot—all while maintaining sterility.

The simplification of pulmonary vein/atrial fibrillation ablation procedures in order to minimize the risks to the patient as well as the risk to the operator of radiation is also under development. A simple, easily deployed system that can rapidly isolate pulmonary veins as well as create linear lines on both the right and left side of heart may help to accomplish this goal. This technology may also be useful for

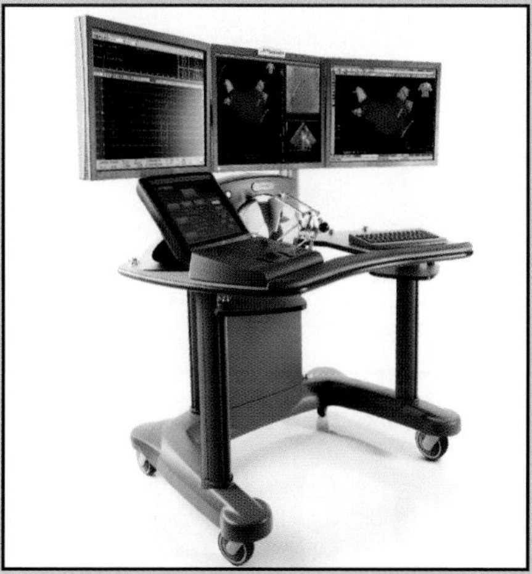

Figure 31.2: The Sensei® Robotic Catheter System is designed to provide the physician with a cost-effective way to remotely perform complex interventional procedures. The mobile physician workstation can be placed in either the cath lab or the control room (courtesy of Hansen Medical Inc., Mountain View, CA).

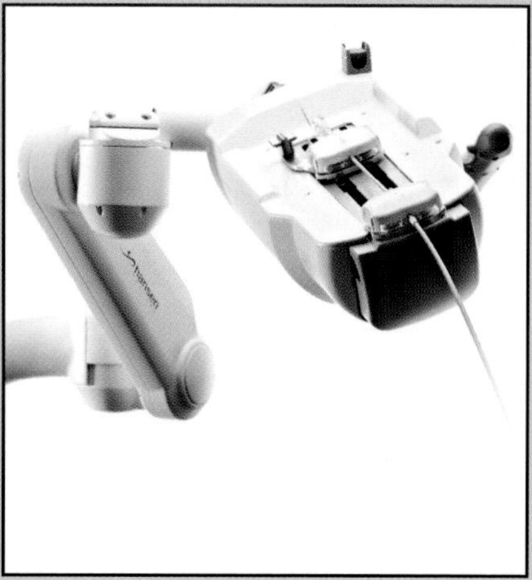

Figure 31.3: The remote catheter manipulator maneuvers the Artisan™ Control Catheter that responds to physician commands from the workstation (courtesy of Hansen Medical Inc., Mountain View, CA).

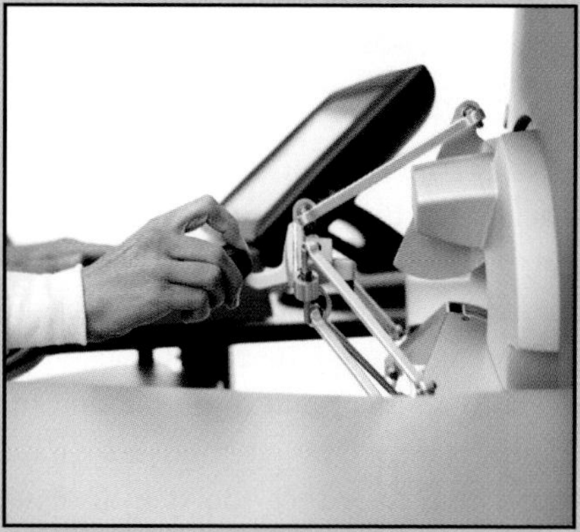

Figure 31.4: The instinctive motion controller allows the physician to control catheter placement in three dimensions (courtesy of Hansen Medical Inc., Mountain View, CA).

catheter ablation of ventricular tachycardia in patients with ischemic and non-ischemic cardiomyopathies. Recently available in Europe is a new catheter ablation system, which utilizes specially shaped catheters and a novel radiofrequency generator that can simultaneously deliver bipolar and unipolar energy to all electrodes (figure 31.6). This approach allows for operators to efficiently create long, contiguous lesions, with operator-controlled lesion depth. This may be particularly useful in facilitating complex ablations, including ablation of atrial fibrillation.

Percutaneous cryoablation to treat atrial fibrillation is still investigational in the United States, though the Arctic Front® percutaneous balloon system (figure 31.7) has received the CE Mark regulatory approval in Europe. The Arctic Front® balloon is available in Europe in two diameters: 23 mm and 28 mm. The balloon's shape allows for anatomical placement of

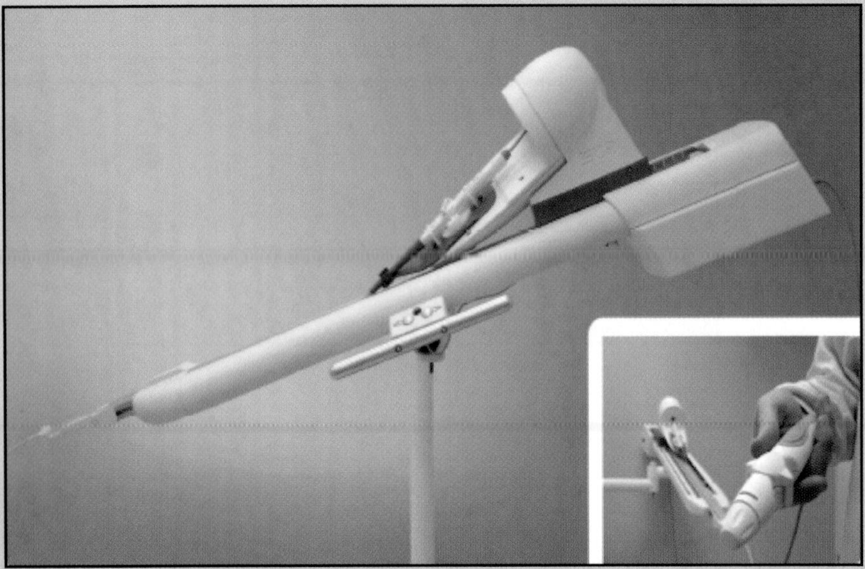

Figure 31.5: Shows the Catheter Robotics Remote Manipulation System. A standard catheter is inserted into the robot and connected to a standard introducer sheath. The system is controlled by a small hand-held remote controller which is similar in size and feel to a standard steerable catheter's handle (see insert). (Reprinted with permission from the *Journal of Invasive of Cardiology* 2008;20:250-253).

the balloon in the antrum or at the ostium of the targeted pulmonary vein. The balloon ablates at contact points with the surrounding tissue. The catheter also features both an inner and outer balloon for enhanced safety. This method may have the potential to reduce the risk of acute thromboembolic complications and atrial esophageal fistula; pulmonary vein stenosis appears to be lower with cryoablation as well. Other modalities for catheter ablation, such as microwave and ultrasound, are being investigated as well.

Prophylactic implantable defibrillator trials (MADIT II, SCD-HeFT, COMPANION, and CARE-HF) have led to global device expansion. In addition, the recently published ACC/AHA/HRS guidelines have expanded pacing, defibrillator, and cardiac resynchronization guidelines (see table 25.1 in Chapter 25, table 26.1 in Chapter 26, and table 27.1 in Chapter 27).

A minimally invasive, subcutaneous implantable defibrillator (S-ICD) continues to be developed by Cameron Health, Inc., located in San Clemente, California (figure 31.8). The S-ICD is currently under investigation in Europe and New Zealand, and is awaiting clinical investigation in the U.S. The clinical trials associated with this system will need to demonstrate consistent arrhythmia detection and discrimination as well as effective defibrillation prior to approval.

Nonexcitatory stimulation in the ventricular refractory period of patients who have

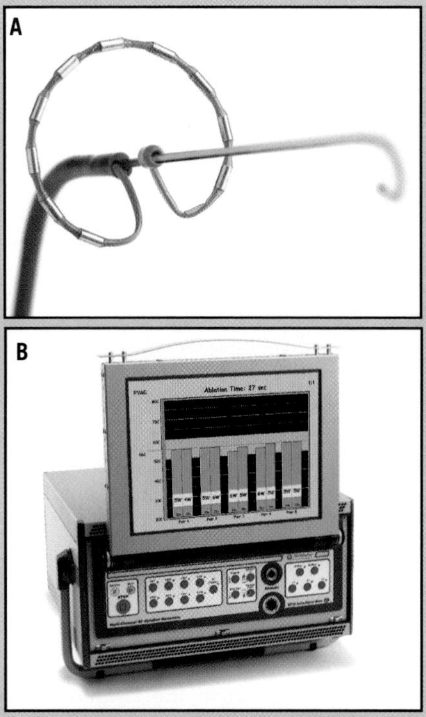

Figure 31.6: (A) The Pulmonary Vein Ablation Catheter (PVAC) features 10 electrodes that each have a thermocouple, allowing for accurate temperature measurement and efficient radiofrequency delivery. (B) The GENius multi-channel radiofrequency generator delivers unipolar and bipolar energy to any or all catheter electrodes simultaneously. This allows for the creation of contiguous lesions up to 70 mm in length. (Reproduced with permission of Medtronic Inc., Minneapolis, MN).

congestive heart failure and a narrow QRS may also be useful in augmenting contractility and improving cardiac performance (OPTIMIZER™ III, Impulse Dynamics N.V., New York) (figure 31.9). The OPTIMIZER™ system is commercially available in Europe (and has received the CE Mark) and is under clinical investigation in the United States.

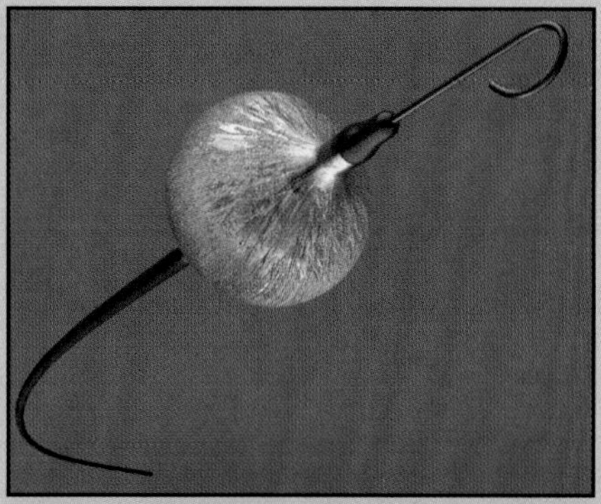

Figure 31.7: The Arctic Front® (Reproduced with permission of Medtronic Inc., Minneapolis, MN).

A percutaneous delivery system for insertion of a moldable pacemaker defibrillator is also under development via a company called InnerPulse, Inc. (located in Research Triangle Park, North Carolina); their system is a percutaneous implantable pacemaker defibrillator system, in which they are developing a quick and easy percutaneous implant technique of a moldable device that would not be visible to the patient from the chest wall or body surface.

Additional hard-wired myocardial systems, in which multiple leads and/or electrodes and/or vectors are deployed, are also under investigation. These multi-lead systems may integrate sensor technology to optimize myocardial performance. Devices will be integrating this type of therapy with Internet (off-site/wireless) monitoring. These systems will have enhanced monitoring, trending, and treatment capabilities for patients with a myriad of cardiac conditions such as congestive heart failure and ischemia in addition to rhythm control. Eventually, drug delivery systems may be incorporated

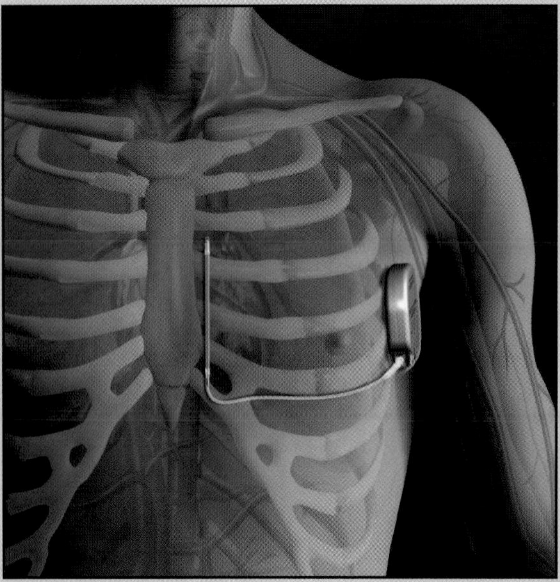

Figure 31.8: A minimally invasive, subcutaneous implantable defibrillator is being studied. This system has several obstacles at this time; however, the possibility of this type of therapy requires further investigation. If these hurdles are overcome, such a system has the potential to avoid the complications associated with having leads in or on the heart and result in a much simplified implant procedure (courtesy of Cameron Health, Inc., San Clemente, CA).

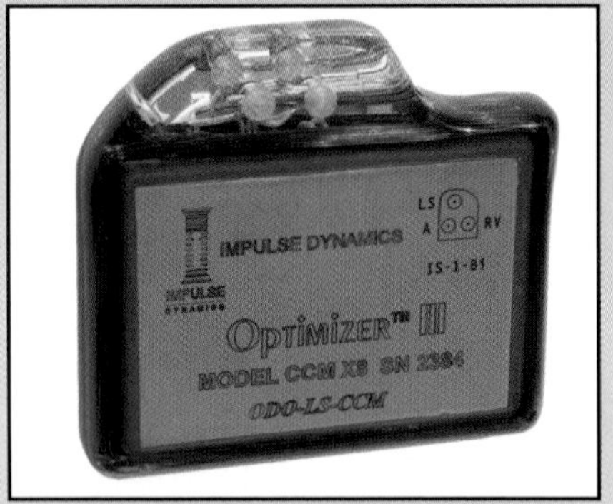

Figure 31.9: The OPTIMIZER™ III (Impulse Dynamics N.V., NY) (Reprinted with permission from *EP Lab Digest* 2006;6:27).

in these devices in order to treat the whole gamut of cardiac conditions remotely in either a manual, semi-automatic, or automatic method.

Magnetic resonance imaging (MRI)-conditional pacemakers are currently under investigation in the United States and await approval by the FDA. The purpose of the EnRhythm MRI SureScan trial is to confirm safety and effectiveness in the clinical magnetic resonance imaging environment of the investigational EnRhythm MRI™ SureScan™ Pacing System. This system was designed and tested to minimize risks from MR, while utilizing the diagnostic capabilities MR may offer. This system is investigational use only (U.S.). Figure 31.10 shows the EnRhythm MRI™ SureScan™ pacemaker, which recently received CE Mark and is now commercially available in select European countries.

There has been impressive growth in the area of genetic causes of sudden death. An enhanced understanding of the role of genetic mutations will undoubtedly provide for important diagnostic and therapeutic advances. Stem cell research

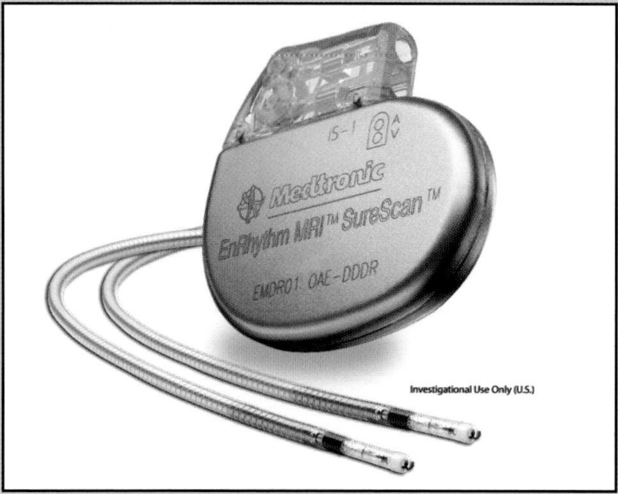

Figure 31.10: The EnRhythm MRI™ SureScan™ pacemaker (Reproduced with permission of Medtronic Inc., Minneapolis, MN).

might also shed light on the utility of this modality for rejuvenating and/or repairing diseased myocardium. Stem cells have the potential for reversing conduction disease and restoring impaired left ventricular function.

Advances in pharmacologic therapies will attempt to augment drug efficacy while decreasing side effects. Dronedarone, an investigational class III antiarrhythmic drug with amiodarone-like properties and purportedly less side effects, was studied in atrial fibrillation patients as part of the ATHENA trial. Patients who received dronedarone had statistically less mortality or hospitalization for cardiac problems when compared to placebo. Dronedarone awaits approval by the U.S. Food and Drug Administration. Other investigational antiarrhythmic drugs are undergoing investigation and may eventually be approved to treat both supraventricular and ventricular arrhythmias.

In summary, the possibilities are endless in the evolving field of electrophysiology. However, the education of both older and newer personnel (EP staff and vendors) needs to be efficiently accomplished in order to help facilitate further growth in this dynamic field. Hopefully, the second edition of *Practical Electrophysiology* will help to accomplish this goal.

Appendix

APPENDIX A:
PRE-ELECTROPHYSIOLOGY PROCEDURE/IMPLANT CHECKLIST

CONSENT COMPLETE/INDICATION DOCUMENTED IN MR AND ADMITTING MD/ASSOC AWARE	
HISTORY AND PHYSICAL ON CHART AND UPDATED	
SOS PRE PROCEDURE ORDERS ON CHART MAR / VS / TEACHING / PAIN SHEET ON CHART AND DOCUMENTED	
DOUBLE ID, NURSING ASSESSMENT	
ALLERGIES CHECKED AND COMPLETED	
IPRO and/or ONET COMPLETED for ICD? IF N/A, DOCUMENT AS SUCH	
PT NPO X 6 HOURS – if Not, document why	
PT VSS AND LAST TEMP < 101.5	Temp=
LAB VALUES MEET OUR CRITERIA T/S ≤ 72 HR IP / DAYS OP K = 3.5 – 5.5	T/S? K=
HGB/HCT ≥ 9/28 WBC<15000-if greater/ or if active infection ID must document clearance for device. PLT > 80,000 INR ≤ 1.5 NON DIALYSIS PT BUN ≤ 60 CRT ≤ 1.8	h/h= WBC= Plt= Inr= BUN/CRT=
HCG NEGATIVE FOR PREGNANCY IN WOMAN OF CHILDBEARING YEARS?	HCG=
ON COUMADIN? ON HEPARIN? ON LOVENOX? DATE/TIME OF LAST DOSE OR WHEN STOPPED	
CHEST X-RAY ≤ 3 MOS AND DISPLAYED IN LAB	
ALL BOLDFACED ITEMS MUST BE MET PRIOR TO PT COMING IN THE LAB The MD needs to be informed of and address any deviations in the chart. When necessary, all issues are to be escalated to the coordinator and then the Director. Please note that the lab should identify any pending blood work and the operator should make a decision to proceed with the procedure prior to receiving the blood work results. Staple this checklist to the super bill for collection.	
RN SIGNATURE:	

APPENDIX B: PATIENT DISCHARGE INSTRUCTIONS

PACEMAKER/DEFIBRILLATOR IMPLANTATION

FIRST 24 HOURS

Activities:

- It is normal to feel tired, slightly uncoordinated and need additional sleep as a result of the medications you received during the procedure.
- Avoid excessive movement, pulling or straining the arm on the side of the incision.
- If discharged before 24 hours, arrange for a care partner to bring you home. Do not drink alcohol or take any sedating drugs.

Care of the incision:

- Keep the protective steri-strips covering the incision dry and open to air. In most cases, no additional dressing is needed.
- Observe incision for signs of bleeding and/or infection; *i.e.,* swelling, increased pain, redness, any drainage, increased temperature, or opening of incision. If any occur, call *(insert phone number)* during work day and after hours call *(insert phone number)* to talk to the covering doctor on call.

24 HOURS THROUGH 2 WEEKS

Activities:

- Avoid any strenuous lifting, straining, housework and exercise with the arm on the side of the incision.
- Avoid any overhead/reaching motion to prevent dislodgement of the leads that have been placed in your heart.

Care of the incision:

- You may shower, lightly pat steri-strips/incision dry. Do not bathe, swim, or soak.
- Allow steri-strips to fall off on their own.
- Incision sutures will dissolve and do not require removal.
- Incision will usually heal over the first two weeks.

Continue to observe incision for signs of bleeding and/or infection as described above. If any occur, call *(insert phone number)* and after hours call *(insert phone number)* to talk to the covering doctor on call.

2 WEEKS THROUGH 6 WEEKS

- Avoid any exercise or repetitive movements that places significant strain on the affected side such as: swimming, golfing, tennis, etc., until the leads are well healed into place in your heart and the incision is healed completely.

MEDICAL FOLLOW UP

Pacemaker implants:

- Two weeks after implant, schedule an office visit at *(insert phone number)*.
- Ongoing Pacemaker follow-up usually includes office visits and telephone evaluation.

Defibrillator implants:

- Two weeks after implant, schedule an office visit at *(insert phone number)*.
- If your device delivers a shock, call the office at *(insert phone number)*.

If your device delivers multiple shocks, call 911 or the local emergency number for immediate assistance.

(Appendix B continued on next page)

APPENDIX B: PATIENT DISCHARGE INSTRUCTIONS *(CONTINUED)*

MEDICATIONS
Continue: all current medications

Coumadin: start_______mg on __________.
Then ____________________________________
New Medication(s): ________________________

Discontinue: _______________________________

Tylenol may be taken as needed for incisional pain.

Additional Instructions: ______________________________

I have received a copy of the above and understand the instructions.

__________________________________ ______________ ________________________________

Patient Signature Date MD/RN Signature

APPENDIX C: INVENTORY MANAGEMENT CHECKLIST

The materials checklist has been updated for the second edition of *Practical Electrophysiology*; however, please note that this checklist is only meant to be a guide for inventory management that could be applied to a new EP lab. Please recheck any descriptive items regarding any of the materials listed before any consideration.

GENERAL STORES

PAR Level		
_______	BX	PACEMAKER PACKS
_______	BX	ELECTROPHYSIOLOGY PKS
_______	BX	STERILE GOWNS
_______	BX	STERILE TOWEL PACK
_______	BX	UNIVERSAL LINEN PACK
_______	BG	ELECTRODE MONITORING FOAM - DOTS
_______	BX	OXISENSOR ADULTS - PULSE OX
_______	BX	SET ADM IV 96″ ADULT - IV TUBING
_______	CS	SHOE COVER LG
_______	CS	SHOE COVER LOW CUT POLY BLUE
_______	CS	BOUFFONT CAPS
_______	CS	SOL DEX 5% 100CC
_______	CS	SOL SOD CHL 0.9% 250CC
_______	CS	SOL SOD CHL 0.9% 500CC IRRIG PLASTIC CONTAINER
_______	CS	SOL SOD CHL 0.9% 500CC PLASTIC BAGS
_______	CS	REM ELECTRO SURG PADS - GROUNDING PAD
_______	BX	NEEDLE 18GA X 1″ REG BEVEL - PINK NEEDLE
_______	BX	TIPPOLISHER - SCRATCH PAD
_______	CS	BULB SYRINGE 50CC
_______	CS	YANKAUER SUCTION
_______	BX	ANGIOSET 22GA X 3/4″
_______	BX	ANGIOSET 20GA X 1″
_______	BX	ELASTOPLAST 3″
_______	BX	ELASTOPLAST 2″
_______	CS	PRESSURE MONITORING KIT
_______	CS	VAMP DIRECT DRAW
_______	CS	STERILE GAUZE 4X4 - INDIV PACKS

(Appendix C continued on next page)

APPENDIX C:

PAR Level		
________	BX	CLAVE CONNECTOR
________	CS	ELECTROSURGICAL HAND TOOL (BOVI)
________		CHLORAPREP 10.5 ML
________		CHLORAPREP 26 ML
________		PRESSURE BAGS IN 8000 VITAL SIGNS INC.
________	EA	SUTURE REMOVAL SET
________	BX	3CC SYRINGE C 22GA X 1 1/2 NEEDLE
________	CS	MAJOR BASINS - SURGICAL BOWLS
________	BX	STERISTRIP (1/2 X 4)
________	BX	10CC SYRINGE C OFFSET BEVEL
________	BX	2.0 SUTURE
________	BX	8 1/2 GLOVES
________	BX	8 GLOVES
________	BX	7 1/2 GLOVES
________	BX	7 GLOVES
________	BX	6 1/2 GLOVES
________	BX	NONSTERILE GLOVES - XLARGE
________	BX	NONSTERILE GLOVES - LG
________	BX	NONSTERILE GLOVES - MED
________	BX	NONSTERILE GLOVES - SM
________	CS	NEEDLE COUNTERS
________	CS	TEMP PACING KIT
________	CS	CENTRAL LINE INSERTION KIT
________	EA	PERICARDIOCENTESIS TRAY
________	BX	VACUTAINER BRAND LUER ADAPTER - BLUE ADAPTER (100/BX)
________	EA	BAER HUGGER
________	BX	SURESTEP GLUCOSE CONTROL SOLUTION - HIGH/LOW
________	BX	12ML SYRINGE 0.9% NAC1 FLUSH - 3ML FILL
________	BX	12ML SYRINGE 0.9% NAC1 FLUSH - 10ML FILL
________	CS	SURGICEL FIBRILLAR (10EA/CA)
________	EA	O2 MASK C TUBING
________	CS	SURGICAL MASK W/O SHIELD

APPENDIX C:

PAR Level		
________	BX	SURESTEP PRO TEST STRIPS
________	BX	BAG PLASTIC - SPECIMEN BIOHAZARD
________	CS	SOLUTION - 0.9% NAC1 - 100ML
________	BX	ID BAND GREEN - ANTICOAGULANT
________	BX	ID BAND RED - ALLERGY
________	BX	ID BAND BLUE
________	BX	TOURNIQUET
________	BX	INSULIN SYRINGE
________	BX	SURGICEL HEMOSTAT
________	BX	BAG - BIOHAZARD (RED BAG)
________	BX	4-0 SUTURE MONOCRYL UNDYED
________	EA	SEMICLOTH PLUS
________	BX	VACUTAINER BLOOD COLLECTION SET 23 3/4GA X 7 (367292)
________	BX	VACUTAINER - LAVENDER TOP (367861)
________	BX	VACUTAINER - 2.7ML - BLUE TOP (363083)
________	BX	VACUTAINER - 3.5ML - ORANGE TOP (367983)
________	BX	VACUTAINER - 10ML - LAVENDER TOP (366457)
________	BG	VACUTAINER ADAPTER
________	CS	SURGIKIT
________	BX	ANGIOCATH 20GA X 1 1/4
________	BX	ANGIOCATH 20GA X 2
________	BX	ANGIOCATH 22GA X 1
________	CS	BAG - PLASTIC PT BELONGING
________	CS	BAG - PLASTIC SOILED LINEN
________	CS	BANDAGE KLING 4" X 5" YARDS
________	BX	BANDAID ADHESIVE STRIP 3" X 1"
________	PK	BASIN EMESIS 9" DISP
________	EA	BATTERY 9 VOLT
________	EA	BATTERY AA
________	CS	BLADE #11
________	BX	BRUSH SCRUB W HIBICLENS
________	EA	CANNULA NASAL
________	CS	CAP DOCTOR SURG DISP
________	BX	DRESSING TEGADERM 2 3/8 X 2 3/4

(Appendix C continued on next page)

APPENDIX C:

PAR Level		
________	BX	DRESSING TEGADERM 4 X 4 3/4
________	PD	FORM CONTROLLED DRUG DISP REC
________	PD	FORM CONTROLLED DRUG REQ
________	PD	FORM LETTERHEAD WUH 8 1/2 X 11
________	PD	FORM PHARMACY STOCK MED SURG
________	PD	FORM REQ MERCHANDISE RETURN
________	PD	FORM SUPPLEMENTAL STOCK REQ
________	PK	LINER WALL SUCTION 1000CC
________	BX	MASK FACE C SHIELD/TIES
________	CS	PAPER WHITE 8 1/2 X 11
________	CS	PAPER WHITE 8 1/2 X 14
________	PT	PEROXIDE HYDROGEN
________	CS	RAZOR PREP
________	CS	SET INFUSION PUMP (IMED)
________	EA	SOLUTION BETADINE 4OZ
________	CS	SPONGE GAUZE 4 X 4 - 12 PLY NONSTERILE
________	CS	SPONGE RAYTEC 4 X 4 (XRAY) STERILE
________	BX	STOPCOCK 3 WAY PLASTIC
________	BX	3-0 SUTURE SILK
________	BX	SYRINGE 10CC
________	BX	SYRINGE 30CC
________	BX	SYRINGE 60CC
________	RL	TAPE DUROPORE 1″
________	RL	TAPE TRANSPORE 1″ X 10″
________	RL	TAPE TRANSPORE 3″ X 10″
________	PK	TISSUES 5 X 8
________	CS	TUBE SUCTION CONN 1/4 X 6
________	EA	URINAL C COVER DISPOSABLE
________	BX	WIPE ALCOHOL PREP 2 PLY MED
________	BX	WIPE - ADHESIVE REMOVER
________	BX	WIPE - SKIN PREP
________	BX	COVER PROBE - ALARIS P850A

APPENDIX C:

PAR
Level

Action
Knee crutch pads - 4340

Alaris
Disposable pulse covers - P840A, P850A

Allegiance
Mobile blood pressure cuff - ref# 7670-04
6734
209-58

Allegiance Healthcare/US Surgical
Oticron precut 3301-62 (22675)
Oticron GS-21 3090-61 (22676)
2-0 suture (in house)
3-0 GS-22 CL829 (22677)
4-0 V-20 GLS-321 (22678)
4-0 Y-426 (in house)
3-0 Silk 224 st. (82848)

Allegiance Healthcare
10 ml offset bevel syringe
mfr# 305482

Allegiance Cardinal

Reg. Clipperhead	# 1918 - case
Spec. Clipperhead	2823 - case
Clippers	39482

ALM
Surgical lighthandle cover - 50258
32951

Amersham (718-193)
Omnipaque 50cc - Y352 (1734)
Omniscan 20cc - J140 (13917)

Armatec Medical
C-arm mobile x-ray drape - AR9951
(104x88 cm) - really big garbage bags (2423)

Arrow (Stepi c Medical)
Cath set fem. Artery
Temp Pacing Catheter c shrouded pins Intr. Kit - A1-07155-KS (21643)

(Appendix C continued on next page)

APPENDIX C:

PAR
Level

Bard

Catheters:

Woven-cnd	- 200574 (04239)
Woven-joseph	- 200624 (04240)
Woven-cnd/deca	- 200355 (23986) (listed as 677)
Dynamic deca	- 201101
Dynamic XT	- 201104
EPXT/8 elect	- 200794 (1427)
Orbiter PV	- 320100 (20765)
Orbiter-st Sml	- 320002 (0120)
Orbiter-st Lg	- 320001 (0119)
Stinger-m F	- 210006m (04352)
DynamicTip-deca	- 6DYNXT002 (23985) (listed as 677)

Cables:

Orbiter PV cable	- 390004P (0123)
Woven-easymate/4	- 200088P (2476)
Woven-deca/10	- ref# 24040 cat# 006590P (24040)
EPXT cable/4	- 200088P (2476)
EPXT cable/8	- 200774P (1461)
Orbiter st cable/24	- 390004P (0123)
Dynamic tip-deca cable	- ref# 24039 cat# 560004P (24039)
Woven josephson Viking soft	- 400504 (677)
cable	- 560002P

Basic instrument tray for cutdown, thoracotomy, thoracentesis, and paracentesis

Ref# MN 52755

Biosense Webster

Lasso/variable	- mfr cat.# D7L202515RT ref# 35T2515R (23987)
Lasso cable	- C6MRMST10SA (0130)

Boston Scientific

Catheters:

Explorer	- 5481 (04280)
Polaris	- 5571 (20296)
Blazer II 6 fr lg	- 5601TK2 (24244)
7 fr sml	- 5031TK1 (24245)
std	- 5031T (20397), 5031TH (#22487)
lg	- 5031TK2 (22650) (677)
xd	- 5031TL (18573)
8 fr sml	- 5086TK1
std	- 5086th
lg	- 5086TK2
xd	- 5086TL

Steelcore 18" guidewire 190cm	- 1003281
Steelcore	- 1003282
Floppy II guidewire 14"/190cm	- 22339M (6648)

APPENDIX C:

PAR
Level

Boston Scientific

Catheters:

Blazer II XP	4500THK2 (24057)
(M004T)	4500TH2
	4500THMK2 (22647)
	4770TH
	4770THM (8771) (677)
	4790THK2 (24243)
	4790THMK2 (22999)
	4500TH (M0044500TH0)
Ultra Ice	9900/M00499000 (21654)
Chilli II/std	- M00490310 (21668)
lg	- M0049031K20 (21669)
Assym	- M0049031N40
Chilli cable	- M004620620 (21672)

Chilli tubing kit	- 2104/m0043521040 (22672)
Fluid dock	- M00499151/9915 (23140)
Convoy Adv Delivery Intr.	- 5662ST/m0045662ST0 (22997)

EPT junction box 1000XP - 822T (25673)

Cables:

Explorer cable	- M0045446S
Polaris cable	- M0045444S
APM to EGM Junction box cable	- 653S (11741)
Thermistor cable	- 651 (M0046510) (04451)
Nontemp cable	- 652 (M0046520) (04301)

Boston Sci/Meditech

Angled guidewire .035/150	- 46151-B
Straight guidewire .035/150	- 46155
Terumo catheter exchange (long) .035/260m	- 46154

Boston Sci/Irvine Biomed

Inquiry Luma cath 7fr XL	- 81961
L	- 81938
6 fr L	- 81960

CardioMedical Products

Hemochron ACT tubes (50/bx)	HRFTCA510 (7564)
(95/bx)	HRFTKACT (20234)

CathEffects

Vector cath	- DVMC-120-4 (23589)
Vector cable	- DVCC-245-5 (23590)

(Appendix C continued on next page)

APPENDIX C:

PAR
Level

Cook

Micropuncture set	- MP1S-501 (04147)
Guidewire .035/145	- TSCF-35-145-3 (04150)
	- THSCF-35-145-3-AES
.032/145	- TSCF-32-145-3
	- THSCF-32-145-3-AES
.032/180	- TSCF-32-180-3 (23907)
	- THSCF-32-180-3-AES
.032/260	- TSCF-32-260-3
	- THSCF-32-26-3-AES
Pericardiocentesis Set	- C-PCS-830-LOCK

Daig/St. Jude

Introducers:

8.5 fr Agilis steerable	- 408304 (21671)
8.5 fr Agilis NXT - 71cm med. Crl	- 408310 (24619)
7fr Fastcath lockdown	- 406702 (13476)
5fr Fastcath	- 406100 (13477)
6fr	- 406104 (8840)
7fr	- 406108 (14680)
8fr	- 406112 (8078)
9fr	- 406116 (13331)
10fr	- 406120 (22150)
5fr Fastcath 23cm long	- 406820
6fr	- 406139
7fr	- 406107
8fr	- 406142
9fr	- 406194
6fr Peelaway 14cm	- 405104
7fr	- 405108 (5959)
9fr	- 405116 (5764)
10fr	- 405120 (15097)
10.5fr	- 405122 (8174)
11fr	- 405124 (5763)
7fr Peelaway 23cm long	- 405269
9fr	- 405254 (20354)
11fr	- 405258
12fr	- 406184
8fr SRO 60cm	- 406820 (22491)
63cm	- 406844 (22151) (677)
81cm	- 407404 (24457)
SR1 63cm	- 406845
8fr SR2	
Ramp	- 406898 (1518)
Sept 60cm	- 406885
SL1 62cm	- 406806 (22152)
81cm	- 407400 (24456)

APPENDIX C:

PAR
Level

Daig/St. Jude

Transeptal Introducers:
10fr Fastcath 60cm - 406901
Lamp 45° Introducer - 407362

Transeptal Needle:
Brk-adult 71cm - 407200 (22492)
89cm - 407205 (24455)
98cm - 407206 (24588)
Brk-1-adult 71cm - 407201 (22493)

Catheters:
Response-5fr - 401222 (04335)
6fr - 401226 (5722)
Pacel-5f - 401762 (04350) (677)
Dec med swp-5f - 401940 (04267)
6fr - 401575
Dec xl crl-6fr - 401915
Duo dec splgcl-7fr - 401904 (20339)
Response-6fr-csl 65cm - 401400 (23348)
120cm - 401392 (23349)
Response Spiral 20cm sm crl-7fr - 402804 (24587)

Safire - 7f/8mm-std - 402839
7fr/8mm-lg - 402840
7fr/4mm-lg - 402811
7fr/4mm-med - 402810

Cables:
Quad 150cm red - 401975
Gy - 401973 (04357)
Bl - 401974 (04336)
Dec 210cm Bk - 401976
20pole spiral cable 150cm Bk - 401661 (24620)

Ethicon (Johnson & Johnson)

Surgiflo - 1991 (40378)
(6ea/bx/cs)

Ethicon (Johnson & Johnson)

Sutures:
VicrylPlus
3.0 - VCP285G
2.0 - VCP259H
3.05H - VCP416H

Vicryl
4.0 - VCP426H
3.0 - VCP232H
(CT-2)

(Appendix C continued on next page)

APPENDIX C:

PAR
Level

Ethicon (Johnson & Johnson)
MonocrylPlus
4.0 - MCP426H
ø silk - 624H

Ethibond
ø sh - X834H
ø CT-1 - X424H
ø percent - X186H

Fingerstick Lancet - 50501

GE
B&W Printing pack-mavigraph(8.5x11) - E8310JG (6223)
(lab1 & 3) - UPC-7021A

GE Healthcare
Quick straps - E6424GK
rolls - 24801

GE Marquette
ECG cable - 2003420-001
ECG leadwires - 2003425-001 (22738)
Instant Print media OEC - E910BP (8.5x10 blue base) not used anymore (04310)
Stim.Input cable 3ft. - 301-00204-03 (amplifier cable)
Pressure cables - 8966 00021 P0250

GE Medical Systems
Arm board - E6412DA
Optical disc 2.6GB - 2003888-001 (22737) Marquette
Fiber optic cable
Prucka keyboard - 2003809-002

GE OEC Med.System-SONY
Blue thermal transparent film MFR# 88-390115-00 (EP2) (22481)
9800+c-arm PO# MK232472
Req# 124694

HP
Toner - Q5949A (21613)
Laserjet toner - C8061Xcc (04197)
Laserjet toner - C4096A (19343)

KOL BIO-Medical
RADPAD - 2214 (20338)

Lynn Medical
CD-R's (100/cs) - Cat# 7MM0A (22673)
- PO# MK291115
148074

APPENDIX C:

PAR
Level

Medex

20″ ext tubing set	- MX450FL (04146)
3 way stopcock	- MX43132
3 way stopcock c MLL	- MX4313L (94355)
3 way stopcock c luerlock	- MX4311L

Medline

Sterile camera laser arm drape 7″x96″	- DYNJE4200
9″x96″	- DYNJE4300 (18164)

Medtronic (Physio-Control)

O2 SAT Sensor cable-LIFEPACK	- DEC-8
ECG paper-LIFEPACK	- 805319-05 (23248)
MDT Massimo Pulse Ox probes (LIFEPACK)	- 11171-000007
Convertors for LIFEPACK	- 11996-000184
Quick combo defib pads	- 11996-000091 (04281)
Internal paddle handles	- 11131-000001
Adult internal defib paddles	- 805355-13 (16332)
Temp pacing cable	- 5433V (12054)
Mdt RFA cable	- 05328

Medtronic

Cougar wire	- CGRXT190HJ (22701)
Fusion wire	- NTLPLJ180 (0116)
Rf Contactr	- 70257533 (202120)
TempTransvenous Pacing System	- 6416-140cm
Templink Extension cable-M	- 210061M (MDT/Bard RFA ext cable) (24145)

Safesheaths:

7fr	- 808700 (23926)
8fr	- 808800 (24670)
9fr	- 808900 (23927)
10fr	- 808100 (24266)
10.5fr	- 808150
11fr	- 808110
12fr	- 808120
12.5fr	- 808125

Mullins Transeptal Introducer-8fr	- ref# EP008591 cat#008552 (24042)
c-valve 8f	- cat# PC08591

Namic

72″ Press. Monitoring line	- 90701722 (3714)
Morse Angio manifold - med pressure	- 70039301 (19447)
Custom AngioKit - collection bag	- 60140233 (3386)
Contrast Injection line - 48″	- 91051482 (14065)
Angiogr. Control Syringe 10cc	- 70085003 (25359)
Morse stopcock - classic	- 70015003

(Appendix C continued on next page)

APPENDIX C:

PAR
Level

Pilling
Beckman Alson Retractors - 165400

7fr safesheath - HLS-1007 (04284)

Pleurovac
Chest drainage ref# A-6000-08LF

Pressure Products

9fr SafeSheath	- HLS-1009 (04238)
10fr SafeSheath	- HLS-1010 (22490)
6fr SafeSheath	- HLS-1006 (23917)
10.5fr SafeSheath	- HLS-1010.5 (4753)
7fr SafeSheath long	- HLS-2507 (22674)
8fr SafeSheath long	- HLS-2508
9fr SafeSheath long	- HLS-2509
11fr SafeSheath long	- HLS-1011

Sealing Adapter - SS-SA-09mm (17362)

Protech Proguard
Radiation Reducing glove - 0498
Size 7 Model RR-1

Sherwood Medical
Genius First temp - 3000A
Tympanic Thermometer

Siemens
ACUSON AcuNav catheter - 08267996

Spectrum
Acuson catheter cover - 956933

St. Jude Medical
EnSite catheter - EC1000 (04283)
NavX patch kit - EN0010 (22386)
Optical disc - 44-02655-001

State of the Art Medical Products
Microlite 8 protective lead goggles - Model FB108G

Sterimed
(bubble bag)

Sterile disposable fluorocover cat no. 4440.332
44"x40" #7493

APPENDIX C:

PAR
Level

Terumo (Medi-tech)
Angled Terumo (.035/150) - GR3506 (2392)

US Surgical (Valleylab)
Electrosurgical pencil c suction tubing (25/cs) - E2516HS (9151)

Vascular Solutions
Hemostat D-Stat Flowable #24843

APPENDIX D: DEPARTMENT OF ELECTROPHYSIOLOGY ACT RECORD

Please note the frequency of ACT measurements has been changed since the previous edition of *Practical Electrophysiology*. The frequency has increased from every 30 minutes to every 20 minutes.

PATIENT NAME____________________ EP MD____________

DATE________________ RN________________________

BASELINE TIME __________ HEPARIN 5000 U IVP____________

BASELINE ACT __________

Then at

20 minutes	______	ACT______	ACTION / RN__________
40 minutes	______	ACT______	ACTION / RN__________
60 minutes	______	ACT______	ACTION / RN__________
80 minutes	______	ACT______	ACTION / RN__________
100 minutes	______	ACT______	ACTION / RN__________
120 minutes	______	ACT______	ACTION / RN__________
140 minutes	______	ACT______	ACTION / RN__________
160 minutes	______	ACT______	ACTION / RN__________
180 minutes	______	ACT______	ACTION / RN__________
200 minutes	______	ACT______	ACTION / RN__________
220 minutes	______	ACT______	ACTION / RN__________
240 minutes	______	ACT______	ACTION / RN__________

NOTES/

Glossary

Ablation: The removal of a body part or destruction of its function through surgical excision. In electrophysiology, ablation means to focally destroy or eliminate a specified area of the myocardium.

Action potential: A rapid change in the membrane potential of an excitable cell, caused by stimulus triggers and selective opening and closing of voltage-sensitive gates in sodium- and potassium-ion channels.

Anterograde: Occurring in the normal or forward direction of conduction or flow, and as it relates to the heart, movement from the atrium to the ventricle.

Antibiotic: A substance, such as penicillin or streptomycin, produced by certain fungi, bacteria, and other organisms or a semisynthetic substance derived from a microorganism, that is able (in a diluted solution) to inhibit or kill another microorganism.

Antihistamine: A medicine used to treat allergies and hypersensitive reactions and colds; works by counteracting the effects of histamine in a receptor site.

Arrhythmia: Any variation from the normal rhythm or rate of the heartbeat.

Atrial fibrillation: Disorder of cardiac rhythm characterized by rapid, irregular atrial impulses and ineffective atrial contractions.

Atrium: A body cavity or chamber, especially of the upper chambers of the heart, that receives blood from the veins and forces it into a ventricle. Also called *auricle*.

Atrial flutter: Rapid, irregular atrial contractions due to an abnormality of atrial excitation. This is a more organized rhythm than atrial fibrillation.

Automaticity: The leakage of ions across the cell membrane during the resting phase, causing a gradual, positively directed change in transmembrane voltage, leading to spontaneous depolarization.

Biventricular pacing: see *Cardiac resynchronization therapy.*

Bradycardia: Excessive slowness in the action of the heart, usually with a heart rate below 60 beats per minute.

Breastbone: see *Sternum.*

Bruit: Any of several generally abnormal sounds heard on auscultation.

Cardiac resynchronization therapy (CRT): A form of therapy for congestive heart failure refractory to drug therapy that uses a specialized pacemaker and/or implantable defibrillator to help coordinate and optimize the contraction of the right and left ventricles. Also called *biventricular pacing.*

Cardiopulmonary resuscitation (CPR): An emergency procedure, often employed after cardiac arrest, in which cardiac massage, artificial respiration, and drugs are used to restore the circulation of oxygenated blood to the heart, brain, and other organs.

Catheter: A hollow, flexible tube for insertion into a body cavity, duct, or vessel to allow the passage of fluids or distend a passageway. Its uses include the drainage of urine from the bladder through the urethra or insertion through a blood vessel into the heart for diagnostic and/or therapeutic purposes.

Catheter ablation: Removal of tissue with electrical current delivered via electrodes positioned at the distal end of a catheter. Energy sources include radiofrequency energy and/or cryothermia (freezing tissue). The technique is used to treat supraventricular and ventricular tachycardias.

Chordae tendineae: Fibrous strands that are attached to the valves and to papillary muscles on the ventricular walls.

Congestive heart failure: A complication of heart diseases; defective cardiac filling and/or impaired contraction and emptying, resulting in the heart's inability to pump a sufficient amount of blood to meet the needs of the body tissues or to be able to do so only with an elevated filling pressure.

Coronary sinus vein: A venous channel that is derived from the sinus venosus, is continuous with the largest of the cardiac veins, receives most of the blood from the walls of the heart, and empties into the right atrium.

Coronary sulcus: The groove separating the atria and the ventricles.

Coronary system: The circulation of blood through the veins and arteries of the heart, which allow for the exchange of nutrients and oxygen within the heart.

Crash cart: A transportable cart with standard emergency medical equipment and intubation tools necessary in cases of emergency.

CRT: see *Cardiac resynchronization therapy.*

Cryoablation: The removal of a body part or tissue or destruction of its function through freezing.

Cusp: A triangular fold or flap of a heart valve; also called *leaflets.*

Defibrillator: An electronic device that administers an electric shock of preset voltage to the heart through the chest wall in an attempt to restore the normal rhythm of the heart during ventricular fibrillation.

Depolarization: Stimulation of the rapid sodium channels in the cell membrane that causes them to open, resulting in a rapid increase in transmembrane potential, viewed as a voltage spike.

Diabetic acidosis: Decreased pH and bicarbonate concentration in the body fluids caused by accumulation of ketone bodies in uncontrolled diabetes mellitus.

ECG: see *Electrocardiogram.*

Electrical conduction system: An impulse-conducting system composed of special cardiac muscle cells and having the power of spontaneous rhythmicity and conduction more highly developed than that of the rest of the heart.

Electrocardiogram (ECG): Recording of the voltages across the entire heart.

Electrophysiologist: One who studies electrophysiology.

Electrophysiology: The branch of cardiology that studies the electrical function of the heart, and in particular, heart rhythm disturbances.

Endocardium: The innermost layer of the heart, made of closely packed endothelial cells that provide a smooth surface for blood flow.

Eustachian valve: Valve of the inferior vena cava.

Excitable cells: Cells that can receive stimulus sequentially and stereotypically.

Fluoroscopy: Examination of an object, such as the human body, by exposing it to x-rays and observing the shadow cast upon a fluorescent screen.

Fulgurate: To destroy (abnormal tissue, for example) by electric current.

Hemoglobin: The protein in red blood cells that transports oxygen as oxyhemoglobin from the lungs to the tissues, where oxygen is readily released and the oxyhemoglobin becomes hemoglobin.

Hemostasis: The process that spontaneously arrests the flow of blood from vessels carrying blood under pressure, accomplished by contraction of the vessels, adhesion and aggregation of formed blood elements, and blood coagulation.

His bundle: Small band of specialized cardiac muscle fibers that originates in the atrioventricular node and extends into the membranous part of the interventricular septum; also called *bundle of His.*

Hypercholesterolemia: The presence of an abnormal amount of cholesterol in the cells and plasma of the blood; associated with the risk of atherosclerosis.

Hypertension: Persistently high arterial blood pressure; currently accepted threshold levels are 140 mmHg systolic and 90 mmHg diastolic pressure.

Hypertrophic cardiomyopathy: A myocardial disease characterized by hypertrophy (an increase in mass or girth), involving mainly the interventricular septum and interfering with left ventricular emptying (but might also include the entire heart).

Hypokalemia: An abnormally low concentration of potassium ions in the blood; also known as *hypopotassemia.*

Hypomagnesemia: An abnormally low level of magnesium in the blood.

Hyponatremia: An abnormally low concentration of sodium ions in the blood.

ICD: see *Implantable cardioverter-defibrillator.*

Iliac crest: The long, curved upper border of the wing of the ilium, or dorsal bone of the pelvis.

Implantable cardioverter-defibrillator (ICD): An implantable device that continuously monitors the electrical activity of the heart and automatically detects and terminates ventricular tachycardia and ventricular fibrillation; it consists of a pulse generator, batteries, and electrodes.

Incisura apicis cordis: A notch near the apex of the heart where the anterior and posterior longitudinal sulci join together.

Intracardiac pacing catheters: Standardly four-poled catheters; also called *quadripolar catheters.*

Intrahisian disease: Disease within the His bundle.

Interatrial groove: The groove separating the two atria in the heart.

Intravenous (IV): Within or administered into a vein.

Ischemia: Lack of blood flow and oxygen delivery to the heart, caused by a constriction or obstruction of its blood vessels.

Isthmus: A contracted anatomical part of passage connecting two larger structures or cavities.

IV: see *Intravenous.*

Leads: Conductors by which one circuit element is electrically connected to another.

Leaflets: see *Cusps.*

Lesion: Any visible abnormal structural change in a bodily part; any break in the skin or an organ caused by violence or surgical incision.

Lown-Ganong-Levine syndrome (LGL syndrome): A preexcitation syndrome characterized by atrial tachycardia together with a short PR interval and a QRS complex of normal duration.

Mines postulate: Hypothesized bidirectional conduction with unidirectional block being the cause of a reentrant arrhythmia.

Monomorphic: Having but a single form; retaining the same consistent form throughout a ventricular tachycardia.

Myocardial infarction: Gross necrosis of the myocardium, as a result of interruption of the blood supply to the area.

Myocardium: The muscle tissue of the heart composed of striated, involuntary muscle known as cardiac muscle; the heart.

Oximeter: A device for measuring the oxygen saturation of arterial blood.

Pacemaker: An electrical device for stimulating or steadying the heartbeat or reestablishing the rhythm of an arrested heart; also called a *pacer.*

Pacemaker-mediated tachycardia: A type of tachycardia that can occur in patients with a dual-chamber pacemaker, in which the device senses the retrograde atrial activity and conducts at the upper rate limit of the device.

Pacemaker syndrome: In which the effects of retrograde conduction are felt, usually by neck pounding or fatigue.

Palpitation: Irregular, rapid beating or pulsation of the heart.

Pectoral: Of or relating to a muscle or organ situated in the breast or the chest.

Percutaneous: Passed, done, or effected through unbroken skin.

Pericardium: The fibroserous sac surrounding the heart and the roots of the great vessels.

Permanent pacemaker: A device designed to stimulate, by electric impulses, contraction of the heart muscles. This device is implanted entirely within the body.

Pharmacotherapy: Treatment of disease through the use of drugs.

Pneumothorax: Accumulation of air or gas in the pleural cavity, as a result of disease or injury to the lung during a subclavian venous stick.

Polymorphic: Having or occurring in several distinct forms; the occurrence of difference forms, stages, or types. Ventricular fibrillation is polymorphic in nature.

Precordium: The part of the ventral surface of the body overlying the heart and the stomach and comprising the epigastrium and the lower median part of the thorax.

Preexcitation: Premature activation of part or all of the cardiac ventricle by an electrical impulse from the atrium that typically is conducted along an accessory pathway (as muscle fibers on the heart surface) bypassing the atrioventricular node and that may produce arrhythmias; is characteristic of Wolff-Parkinson-White syndrome.

Pulmonary: Relating to, functioning like, or associated with the lungs.

Refractory period: The period of time following depolarization in which heart tissue fails to respond to a premature stimuli.

Repolarization: The process of getting the ions back to where they started after depolarization.

Resting phase: The period of time between the action potentials; no net movement of ions across the cell membrane.

Retrograde: To move, or seem to move, backward. Typically from the ventricle to the atrium.

Semilunar: The valves at the beginning of the aorta and the pulmonary artery, which prevent the blood from flowing back into the ventricle.

Septal: Of or relating to a septum or septa.

Septum: A thin partition or membrane that divides two cavities such as the atria or ventricles.

Sheath: An enveloping tubular structure; usually used to introduce a lead or catheter.

Sternum: A long, flat bone that is situated along the ventral midline of the thorax and articulates with the ribs; the manubrium of the sternum articulates with the clavicle; also called the *breastbone.*

Subclavian crush syndrome: In which pacemaker or defibrillator lead damage occurs due to pressure between the first rib and the clavicle. Typically the result of the lead placed via the subclavian venous approach.

Sulcus: A deep, narrow furrow or groove, as in an organ or a tissue.

Supraventricular tachycardia (SVT): Relating to or being a rhythmic abnormality of the heart caused by impulses originating above the ventricles (as in the atrioventricular node). Examples include atrial tachycardia and AV-node reentrant tachycardia.

SVT: see *Supraventricular tachycardia.*

Symphysis pubis: The rather rigid articulation of the two pubic bones in the midline of the lower anterior part of the abdomen; also called the *pubic symphysis.*

Syncope: A transient loss of consciousness and postural tone caused by diminished blood flow to the brain (brain ischemia); *presyncope* refers to the sensation of lightheadedness and loss of strength that precedes a syncopal event or accompanies an incomplete syncope.

Tachycardia: Abnormally rapid heart rate, typically greater than 100 beats per minute.

Thebesian valve: A valve of the coronary sinus.

Thoracic cavity: The region of the thorax that includes the pleural cavity and the mediastinum.

Threshold potential: The increase of voltage obtained by stimulus opening some of the sodium gates; the stimulus for all the sodium channels to be opened, and the start of depolarization.

Torsades de pointes: Ventricular tachycardia characterized by fluctuation of the QRS complexes around the electrocardiographic baseline and typically caused by a long QT interval.

Transmembrane potential: The voltage difference across the cell membrane between the inside of a cardiac cell, which has a negative electrical charge, and the outside of the cell, which has a positive charge; the resting transmembrane potential (which is -80 mV to -90 mV in cardiac muscle) is the result of an accumulation of negatively charged molecules (ions) within the cell.

Transseptal: Passing through a septum.

Trendelenburg: Tilting the head downward below the feet in order to enhance blood flow to the heart and brain.

Tricuspid valve: The atrioventricular valve on the right side of the heart.

Vasovagal syncope: A usually transitory condition marked by anxiety, nausea, respiratory distress, and fainting believed to be due to vasomotor and vagal disturbances; also called *vasodepressor syncope* or *neurocardiogenic syncope.*

Vaughn Williams classification of antiarrhythmic drugs: Classification of antiarrhythmic drugs proposed by Vaughn Williams that organizes drugs according to their effects on action potentials in individual cells.

Ventricle: A chamber of the heart that receives blood from the atrium and propels blood either to the lungs (right ventricle) or the body (left ventricle).

Ventricular fibrillation: Another often fatal (if left untreated) form of arrhythmia characterized by rapid, irregular fibrillar twitching of the ventricles of the heart in place of normal contractions, resulting in a loss of pulse.

Ventricular tachycardia: An abnormally rapid ventricular rhythm with wide QRS complexes, usually in excess of 120 beats per minute; it is generated within the ventricle, below the His bundle, and is most commonly associated with atrioventricular dissociation.

Wolff-Parkinson-White (WPW) syndrome: An electrocardiographic pattern sometimes associated with paroxysmal tachycardia, characterized by a short PR interval and a delta wave (slurred segment between the P wave and QRS complex).

Index

A

B

C

D

E

F

G

H

I

J

K

L

M

N

S

T

U

V

W

X

Y

Z

Bibliography

1. Abraham WT, Fisher WG, Smith AL, et al. Cardiac resynchronization in chronic heart failure. *N Engl J Med* 2002;346:1845–1853.

2. Aizawa Y, Chinushi M, Naitoh N, et al. Catheter ablation of ventricular tachycardia with radiofrequency currents, with special reference to the termination and minor morphologic change of reinduced ventricular tachycardia. *Am J Cardiol* 1995;76:574–579.

3. Akhtar M, Breithardt G, Camm AJ, et al. CAST and Beyond: Implications of the Cardiac Arrhythmia Suppression Trial. Task Force of the Working Group on Arrhythmias of the European Society of Cardiology. *Circulation* 1990;81:1123–1127.

4. Akhtar M, Shenasa M, Jazayeri M, et al. QRS complex tachycardia: Wide QRS complex tachycardia. Reappraisal of a common clinical problem. *Ann Intern Med* 1988;109:905–912.

5. Almquist A, Goldenberg IF, Milstein S, et al. Provocation of bradycardia and hypotension by isoproterenol and upright posture in patients with unexplained syncope. *N Engl J Med* 1989;320:346–351.

6. American Cancer Society, Inc., Surveillance Research, Cancer Facts and Figures, 2001.

7. American Heart Association. 2002 Heart and Stroke Statistical Update.

8. Aminoff MJ, Scheinman MM, Griffin JC, et al. Electrocerebral accompaniments of syncope associated with malignant ventricular arrhythmias. *Ann Intern Med* 1988;108:791–796.

9. Amiodarone vs. Sotalol Study Group. Multicentre randomized trial of sotalol vs. amiodarone for chronic malignant ventricular tachyarrhythmias. *Eur Heart J* 1989;10:685–694.

10. Anderson JL, Pritchett ELC. International symposium on supraventricular arrhythmias: Focus on flecainide. *Am J Cardiol* 1988;62:1D–67D.

11. Anderson KP, Walker R, Dustman T, et al. Rate-related electrophysiologic effects of long-term administration of amiodarone on

canine ventricular myocardium in vivo. *Circulation* 1989;79:948–958.

12. Antman EM, Beamer AD, Cantillon C, et al. Long-term oral propafenone therapy for suppression of refractory symptomatic atrial fibrillation and atrial flutter. *J Am Coll Cardiol* 1988;12:1005–1011. (Published erratum appears in *J Am Coll Cardiol* 1989;13:264.)

13. Antonaccio MJ, Gomoll AW. Sotalol—Pharmacological and antiarrhythmic effects. *Cardiovasc Drug Rev* 1988;6:239.

14. Antonelli D, Turgeman Y, Kaveh Z, et al. Short-term thrombosis after transvenous permanent pacemaker insertion. *Pacing Clin Electrophysiol* 1989;12:280–282.

15. Arnold AZ, Mick MJ, Mazurek RP, et al. Role of prophylactic anticoagulation for direct current cardioversion in patients with atrial fibrillation or atrial flutter. *J Am Coll Cardiol* 1992;19:851–855.

16. Atrial fibrillation follow-up investigation of rhythm management—The AFFIRM study design. The Planning and Steering Committees of the AFFIRM study for the NHLBI AFFIRM investigators. *Am J Cardiol* 1997;79:1198–1202.

17. Bacaner MB, Clay JR, Shrier A, Brochi RM. Potassium channel blockade: A mechanism for suppressing ventricular fibrillation. *Proc Natl Acad Sci* 1986;83:2223–2227.

18. Baddour LM, Bettmann MA, Bolger AF, et al. AHA Scientific Statement. Nonvalvular cardiovascular device–related infections. *Circulation* 2003;108:2015.

19. Bahnson TD. Catheter ablation of ventricular tachycardia late after myocardial infarction: Techniques, indications, and recent advances. *EP Lab Digest* 2003;3:24–30.

20. Bailie DS, Inoue H, Kaseda S, et al. Magnesium suppresses early afterdepolarizations and ventricular tachyarrhythmias induced by cesium in dogs. *Circulation* 1988;77:1395–1402.

21. Bardy GH, Ivey TD, Coltorti F, et al. Developments, complications and limitations of catheter-mediated electrical ablation of posterior accessory atrioventricular pathways. *Am J Cardiol* 1988;61:309–316.

22. Bardy GH, Lee KL, Mark DB, et al., and the Sudden Cardiac Death in Heart Failure Trial (SCD-HeFT) Investigators. Amiodarone or an implantable cardioverter-defibrillator for congestive heart failure. *N Engl J Med* 2005;352:225–237.

23. Barold SS, Schoenfeld MH. Pacemaker elective replacement indicators. *Pacing Clin Electrophysiol* 1989;12:990–995.

24. Barold SS, Wyndham CR, Kappenberger L, et al. Implanted atrial pacemakers for paroxysmal atrial flutter. Long-term efficacy. *Ann Intern Med* 1987;107:144–149.

25. Bartecchi CE. Temporary pacing catheter electrodes. In Bartecchi CE and Mann DE (eds). *Temporary Cardiac Pacing.* Chicago: Precept Press, Inc., 1990, p.168.

26. Bauer LA, Black D, Gensler A, Sprinkle J. Influence of age, renal function and heart failure on procainamide clearance and N-acetylprocainamide serum concentrations. *Int J Clin Pharmacol Ther Toxicol* 1989;27:213–216.

27. Belardinelli L, Berne RM. The cardiac effects of adenosine. *Prog Cardiovasc Dis* 1989;32:73–97.

28. Belhassen B, Glick A, Laniado S. Comparative clinical and electrophysiologic effects of adenosine triphosphate and verapamil on paroxysmal reciprocating junctional tachycardia. *Circulation* 1988;77:795–805.

29. Belardinelli L, Pelleg A. Cardiac electrophysiology and pharmacology of

adenosine. *J Cardiovasc Electrophysiol* 1990;1:327.

30. Berger MD, Waxman HL, Buxton AE, et al. Spontaneous compared with induced onset of sustained ventricular tachycardia. *Circulation* 1988;78:885–892.

31. Bernstein AD, Camm AJ, Fletcher RD, et al. The NASPE/BPEG generic pacemaker code for antibradyarrhythmias and adaptive-rate pacing and antitachyarrhythmia devices. *Pacing Clin Electrophysiol* 1987;10:794–799.

32. Bharati S, Lev M. *Cardiac Conduction System in Unexplained Sudden Death.* Mt. Kisco, NY: Futura Publishing Company, 1990.

33. Bharati S, Lev M. Histopathologic changes in the heart including the conduction system after catheter ablation. *Pacing Clin Electrophysiol* 1989;12:159–169.

34. Bianconi L, Boccadamo R, Pappalardo A, et al. Effectiveness of intravenous propafenone for conversion of atrial fibrillation and flutter of recent onset. *Am J Cardiol* 1989;64:335–338.

35. Bigger JT Jr, Sahar DI. Clinical types of proarrhythmic response to antiarrhythmic drugs. *Am J Cardiol* 1987;59:2E–9E.

36. Bigger JT Jr. The events surrounding the removal of encainide and fecainide for the Cardiac Arrhythmias Suppression Trial (CAST) and why CAST is continuing with moricizine. *J Am Coll Cardiol* 1990;15:243–245.

37. Billman GE, Hoskins RS. Time-series analysis of heart rate variability during sub maximal exercise. Evidence for reduced cardiac vagal tone in animals susceptible to ventricular fibrillation. *Circulation* 1989;80:146–157.

38. Blackburn T, Dunn M. Pacemaker-induced superior vena cava syndrome. Consideration of management. *Am Heart J* 1988;116:893–896.

39. Blomström-Lundqvist C, Scheinman MM, et al. ACC/AHA/ESC guidelines for the management of patients with supraventricular arrhythmias—executive summary: A report of the American College of Cardiology/American Heart Association Task Force on Practice Guidelines and the European Society of Cardiology Committee for Practice Guidelines (Writing Committee to Develop Guidelines for the Management of Patients With Supraventricular Arrhythmias). *Circulation* 2003;108:1871-1909.

40. Bocka JJ. External transcutaneous pacemakers. *Ann Emerg Med* 1989;18:1280–1286.

41. Boineau JP, Canavan TE, Schuessler RB, et al. Demonstration of a widely distributed atrial pacemaker complex in the human heart. *Circulation* 1988;77:1221–1237.

42. Borggrefe M, Breithardt G, Podozeck A, et al. Catheter ablation of ventricular tachycardia using defibrillator pulses: Electrophysiological findings and long-term results. *Eur Heart J* 1989;10:591–601.

43. Borggrefe M, Hindricks G, Haverkamp W, et al. Radiofrequency ablation. In Zipes DP, Jalife J (eds). *Cardiac Electrophysiology: From Cell to Bedside.* Philadelphia, PA: W. B. Saunders Company, 1990, p.997.

44. Borggrefe MM, Lawo T, Butter C, et al. Randomized, double blind study of non-excitatory, cardiac contractility modulation electrical impulses for symptomatic heart failure. *Eur Heart J* 2008;29:1019-1028.

45. Borggrefe M, Trampisch HJ, Breithardt G. Reappraisal of criteria for assessing drug efficacy in patients with ventricular tachyarrhythmias: Complete versus partial suppression of inducible

arrhythmias. *J Am Coll Cardiol* 1988;12:140–149.

46. Boudoulas H, Kolibash AJ Jr, Baker P, et al. Mitral valve prolapse and the mitral valve prolapse syndrome: A diagnostic classification and pathogenesis of symptoms. *Am Heart J* 1989;118:796–818.

47. Brandt J, Fahraeus T, Schuller H. Rate adaptive atrial pacing (AAIR). Clinical aspects. In Barold SS, Mugica J (eds). *New Perspectives in Cardiac Pacing.* 2. Mt. Kisco, NY: Futura Publishing Co., 1991, p.303.

48. Braunwald E, Zipes DP, Libby P, Bonow R. *Braunwald's Heart Disease, 7th edition.* Philadelphia: W. B. Saunders Company, 2004.

49. Breithardt G, Borggrefe M, Karbenn U, Schwarzmaier J. Effects of pharmacological and non-pharmacological interventions on ventricular late potentials. *Eur Heart J* 1987;8(Suppl A):97–104.

50. Breithardt G, Borggrefe M, Martinez-Rubio A, Podczeck A. Signal averaging. *Prog Cardiol* 1988;257.

51. Bristow MR, Saxon LA, Boehmer J, et al. Cardiac-resynchronization therapy with or without an implantable defibrillator in advanced chronic heart failure. *N Engl J Med* 2004;350:2140–2150.

52. Brodsky MA, Allen BJ, Capparelli EV, et al. Factors determining maintenance of sinus rhythm after chronic atrial fibrillation with left atrial dilatation. *Am J Cardiol* 1989;63:1065–1068.

53. Brodsky MA, Allen BJ, Luckett CR, et al. Antiarrhythmic efficacy of solitary beta-adrenergic blockade for patients with sustained ventricular tachyarrhythmias. *Am Heart J* 1989;118:272–280.

54. Bromberg BI, Dick M II, Scott WA, Morady F. Transcatheter electrical ablation of accessory pathways in children. *Pacing Clin Electrophysiol* 1989;12:1787–1796.

55. Brooks R, Garan H, McGovern BA, Ruskin JN. The automatic implantable cardioverter/defibrillator. In Braunwald E (ed). *Heart Disease: A Textbook of Cardiovascular Medicine, 3rd edition.* Philadelphia: W. B. Saunders Company. Update No. 9, 1990, p.193.

56. Brooks R, Garan H, Ruskin JN. Evaluation of the patient with unexplained syncope. In Zipes DP, and Jalife J (eds). *Cardiac Electrophysiology: From Cell to Bedside.* Philadelphia, PA: W. B. Saunders Company, 1990, p.646.

57. Brugada P, deSwart H, Smeets JL, Wellens HJ. Transcoronary chemical ablation of ventricular tachycardia. *Circulation* 1989;79:475–482.

58. Brugada P, Talajic M, Smeets J, et al. The value of the clinical history to assess prognosis of patients with ventricular tachycardia or ventricular fibrillation after myocardial infarction. *Eur Heart J* 1989;10:747–752.

59. Buja GF, Nava A, Martini B, et al. Right ventricular dysplasia: A familial cardiomyopathy? *Eur Heart J* 1989;10(Suppl. D):13–15.

60. Burkart F, Pfisterer M, Kiowski W, et al. Improved survival of patients with asymptomatic ventricular arrhythmias after myocardial infarction with amiodarone: A randomized controlled trial. *Circulation* 1989;80(Suppl. II):II119.

61. Buxton AE. Ongoing risk stratification trials: The primary prevention of sudden death. *Control Clin Trials* 1996;17:47S–51S.

62. Buxton AE, Fisher JD, Josephson ME, et al. Prevention of sudden death in patients with coronary artery disease: The Multicenter Unsustained Tachycardia Trial

(MUSTT). *Prog Cardiovasc Dis* 1993;36:215–226.

63. Buxton AE, Lee KL, Fisher JD, et al., for the Multicenter Unsustained Tachycardia Trial Investigators. A randomized study of the prevention of sudden death in patients with coronary artery disease. *N Engl J Med* 1999;341:1882–1890.

64. Buxton AE, Marchlinski FE, Flores BT, et al. Nonsustained ventricular tachycardia in patients with coronary artery disease: Role of electrophysiologic study. *Circulation* 1987;75:1178–1185.

65. Buxton AE, Simson MB, Falcone RA, et al. Results of signal-averaged electrocardiography and electrophysiologic study in patients with nonsustained ventricular tachycardia after healing of acute myocardial infarction. *Am J Cardiol* 1987;60:80–85.

66. Byrd CL, Schwartz SJ, Gonzales M, et al. DDD pacemakers maximize hemodynamic benefits and minimize complications for most patients. *Pacing Clin Electrophysiol* 1988;11:1911–1916.

67. Caceres J, Jazayeri M, McKinnie J, et al. Sustained bundle branch reentry as a mechanism of clinical tachycardia. *Circulation* 1989;79:256–270.

68. Calkins H, Brugada J, Packer DL, et al. HRS/EHRA/ECAS expert Consensus Statement on catheter and surgical ablation of atrial fibrillation: recommendations for personnel, policy, procedures and follow-up. A report of the Heart Rhythm Society (HRS) Task Force on catheter and surgical ablation of atrial fibrillation. *Heart Rhythm* 2007;4:816-861.

69. Calkins H, Kim Y, Schmaltz S, et al. Electrogram criteria for identification of appropriate target sites for radiofrequency catheter ablation of accessory atrioventricular connections. *Circulation* 1992;85:565–573.

70. Calkins H, Sousa J, el-Atassi R, et al. Diagnosis and cure of the Wolff-Parkinson-White syndrome or paroxysmal supraventricular tachycardias during a single electrophysiologic test. *N Engl J Med* 1991;324:1612–1618.

71. Camm AJ, Davies DW, Ward DE. Tachycardia recognition by implantable electronic devices. *Pacing Clin Electrophysiol* 1987;10:1175–1190.

72. Camm AJ, Lau CP. Syncope of undetermined origin: Diagnosis and management. *Prog Cardiol* 1988;1:139–156.

73. Cannom DS, Winkle RA. Implantation of the automatic implantable cardioverter defibrillator (AICD): Practical aspects. *Pacing Clin Electrophysiol* 1986;9:793–809.

74. Capparelli EV, Kluger J, Regnier JC, Chow MS. Clinical and electrophysiologic effects of flecainide in patients with refractory ventricular tachycardia. *J Clin Pharmacol* 1988;28:268–275.

75. Cardinal R, Janse MJ, van Eeden I, et al. The effects of lidocaine on intracellular and extracellular potentials, activation, and ventricular arrhythmias during acute regional ischemia in the isolated porcine heart. *Circ Res* 1981;49:792–806.

76. Chakko S, de Marchena E, Kessler KM, Myerburg RJ. Ventricular arrhythmias in congestive heart failure. *Clin Cardiol* 1989;12:525–530.

77. Chang MS, Zipes DP. Differential sensitivity of sinus node, atrioventricular node, atrium, and ventricle to propranolol. *Am Heart J* 1988;116:371–378.

78. Charos GS, Haffajee CI, Gold RL, et al. A theoretically and practically more effective method for interruption of ventricular tachycardia: Self-adapting autodecremental overdrive pacing. *Circulation*

1986;73:309–315.

79. Chen MY, Goldenberg IF, Milstein S, et al. Cardiac electrophysiologic and hemodynamic correlates of neurally mediated syncope. *Am J Cardiol* 1989;63:66–72.

80. Chung ES, Leon AR, Tavazzi L, et al. Results of the Predictors of Response to CRT (PROSPECT) trial. *Circulation* 2008;117:2608-2616.

81. Cleland JG, Daubert JC, Erdmann E, et al; the Cardiac Resynchronization-Heart Failure (CARE-HF) Study Investigators. The effect of cardiac resynchronization on morbidity and mortality in heart failure. *N Engl J Med* 2005;352:1539–1549.

82. Clinical competence in invasive cardiac electrophysiological studies. ACP/ACC/AHA Task Force on Clinical Privileges in Cardiology. *J Am Coll Cardiol* 1994;23:1258–1261.

83. Coggins DL, Randall JL, Sweeney J, et al. Radiofrequency catheter ablation as a cure for idiopathic tachycardia of both left and right ventricular origin. *J Am Coll Cardiol* 1994;23:1333–1341.

84. Cohen MB, Snow JS, Grasso V, et al. Efficacy of pindolol for treatment of vasovagal syncope. *Am Heart J* 1995;130:786–790.

85. Cohen TJ. Results of the COMPANION trial—Another breakthrough in electrophysiology. *J Invasive Cardiol* 2003;15:171.

86. Cohen TJ. QT dispersion: A simple and cheap method for predicting ventricular tachycardia susceptibility. *J Invasive Cardiol* 1997;9:39.

87. Cohen TJ, Zadeh H, Fruauff A, Klein J. Arrhythmogenic right ventricular dysplasia and the implantable cardioverter-defibrillator: A case report and review of the literature. *J Invasive Cardiol* 2000;12:422–424.

88. Cohen TJ, Chien WW, Lurie KG, et al. Radiofrequency catheter ablation for treatment of bundle branch reentrant ventricular tachycardia: Results and long-term follow-up. *J Am Coll Cardiol* 1991;18:1767–1773.

89. Cohen TJ, Goldner BG, Jadonath R, et al. Development of an interactive computer-guided method for radiofrequency catheter ablation of ventricular tachycardia. *Pacing Clin Electrophysiol* 1996;19[Pt.I]:472–476.

90. Cohen TJ, Liem LB. A hemodynamically responsive antitachycardia system. Development and basis for design in humans. *Circulation* 1990;82:394–406.

91. Cohen TJ, Noubani H, Goldner BG, et al. Active compression-decompression provides effective defibrillation during cardiopulmonary resuscitation. *Am Heart J* 1995;130:186–187.

92. Cohen TJ, Tucker KJ, Abbott JA, et al. Usefulness of adenosine in augmenting ventricular preexitation for noninvasive localization of accessory pathways. *Am J Cardiol* 1992;69:1178–1185.

93. Cohen TJ, Quan C, Ibrahim B, et al. A blind comparison of four non-invasive twelve-lead electrocardiogram algorithms for predicting susceptibility to ventricular tachycardia. *J Invasive Cardiol* 2002;14:535–540.

94. Cohen TJ. Innovative emergency defibrillation methods for refractory ventricular fibrillation in a variety of hospital settings. *Am Heart J* 1993;126:962–968.

95. Cohen TJ, Liem LB. A hemodynamic responsive antitachycardia system. Development and basis for design in humans. *Circulation* 1990;82:394–406.

96. Colatsky TJ. Mechanisms of action of lidocaine and quinidine on action potential duration in rabbit cardiac Purkinje fibers. An effect on steady state sodium currents?

Circ Res 1982;50:17–27.

97. Colavita PG, Packer DL, Pressley JC, et al. Frequency, diagnosis and clinical characteristics of patients with multiple accessory atrioventricular pathways. *Am J Cardiol* 1987;59:601–606.

98. Connolly SJ, Gent M, Roberts RS, et al. Canadian Implantable Defibrillator Study (CIDS): A randomized trial of the implantable cardioverter defibrillator against amiodarone. *Circulation* 2000;101:1297–1302.

99. Cooper MJ, Hunt LJ, Palmer KJ, et al. Quantitation of day to day variability in mode of induction of ventricular tachyarrhythmias by programmed stimulation. *J Am Coll Cardiol* 1988;11:101–108.

100. Cooper MJ, Hunt LJ, Richards DA, et al. Effect of repetition of extrastimuli on sensitivity and reproducibility of mode of induction of ventricular tachycardia by programmed stimulation. *J Am Coll Cardiol* 1988;11:1260–1267.

101. Coplen SE, Antman EM, Berlin JA, et al. Efficacy and safety of quinidine therapy for maintenance of sinus rhythm after cardioversion. A meta-analysis of randomized trials. *Circulation* 1990;82:1106–1116.

102. Crawford MH, Bernstein SJ, Deedwania PC, et al. ACC/AHA Practice Guidelines. ACC/AHA Guidelines for ambulatory electrocardiography: Executive summary and recommendations. A Report of the American College of Cardiology/American Heart Association Task Force on Practice Guidelines (Committee to Revise the Guidelines for Ambulatory Electrocardiography) Developed in Collaboration With the North American Society for Pacing and Electrophysiology. *Circulation* 1999;100:886–893.

103. Cripps T, Bennett D, Camm J, Ward D. Prospective evaluation of clinical assessment, exercise testing and signal-averaged electrocardiogram in predicting outcome after acute myocardial infarction. *Am J Cardiol* 1988;62:995–999.

104. Cripps T, Bennett ED, Camm AJ, Ward DE. Inducibility of sustained monomorphic ventricular tachycardia as a prognostic indicator in survivors of recent myocardial infarction: A prospective evaluation in relation to other prognostic variables. *J Am Coll Cardiol* 1989;14:289–296.

105. Critelli G, Gallagher JJ, Thiene G, et al. Electrophysiologic and histopathologic correlations in a case of permanent form of reciprocating tachycardia. *Eur Heart J* 1985;6:130–137.

106. Davidenko JM, Cohn L, Goodrow R, Antzelevitch C. Quinidine-induced action potential prolongation, early afterdepolarizations, and triggered activity in canine Purkinje fibers. Effects of stimulation rate, potassium, and magnesium. *Circulation* 1989;79:674–686.

107. Davies DW, Butrous GS, Spurrell RA, Camm AJ. Pacing techniques in the prophyaxis of junctional reentry tachycardia. *Pacing Clin Electrophysiol* 1987;10:519–532.

108. Davis JC, Finkebeiner W, Ruder MA, et al. Histologic changes and arrhythmogenicity after discharge through transseptal catheter electrode. *Circulation* 1986;74:637–644.

109. De Marneffe M, Jacobs P, Haardt R, et al. Variations of normal sinus node function in relation to age: Role of autonomic influence. *Eur Heart J* 1986;7:662–672.

110. de Belder MA, Camm AJ. Devices for tachycardia termination. *Am J Cardiol* 1989;64:70J–74J.

111. de Belder MA, Camm AJ. Implantable cardioverter-defibrillators

(ICDs) 1989: How close are we to the ideal device? *Clin Cardiol* 1989;12:339–345.

112. de Belder MA, Malik M, Ward DE, et al. Pacing modalities for tachycardia termination. *Pacing Clin Electrophysiol* 1990;13:231–248.

113. de Vreede-Swagemakers JJ, Gorgels AP, Dubois-Arbouw WI, et al. Out-of-hospital cardiac arrest in the 1990's: A population-based study in the Maastricht area on incidence, characteristics and survival (abstract). *J Am Coll Cardiol* 1997;30:1500–1505.

114. den Dulk K, Bertholet M, Brugada P, et al. A versatile pacemaker system for termination of tachycardias. *Am J Cardiol* 1983;52:731–738.

115. den Dulk K, Brugada P, Smeets JLRM, Wellens HJ. Long-term antitachycardia pacing experience for supraventricular tachycardia. *Pacing Clin Electrophysiol* 1990:13:1020–1030.

116. den Dulk K, Kersschot IE, Brugada P, Wellens HJ. Is there a universal antitachycardia pacing mode? *Am J Cardiol* 1986;57:950–955.

117. Denes P, Kehoe R, Rosen KM. Multiple reentrant tachycardias due to retrograde conduction of dual atrioventricular bundles with atrioventricular nodal-like properties. *Am J Cardiol* 1979;44:162–170.

118. Denniss AR, Richards DA, Cody DV, et al. Prognostic significance of ventricular tachycardia and fibrillation induced at programmed stimulation and delayed potentials detected on the signal-averaged electrocardiograms of survivors of acute myocardial infarction. *Circulation* 1986;74:731–745.

119. Desai JM, Nyo H, Vera Z, et al. Orthogonal electrode catheter array for mapping of endocardial focal site of ventricular activation. *Pacing Clin Electrophysiol* 1991;14:557–576.

120. Desai JM, Nyo H, Vera Z, Tesluk H. Two phase radiofrequency catheter ablation of isolated ventricular endomyocardium. *Pacing Clin Electrophysiol* 1991;14:1179–1194.

121. Dewey RC, Capeless MA, Levy AM. Use of ambulatory electrocardiographic monitoring to identify high risk patients with congenital complete heart block. *N Engl J Med* 1987;316:835–839.

122. DiMarco JP, Miles W, Akhtar M, et al. Adenosine for paroxysmal supraventricular tachycardia: Dose ranging and comparison with verapamil: Assessment in placebo-controlled, multicenter trials. *Ann Intern Med* 1990;113:104–110.

123. DiMarco JP. Electrophysiology of adenosine. *J Cardiovasc Electrophysiol* 1990;1:340–348.

124. Dorian P, Cass D, Schwartz B, et al. Amiodarone as compared with lidocaine for shock-resistant ventricular fibrillation. *N Engl J Med* 2002:346:884–890.

125. Drew BJ, Califf RM, Funk M, et al. AHA Scientific Statement. Practice standards for electrocardiographic monitoring in hospital settings. An American Heart Association Scientific Statement From the Councils on Cardiovascular Nursing, Clinical Cardiology, and Cardiovascular Disease in the Young: Endorsed by the International Society of Computerized Electrocardiology and the American Association of Critical-Care Nurses. *Circulation* 2004;110:2721–2746.

126. Duff HJ, Mitchell LB, Wyse DG. Antiarrhythmic efficacy of propranolol: Comparison of low and high serum concentrations. *J Am Coll Cardiol* 1986;8:959–965.

127. Duffin E, Zipes DP. Chronic electrical control of tachyarrhythmias. In Mandel

WJ (ed). *Cardiac Arrhythmias: Their Mechanism, Diagnosis, and Management.* Philadelphia: J.B. Lippincott Co., 1987, p.764.

128. Dusman RE, Stanton MS, Miles WM, et al. Clinical features of amiodarone-induced pulmonary toxicity. *Circulation* 1990;82:51–59.

129. Eisenberg MS, Mengert TJ. Cardiac resuscitation. *N Engl J Med* 2001;344:1304–1313.

130. Eldar M, Griffin JC, Abbott JA, et al. Permanent cardiac pacing in patients with the long QT syndrome. *J Am Coll Cardiol* 1987;10:600–607.

131. Ellenbogen KA, O'Callaghan WG, Colavita PG, et al. Catheter atrioventricular junction ablation for recurrent supraventricular tachycardia with nodoventricular fibers. *Am J Cardiol* 1985;55:1277-1279.

132. Ellenbogen KA, Ramirez NM, Packer DL, et al. Accessory node ventricular (Mahaim) fibers: A clinical review. *Pacing Clin Electrophysiol* 1986;9:868–884.

133. Elmqvist R. Review of early pacemaker development. *Pacing Clin Electrophysiol* 1978;1:535–536.

134. El-Sherif N, Bekheit SS, Henkin R. Quinidine-induced long QTU interval and torsades de pointes: Role of bradycardia-dependent early afterdepolarizations. *J Am Coll Cardiol* 1989;14:252–257.

135. El-Sherif N, Ursell SN, Bekheit S, et al. Prognostic significance of the signal-averaged ECG depends on the time of recording in the postinfarction period. *Am Heart J* 1989;118:256–264.

136. Epstein AE, DiMarco J, Ellenbogen K, et al. ACC/AHA/HRS 2008 Guidelines for Device-Based Therapy of Cardiac Rhythm Abnormalities: A report of the American College of Cardiology/American Heart Association Task Force on Practice Guidelines (Writing Committee to Revise the ACC/AHA/NASPE 2002 Guideline Update for Implantation of Cardiac Pacemakers and Antiarrhythmia Devices) developed in collaboration with the American Association for Thoracic Surgery and Society of Thoracic Surgeons. *J Am Coll Cardiol* 2008;51:e1-62.

137. Epstein AE, Miles WM, Benditt DG, et al. Personal and public safety issues related to arrhythmias that may affect consciousness: Implications for regulation and physician recommendations. A Medical/Scientific Statement From the American Heart Association and the North American Society of Pacing and Electrophysiology. *Circulation* 1996;94:1147–1166.

138. Epstein LM, Scheinman MM, Langberg JJ, et al. Percutaneous catheter modification of the atrioventricular node. A potential cure for atrioventricular nodal reentrant tachycardia. *Circulation* 1989;80:757–768.

139. ECC Committee, Subcommittees and Task Forces of the American Heart Association. 2005 American Heart Association Guidelines for Cardiopulmonary Resuscitation and Emergency Cardiovascular Care. *Circulation* 2005;112[Suppl I]:IV-19-IV-34.

140. ECC Committee, Subcommittees and Task Forces of the American Heart Association. 2005 American Heart Association Guidelines for Cardiopulmonary Resuscitation and Emergency Cardiovascular Care. *Circulation* 2005;112[Suppl I]:IV-67-IV-77.

141. Estes NA 3rd, Halperin JL, Calkins H, et al. ACC/AHA/Physician Consortium 2008 Clinical Performance Measures for

Adults with Nonvalvular Atrial Fibrillation or Atrial Flutter: A report of the American College of Cardiology/American Heart Association Task Force on Performance Measures and the Physician Consortium for Performance Improvement (Writing Committee to Develop Clinical Performance Measures for Atrial Fibrillation) Developed in Collaboration with the Heart Rhythm Society. *J Am Coll Cardiol* 2008;51:865-884.

142. Estes NA III, Manolis AS, Greenblatt DJ, et al. Therapeutic serum lidocaine and metabolite concentrations in patients undergoing electrophysiologic study after discontinuation of intravenous lidocaine infusion. *Am Heart J* 1989;117:1060–1064.

143. Estes NA III, Deering TF, Manolis AS, et al. External cardiac programmed stimulation for noninvasive termination of sustained supraventricular and ventricular tachycardia. *Am J Cardiol* 1989;63:177–183.

144. Evans GT, Scheinman MM, Bardy G, et al. Predictors of in-hospital mortality after direct current catheter ablation of the atrioventricular junction: Results of a prospective, international, multicenter study. *Circulation* 1991;84:1924–1937.

145. Evans GT, Scheinman MM, Zipes DP, et al. The percutaneous cardiac mapping and ablation registry: Final summary of results. *Pacing Clin Electrophysiol* 1988;11:1621–1626.

146. Fain ES, Lee JT, Winkle RA. Effect of acute intravenous and chronic oral amiodarone on defibrillation energy requirements. *Am Heart J* 1987;114:8–17.

147. Falk RH. Flecainide-induced ventricular tachycardia and fibrillation in patients treated for atrial fibrillation. *Ann Intern Med* 1989;111:107–111.

148. Falkoff MD, Barold SS, Goodfriend MA, et al. Long-term management of ventricular tachycardia by implantable automatic burst tachycardia-terminating pacemakers. *Pacing Clin Electrophysiol* 1986;9:885–896.

149. Fananapazir L, German LD, Gallagher JJ, et al. Importance of preexcited QRS morphology during induced atrial fibrillation to the diagnosis and localization of multiple accessory pathways. *Circulation* 1990;81:578–585.

150. Fananapazir L, Packer DL, German LD, et al. Procainamide infusion test: Inability to identify patients with Wolff-Parkinson-White syndrome who are potentially at risk of sudden death. *Circulation* 1988;77:1291–1296.

151. Fauchier JP, Cosnay P, Moquet B, et al. Late ventricular arrhythmias in dilated or hypertrophy cardiomyopathies. A prospective study of about 83 patients. *Pacing Clin Electrophysiol* 1988;11:1974–1983.

152. Feld GK, Nademanee K, Stevenson W, et al. Clinical and electrophysiologic effects of amiodarone in patients with atrial fibrillation complicating the Wolff-Parkinson-White syndrome. *Am Heart J* 1988;115:102–107.

153. Feuer JM, Shandling AH, Messenger JC. Influence of cardiac pacing mode on the long-term development of atrial fibrillation. *Am J Cardiol* 1989;64:1374–1379.

154. Fiandra O. The first pacemaker implant in America. *Pacing Clin Electrophysiol* 1988;11:1234–1238.

155. Fisch C. Clinical competence in electrocardiography: A statement for physicians from the ACP/ACC/AHA Task Force on Clinical Privileges in Cardiology. *J Am Coll Cardiol* 1995;25:1465–1469.

156. Fisher JD, Brodman RF, Kim SG, et

al. VT/VF: 60/60 protection. *Pacing Clin Electrophysiol* 1990;13:218–222.

157. Fisher JD, Kim SH, Mercando AD. Electrical devices for treatment of arrhythmias. *Am J Cardiol* 1988;61:45A–57A.

158. Fisher JD, Teichman SL, Ferrick A, et al. Antiarrhythmic effects of VVI pacing at physiologic rates: A crossover controlled evaluation. *Pacing Clin Electrophysiol* 1987;10[Pt.1]:822–830.

159. Fisher JD. Clinical results with antitachycardia pacemakers. In Saksena S, and Goldschlager N (eds). *Electrical Therapy for Cardiac Arrhythmias. Pacing, Antitachycardia Devices, Catheter Ablation.* Philadelphia: W. B. Saunders Company, 1990, p.525.

160. Fitzgerald DM, Friday KJ, Wah JA, et al. Electrogram patterns predicting successful catheter ablation of ventricular tachycardia. *Circulation* 1988;77:806–814.

161. Fleg JL. Ventricular arrhythmias in the elderly: Prevalence, mechanisms, and therapeutic implications. *Geriatrics* 1988;43:23–29.

162. Floresco N. Pince Excitatrice. *J Physiol Path General* 1905;7:785–786.

163. Floresco N. Rappel a la Vie Par L'Escitation Directe du Coeur. *J Physiol Path General* 1905;7:797–803.

164. Fogoros RM, Elson JJ, Bonnet CA, et al. Efficacy of the automatic implantable cardioverter-defibrillator in prolonging survival in patients with severe underlying cardiac disease. *J Am Coll Cardiol* 1990;16:381–386.

165. Fogoros RM, Fiedler SB, Elson JJ. The automatic implantable cardioverter-defibrillator in drug-refractory ventricular tachyarrhythmias. *Ann Intern Med* 1987;107:635–641.

166. Fontaine G, Frank R, Rougier I, et al. Electrode catheter ablation of resistant ventricular tachycardia in arrhythmogenic right ventricular dysplasia: Experience of 13 patients with a mean follow-up of 45 months. *Eur Heart J* 1989;10(Suppl D):74–81.

167. Fontaine G, Tonet J, Frank R, et al. Clinical experience with fulguration and antiarrhythmic therapy for the treatment of ventricular tachycardia. Long-term follow-up of 43 patients. *Chest* 1989;95:785–797.

168. Forssmann W. Die sondierung des rechten herzens. *Klinische Wochenschrift* 1929;8:2085–2087.

169. Frame LH, Page RL, Hoffman BF. Atrial reentry around an anatomic barrier with a partially refractory excitable gap: A canine model of atrial flutter. *Circ Res* 1986;58:495–511.

170. Friedman PL. Cryotherapy: Treating arrhythmias safely and effectively. *EP Lab Digest* 2003;3:1,6,7.

171. Fromer M, Gloor H, Kus T, et al. Clinical experience with a new software-based antitachycardia pacemaker for recurrent supraventricular and ventricular tachycardias. *Pacing Clin Electrophysiol* 1990;13:890–899.

172. Fujimura O, Yee R, Klein GJ, et al. The diagnostic sensitivity of electrophysiologic testing in patients with syncope caused by transient bradycardia. *N Engl J Med* 1989;321:1703–1707.

173. Funk-Brentano C, Kroemer HK, Lee JT, Roden DM. Propafenone. *N Engl J Med* 1990;322:518–525.

174. Funk-Brentano C, Lights RT, Lineberry MD, et al. Pharmacokinetic and pharmacodynamic interaction of N-acetyl procainamide and procainamide in humans. *J Cardiovasc Pharmacol* 1989;14:364–373.

175. Furberg CD, Byington RP. Beta-adrenergic blockers in patients with acute

myocardial infarction. *Cardiovasc Clin* 1989;20:235–248.

176. Furlanello F, Bettini R, Bertoldi A, et al. Arrhythmia patterns in athletes with arrhythmogenic right ventricular dysplasia. *Eur Heart J* 1989;10(Suppl D):16–19.

177. Furman S, Hayes DL, Holmes DR. *A Practice of Cardiac Pacing (Third Edition).* Mt. Kisco, NY: Futura Publishing Co., 1993.

178. Furman S. AICD benefit. *Pacing Clin Electrophysiol* 1989;12:399–400.

179. Furman S. Implantable cardioverter defibrillator statistics. *Pacing Clin Electrophysiol* 1990;13:1–2.

180. Fuster V, Rydén LE, Asinger RW, et al. ACC/AHA/ESC guidelines for the management of patients with atrial fibrillation. A report of the American College of Cardiology/American Heart Association Task Force on Practice Guidelines and the European Society of Cardiology Committee for Practice Guidelines and Policy Conferences (Committee to develop guidelines for the management of patients with atrial fibrillation) developed in collaboration with the North American Society of Pacing and Electrophysiology. *Eur Heart J* 2001;22:1852-1923.

181. Fuster V, Rydén LE, Asinger RW, et al. ACC/AHA/ESC Guidelines for the Management of Patients With Atrial Fibrillation: Executive Summary. A Report of the American College of Cardiology/American Heart Association Task Force on Practice Guidelines and the European Society of Cardiology Committee for Practice Guidelines and Policy Conferences (Committee to Develop Guidelines for the Management of Patients With Atrial Fibrillation). Developed in Collaboration With the North American Society of Pacing and Electrophysiology. *Circulation* 2001;104:2118-2150.

182. Fuster V, Rydén LE, Cannom, DS, et al. ACC/AHA/ESC 2006 Guidelines for the Management of Patients With Atrial Fibrillation. A Report of the American College of Cardiology/American Heart Association Task Force on Practice Guidelines and the European Society of Cardiology Committee for Practice Guidelines (Writing Committee to Revise the 2001 Guidelines for the Management of Patients With Atrial Fibrillation): Developed in Collaboration With the European Heart Rhythm Association and the Heart Rhythm Society. *Circulation* 2006;114:e257-e354.

183. Gabry MD, Brodman R, Johnston D, et al. Automatic implantable cardioverter-defibrillator: Patient survival, battery longevity and shock delivery analysis. *J Am Coll Cardiol* 1987;9:1349.

184. Gage BF, Cardinalli AB, Albers GW, Owens DK. Cost-effectiveness of warfarin and aspirin for prophylaxis of stroke in patients with nonvalvular atrial fibrillation. *JAMA* 1995;274:1839–1845.

185. Gallagher JD, Bianchi J, Gessman LJ. A comparison of the electrophysiologic effects of acute and chronic amiodarone administration on canine Purkinje fibers. *J Cardiovasc Pharmacol* 1989;13:723–729.

186. Gallagher JJ, Sealy WC, Kasell J, et al. Multiple accessory pathways in patients with the pre-excitation syndrome. *Circulation* 1976;54:571–591.

187. Gallagher JJ, Sealy WC. The permanent form of junctional reciprocating tachycardia: Further elucidation of the underlying mechanism. *Eur Heart J* 1978;8:413–430.

188. Gallagher JJ, Smith WM, Kasell JH, et al. Role of Mahaim fibres in cardiac arrhythmias in man. *Circulation*

1981;64:176–189.

189. Gallagher JJ, Svenson RH, Kasell JH, et al. Catheter technique for closed chest ablation of the atrioventricular system. *N Engl J Med* 1982;306:194–200.

190. Gang ES, Lew AS, Hong M, et al. Decreased incidence of ventricular late potentials after successful thrombolytic therapy for acute myocardial infarction. *N Engl J Med* 1989;321:712–716.

191. Garan H, Kuchar D, Freeman C, et al. Early assessment of the effect of map-guided transcatheter intracardiac electric shock on sustained ventricular tachycardia secondary to coronary artery disease. *Am J Cardiol* 1988;61:1018–1023.

192. Garratt C, Antoniou A, Ward D, Camm AJ. Misuse of verapamil in pre-excited atrial fibrillation. *Lancet* 1989;1:367–369.

193. Giardine EG, Wechsler ME. Low dose quinidine-mexiletine combination therapy versus quinidine monotherapy for treatment of ventricular arrhythmias. *J Am Coll Cardiol* 1990;15:1138–1145.

194. Gillette PC, Garson A Jr, Cooley DA, et al. Prolonged and decremental antegrade conduction properties in right anterior accessory connections: Wide QRS antidromic tachycardia of left bundle branch block pattern without Wolff-Parkinson-White configuration in sinus rhythm. *Am Heart J* 1982;103:66–74.

195. Ginsburg W. Prepare to be shocked: The evolving standard of care in treating sudden cardiac arrest. *Am J Emerg Med* 1998;16:315-319.

196. Gleadhill IC, Wise RA, Schonfeld SA, et al. Serial lung function testing in patients treated with amiodarone: A prospective study. *Am J Med* 1989;84:4–10.

197. Glikson M, Suleiman M, Luria DM, et al. Do abandoned leads pose risk to implantable cardioverter-defibrillator patients? *Heart Rhythm* 2009;6:65-68.

198. Goldberger JJ, Cain ME, Hohnloser SH, et al. American Heart Association/American College of Cardiology Foundation/Heart Rhythm Society scientific statement on noninvasive risk stratification techniques for identifying patients at risk for sudden cardiac death: a scientific statement from the American Heart Association Council on Clinical Cardiology Committee on Electrocardiography and Arrhythmias and Council on Epidemiology and Prevention. *Circulation* 2008;118:1497-1518.

199. Goldner B, Jadonath R, Merkatz K, et al. Radiofrequency catheter ablation as primary therapy for supraventricular tachycardia. *J Invasive Cardiol* 1995;7:107–112.

200. Gomes JA, Winters SL, Martinson M, et al. The prognostic significance of quantitative signal-averaged variables relative to clinical variables, site of myocardial infarction, ejection fraction and ventricular premature beats: A prospective study. *J Am Coll Cardiol* 1989;13:377–384.

201. Goodman LR, Almassi GH, Troup PJ, et al. Complications of automatic implantable cardioverter defibrillators: Radiographic, CT, and echocardiographic evaluation. *Radiology* 1989;170:447–452.

202. Gorgels AP, van den Dool A, Hofs A, et al. Procainamide is superior to lidocaine in terminating sustained ventricular tachycardia. *Circulation* 1989;80(Suppl II):652.

203. Gottlieb SS, Kukin ML, Medina N, et al. Comparative hemodynamic effects of procainamide, tocainide, and encainide in severe chronic heart failure. *Circulation*

1990;81:860–864.

204. Goy JJ, Fromer M, Schlaepfer J, et al. Clinical efficacy of radiofrequency current in the treatment of patients atrioventricular node reentrant tachycardia. *J Am Coll Cardiol* 1990;16:418–423.

205. Graber HL, Unverferth DV, Baker PB, et al. Evolution of a hereditary cardiac conduction and muscle disorder: A study involving a family with six generations affected. *Circulation* 1986;74:21–35.

206. Gradman A, Deedwania P, Cody R, et al. Predictors of total mortality and sudden death in mild to moderate heart failure. Captopril-Digoxin Study Group. *J Am Coll Cardiol* 1989;14:564–570.

207. Greenberg ML, Lerman BB, Haines DE, et al. Stability of electrophysiological parameters after acute amiodarone loading: Implications for patient management. *Pacing Clin Electrophysiol* 1989;12:1038–1043.

208. Greenspon AJ, Volosin KJ, Greenberg RM, et al. Amiodarone therapy: Role of early and late electrophysiologic studies. *J Am Coll Cardiol* 1988;11:117–123.

209. Gregoratos G, Abrams J, Freedman RA, et al. ACC/AHA/NASPE Practice Guidelines—Full Text. ACC/AHA/NASPE 2002 Guideline Update for Implantation of Cardiac Pacemakers and Antiarrhythmia Devices. A Report of the American College of Cardiology/American Heart Association Task Force on Practice Guidelines (ACC/AHA/NASPE Committee on Pacemaker Implantation). 2002.

210. Gregoratos G, Abrams J, Freedman RA, et al. ACC/AHA Practice Guidelines. ACC/AHA/NASPE 2002 guideline update for implantation of cardiac pacemakers and antiarrhythmia devices: Summary article. A Report of the American College of Cardiology/American Heart Association Task Force on Practice Guidelines (ACC/AHA/NASPE Committee to Update the 1998 Pacemaker Guidelines). *Circulation* 2002;106:2145-2161.

211. Gregoratos G, Cheitlin MD, Conill A, et al. ACC/AHA Practice Guidelines. ACC/AHA guidelines for implantation of cardiac pacemakers and antiarrhythmia devices: Executive summary. A Report of the American College of Cardiology/American Heart Association Task Force on Practice Guidelines (Committee on Pacemaker Implantation). *Circulation* 1998;97:1325–1335.

212. Greve H, Koch T, Gulker H, et al. Termination of malignant ventricular tachycardias by use of an automatic defibrillator (AICD) in combination with an antitachycardial pacemaker. *Pacing Clin Electrophysiol* 1988;11:2040–2044.

213. Griffin JC, Schuenemeyer TD, Hess KR, et al. Pacemaker follow-up: Its role in the detection and correction of pacemaker system malfunction. *Pacing Clin Electrophysiol* 1986;9:387–391.

214. Griffin JC, Sweeney M. The management of paroxysmal tachycardias using the Cybertach-60. *Pacing Clin Electrophysiol* 1984;7:1291–1295.

215. Griffin JC. The optimal pacing mode for the individual patient: The role of DDDR. In Barold SS, and Mugica J (eds). *New Perspectives in Cardiac Pacing, 2*. Mt. Kisco, NY: Futura Publishing Co., 1991, p.325.

216. Griffith MJ, Linker NJ, Ward DE, Camm AJ. Adenosine in the diagnosis of broad complex tachycardia. *Lancet* 1988;1:672–675.

217. Grossman DS, Cohen TJ, Goldner B, Jadonath R. Pseudorecurrence of paroxysmal supraventricular tachycardia after

radiofrequency catheter ablation. *Am Heart J* 1994;128:516–519.

218. Guarnieri T, Levine JH, Veltri EP, et al. Success of chronic defibrillation and the role of antiarrhythmic drugs with the automatic implantable cardioverter/defibrillator. *Am J Cardiol* 1987;60:1061–1064.

219. Guidelines for clinical intracardiac electrophysiologic studies. A report of the American College of Cardiology/American Heart Association Task Force on Assessment of Diagnostic and Therapeutic Cardiovascular Procedures (Subcommittee to Assess Clinical Intracardiac Electrophysiologic Studies). *J Am Coll Cardiol* 1989;14:1827–1842 and *Circulation* 1989;80:1925–1939.

220. Guiraudon GM, Klein GJ, van Hemel N, et al. Atrial flutter: Lessons from surgical interventions (musing on atrial flutter mechanism). *Pacing Clin Electrophysiol* 1996;19[Pt.II]:1933–1938.

221. Guize L, Soria R, Chaouat JC, et al. Prévalence et évolution du syndrome de Wolff-Parkinson-White dans une population de 138,048 sujets. *Ann Med Intern* 1985;136:474–478.

222. Haberman RJ, Veltri EP, Mower MM. The effects of amiodarone on defibrillation threshold. *J Electrophysiol* 1988;2:415–423.

223. Haines DE, Lerman BB, Kron IL, DiMarco JP. Surgical ablation of ventricular tachycardia with sequential map-guided subendocardial resection: Electrophysiologic assessment of long-term follow-up. *Circulation* 1988;77:131–141.

224. Haines DE, Verow AF. Observations on electrode-tissue interface temperature and effect on electrical impedance during radiofrequency ablation of ventricular myocardium. *Circulation* 1990;82:1034–1038.

225. Haissaguerre M, Fischer B, Labbe T, et al. Frequency of recurrent atrial fibrillation after catheter ablation of overt accessory pathways. *Am J Cardiol* 1992;69:493–497.

226. Haissaguerre M, Jais P, Shah DC, et al. Electrophysiological end point for catheter ablation of atrial fibrillation initiated from multiple pulmonary venous foci. *Circulation* 2000;101:1409–1417.

227. Haissaguerre M, Warin JF, LeMetayer P, et al. Catheter ablation of Mahaim fibers with preservation of atrioventricular nodal conduction. *Circulation* 1990;82:418–427.

228. Haissaguerre M, Warin JF, Lemetayer P, et al. Closed-chest ablation of retrograde conduction in patients with atrioventricular nodal reentrant tachycardia. *N Engl J Med* 1989;320:426–433.

229. Hargrove WC III, Josephson ME, Marchlinski FE, Miller JM. Surgical decisions in the management of sudden cardiac death and malignant ventricular arrhythmias. Subendocardial resection, the automatic internal defibrillator, or both. *J Thorac Cardiovasc Surg* 1989;97:923–928.

230. Harris L, Mickleborough LL, Shaikh N, et al. Electrical ablation with a balloon electrode array: Chronic electrophysiologic response. *Pacing Clin Electrophysiol* 1988;11:1262–1266.

231. He DS, Zimmer JE, Hynynen K, et al. Preliminary results using ultrasound energy for ablation of the ventricular myocardium in dogs. *Am J Cardiol* 1994;73:1029–1031.

232. Heald SC, Davies DW, Ward DE, et al. Radiofrequency catheter ablation of Mahaim tachycardia by targeting Mahaim potentials at the tricuspid annulus. *Br Heart J* 1995;73:250–257.

233. Heinz G, Siostrzonek P, Kreiner G,

Gossinger H. Improvement in left ventricular systolic function after successful radiofrequency His bundle ablation for drug refractory, chronic atrial fibrillation and recurrent atrial flutter. *Am J Cardiol* 1992;69:489–492.

234. Henthorn RW, Waldo AL, Anderson JL, et al. Flecainide acetate prevents recurrent of symptomatic paroxysmal supraventricular tachycardia. The Flecainide Supraventricular Tachycardia Study Group. *Circulation* 1991;83:119–125.

235. Herre JM, Sauve MJ, Malone P, et al. Long-term results of amiodarone therapy in patients with recurrent sustained ventricular tachycardia or ventricular fibrillation. *J Am Coll Cardiol* 1989;13:442–449.

236. Hirsh J, Anand SS, Halperin JL, Fuster V. AHA Scientific Statement. Guide to anticoagulant therapy: Heparin. A Statement for Healthcare Professionals From the American Heart Association. *Circulation* 2001;103:2994.

237. Hirsh J, Fuster V, Ansell J, Halperin JL. AHA/ACC Scientific Statement. American Heart Association/American College of Cardiology Foundation guide to warfarin therapy. *Circulation* 2003;107:1692.

238. Hiss RG, Lamb LE. Electrocardiographic findings in 122,043 individuals. *Circulation* 1962;25:947–961.

239. Hjalmarson A. International betablocker review in acute and postmyocardial infraction. *Am J Cardiol* 1988;61:26B–29B.

240. Hoff PI, Tronstad A, Oie B, Ohm OJ. Electrophysiologic and clinical effects of flecainide for recurrent paroxysmal supraventricular tachycardia. *Am J Cardiol* 1988;62:585–589.

241. Hoffa M, Ludwig C. *Ztschrft Rat Med* 1850;9:107.

242. Hoffman BF, Dangman KH. The role of antiarrhythmic drugs in sudden cardiac death. *J Am Coll Cardiol* 1986;8:104A–109A.

243. Hoffman BF. The genesis of cardiac arrhythmias. *Prog Cardiovasc Dis* 1966;8:319–329.

244. Hohnloser SH, Crijns HJ, van Eickels M, et al, for the ATHENA Investigators. Effect of dronedarone on cardiovascular events in atrial fibrillation. *N Engl J Med* 2009;360:668-678.

245. Hohnloser SH, Woosley RL. Sotalol. *N Engl J Med* 1994:331:31–38.

246. Holley LK, Cooper M, Uther JB, Ross DA. Safety and efficacy of pacing for ventricular tachycardia. *Pacing Clin Electrophysiol* 1986;9(Pt.II):1316–1319.

247. Hondeghem LM, Snyders DJ. Class III antiarrhythmic agents have a lot of potential but a long way to go. Reduced effectiveness and dangers of reverse use dependence. *Circulation* 1990;81:686–690.

248. Hondeghem LM. Molecular interactions of antiarrhythmic agents with receptor sites. In Zipes DP, and Jalife J (eds). *Cardiac Electrophysiology: From Cell to Bedside.* Philadelphia, PA: W. B. Saunders Company, 1990, p.865.

249. Horowitz LN. Safety of electrophysiologic studies. *Circulation* 1986;73:II28–II31.

250. Horowitz LN, Zipes DP, Bigger JT Jr, et al. Proarrhythmia, arrhythmogenesis or aggrevation of arrhythmia—A status report, 1987. *Am J Cardiol* 1987;59:54E–56E.

251. Hosenpud JD, Greenberg BH. *Congestive Heart Failure. Pathophysiology, Diagnosis, and Comprehensive Approach to Management. 2nd edition.* Philadelphia, PA: Lippincott Williams & Wilkins, 2000.

252. Huang SK, Bharati S, Graham AR, et al. Chronic incomplete atrioventricular block induced by radiofrequency catheter ablation. *Circulation* 1989;80:951–961.

253. Huang SK, Graham AR, Wharton K. Radiofrequency catheter ablation of the left and right ventricles: Anatomic and electrophysiologic observations. *Pacing Clin Electrophysiol* 1988;11:449–459.

254. Hunt SA, Abraham WT, Chin MH, et al. ACC/AHA Practice Guidelines. ACC/AHA 2005 Guideline Update for the Diagnosis and Management of Chronic Heart Failure in the Adult: A Report of the American College of Cardiology/American Heart Association Task Force on Practice Guidelines (Writing Committee to Update the 2001 Guidelines for the Evaluation and Management of Heart Failure): Developed in collaboration with the American College of Chest Physicians and the International Society for Heart and Lung Transplantation: Endorsed by the Heart Rhythm Society. *Circulation* 2005;112:e154-235.

255. Huycke EC, Sung RJ, Dias VC, et al. Intravenous diltiazem for termination of reentrant supraventricular tachycardia: A placebo-controlled, randomized, double-blind multicenter study. *J Am Coll Cardiol* 1989;13:538–544.

256. Iesaka Y, Aonuma K, Nitta J, et al. Effects of procainamide and lidocaine on electrically inducible ventricular tachycardia studied with programmed ventricular stimulation in post myocardial infarction. *Jpn Circ J* 1988;52:262–271.

257. Imaizumi Y, Giles WR. Quinidine-induced inhibition of transient outward current in cardiac muscle. *Am J Physiol* 1987;253(*Heart Circ Physiol* 22):H704–H708.

258. Inoue H, Zipes DP. Results of sympathetic denervation in the canine heart: Supersensitivity that may be arrhythmogenic. *Circulation* 1987;75:877–887.

259. Inoue S, Shinohara F, Sakai T, et al. Myocarditis and arrhythmia: A clinicopathological study of conduction system based on serial section in 65 cases. *Jpn Circ J* 1989;53:49–57.

260. Jackman WM, Wang XZ, Friday KJ, et al. Catheter ablation of accessory atrioventricular pathways (Wolff-Parkinson-White syndrome) by radiofrequency current. *N Engl J Med* 1991;324:1605–1611.

261. Jackman WM, Friday KJ, Fitzgerald DM, et al. Localization of left free-wall and posteroseptal accessory atrioventricular pathways by direct recording of accessory pathway activation. *Pacing Clin Electrophysiol* 1989;12:204–214.

262. Jackman WM, Friday KJ, Scherlag BJ, et al. Direct endocardial recording from an accessory atrioventricular pathway: Localization of the site of block, effect of antiarrhythmic drugs, and attempt at non-surgical ablation. *Circulation* 1983;68:906–916.

263. Jackman WM, Friday KJ, Yeung-Lai-Wah JA, et al. New catheter technique for recording left free-wall accessory atrioventricular pathway activation: Identification of pathway fiber orientation. *Circulation* 1988;78:598–611.

264. Jackman WM, Wang XZ, Friday KJ, et al. Catheter ablation of atrioventricular junction using radiofrequency current in 17 patients. Comparison of standard and large-tip catheter electrodes. *Circulation* 1991;83:1562–1576.

265. Jadonath RL, Schwartzman DS, Preminger MW, et al. Utility of the 12-lead electrocardiogram in localizing the origin of right ventricular outflow tract tachycardia. *Am Heart J* 1995;130:1107–1113.

266. Jadvar H, Arzbaecher R. Temporary esophageal pacing. In Bartecchi CE, and Mann DE (eds). *Temporary Cardiac Pacing.*

Chicago: Precept Press, Inc., 1990, p.146.

267. Janosik DL, Redd RM, Buckingham TA, et al. Utility of ambulatory electrocardiography in detecting pacemaker dysfunction in the early postimplantation period. *Am J Cardiol* 1987;60:1030–1035.

268. Jazayeri MR, Van Wyhe G, Avitall B, et al. Isoproterenol reversal of antiarrhythmic effects in patients with inducible sustained ventricular tachyarrhythmias. *J Am Coll Cardiol* 1989;14:705–711.

269. Jessup M, Abraham WT, Casey DE, et al. Focused Update: ACCF/AHA Guidelines for the Diagnosis and Management of Heart Failure in Adults. A Report of the American College of Cardiology Foundation/American Heart Association Task Force on Practice Guidelines. *Circulation* 2009 Mar 26.

270. Johnston FA, Robinson JR, Fyfe T. Exercise testing in the diagnosis of sick sinus syndrome in the elderly: Implications for treatment. *Pacing Clin Electrophysiol* 1987;10:831–838.

271. Josephson ME. *Clinical Cardiac Electrophysiology: Techniques and Interpretations (Third Edition).* Philadelphia, PA: Lippincott Williams & Wilkins. 2002.

272. Josephson ME. Antiarrhythmic agents and the danger of proarrhythmic events. *Ann Intern Med* 1989;111:101–103.

273. Josephson ME. New approaches to the management of atrial fibrillation: The role of the atrial defibrillator. *Circulation* 1998;98:1594–1596.

274. Kadish AH, Buxton AE, Kennedy HL, et al. ACC/AHA clinical competence statement on electrocardiography and ambulatory electrocardiography: A report of the ACC/AHA/ACP–ASIM task force on clinical competence (ACC/AHA Committee to develop a clinical competence statement on electrocardiography and ambulatory electrocardiography) endorsed by the International Society for Holter and Noninvasive Electrocardiology. *Circulation* 2001;104:3169–3178.

275. Kadish AH, Morady F. Torsades de pointes. In Zipes DP, and Jalife J (eds). *Cardiac Electrophysiology: From Cell to Bedside.* Philadelphia, PA: W. B. Saunders Company, 1990, p.605.

276. Kalbfleisch SJ, Williamson B, Man C, et al. A randomized comparison of the right- and left-sided approaches to ablation of the atrioventricular junction. *Am J Cardiol* 1993;72:1406–1410.

277. Kannel WB, Abbott RD, Savage DD, McNamara PM. Epidemiologic features of chronic atrial fibrillations: The Framingham Study. *N Engl J Med* 1982;306:1018–1022.

278. Kapoor WN, Hammill SC, Gersh BJ. Diagnosis and natural history of syncope and the role of invasive electrophysiological testing. *Am J Cardiol* 1989;63:730–734.

279. Kappenberger L, Valin H, Sowton E. Multicenter long-term results of antitachycardia pacing for supraventricular tachycardias. *Am J Cardiol* 1989;63:191–193.

280. Kasanuki H, Ohnishi S, Hosoda S. Differentiation and mechanisms of prevention and termination of verapamil sensitive sustained ventricular tachycardia. *Am J Cardiol* 1989;64:46J–49J.

281. Kaseda S, Glimour RF Jr, Zipes DP. Depressant effects of magnesium on early afterdepolarizations and triggered activity induced by cesium quinidine and 4-amino pyridine in canine cardiac Purkinje fibers. *Am Heart J* 1989;118:458–466.

282. Kay GN, Epstein AE, Plumb VJ. Preferential effect of procainamide on the reentrant circuit of ventricular tachycardia. *J Am Coll Cardiol* 1989;14:382–390.

283. Kay GN, Vance JP, Dailey SM, Epstein AE. Current role of the automatic implantable cardioverter-defibrillator in the treatment of life-threatening ventricular arrhythmias. *Am J Med* 1990;88:25N–34N.

284. Kelly P, Ruskin JN, Blahakes GJ, et al. Surgical coronary revascularization in survivors of prehospital cardiac arrest: Its effect on inducible ventricular arrhythmias and long-term survival. *J Am Coll Cardiol* 1990;15:267–273.

285. Kelly PA, Cannom DS, Garan H, et al. Predictors of automatic implantable cardioverter-defibrillator discharge for life-threatening ventricular arrhythmias. *Am J Cardiol* 1988;62:83–87.

286. Kelly PA, Cannom DS, Garan H, et al. The automatic implantable cardioverter-defibrillator: Efficacy, complications and survival in patients with malignant ventricular arrhythmias. *J Am Coll Cardiol* 1988;11:1278–1286.

287. Kelly PA, Wallace S, Tucker B, et al. Postoperative infection with the automatic implantable cardioverter defibrillator: Clinical presentation and use of the gallium scan in diagnosis. *Pacing Clin Electrophysiol* 1988;11:1220-1225.

288. Kenney RA, Ingram A, Bayliss J, Sutton R. Head-up tilt: A useful test for investigating unexplained syncope. *Lancet* 1986;1:1352–1355.

289. Keren A, Syrris P, McKenna WJ. Hypertrophic cardiomyopathy: The genetic determinants of clinical disease expression. *Nat Clin Pract Cardiovasc Med* 2008;5:158–168.

290. Kerver RE. External direct current defibrillation and cardioversion. In Zipes DP, and Jalife J (eds). *Cardiac Electrophysiology: From Cell to Bedside.* Philadelphia, PA: W. B. Saunders Company, 1990, p.954.

291. Kessler KM, McAuliffe D, Kozlovskis P, et al. QRS morphology-dependent pharmacodynamics in multiform ventricular ectopic activity. *Am J Cardiol* 1988;61:563–569.

292. Kinoshita K, Hearse DJ, Braimbridge MV, Manning AS. Ischemia and reperfusion-induced arrhythmias in conscious rate—Studies with prazosin and atenolol. *Jpn Circ J* 1988;52:1334–1394.

293. Kleiger RE, Miller JP, Bigger JT Jr, Moss AJ. Decreased heart rate variability and its association with increased mortality after acute myocardial infarction. *Am J Cardiol* 1987;59:256–262.

294. Kleiman RB, Miller JM, Buxton AE, et al. Prognosis following sustained ventricular tachycardia occurring early after myocardial infarction. *Am J Cardiol* 1988;62:528–533.

295. Klein GJ, Bashore TM, Sellers TD, et al. Ventricular fibrillation in the Wolff-Parkinson-White syndrome. *N Engl J Med* 1979;301:1080–1085.

296. Klein GJ, Guiraudon GM, Kerr CR, et al. "Nodoventricular" accessory pathway: Evidence for a distinct accessory AV pathway with atrioventricular node-like properties. *J Am Coll Cardiol* 1988;11:1035–1040.

297. Klein GJ, Hackel DB, Gallagher JJ. Anatomic substrate of impaired antegrade conduction over an accessory atrioventricular pathway in the Wolff-Parkinson-White syndrome. *Circulation* 1980;61:1249–1256.

298. Klein GJ, Prystowsky EN, Pritchett ELC, et al. Atypical patterns of retrograde conduction over accessory atrioventricular pathways in the Wolff-Parkinson-White syndrome. *Circulation* 1979;60:1477–1486.

299. Klein LS, Fineberg N, Heger JJ, et al. Prospective evaluation of a discriminant

function for prediction of recurrent symptomatic ventricular tachycardia or ventricular fibrillation in coronary artery disease patients receiving amiodarone and having inducible ventricular tachycardia at electrophysiologic study. *Am J Cardiol* 1988;61:1024–1030.

300. Klein LS, Miles WM, Heger JJ, Zipes DP. Transcutaneous pacing: Patient tolerance, strength-interval relations and feasibility for programmed electrical stimulation. *Am J Cardiol* 1988;62:1126–1129.

301. Klein RC, Machell C, Rushforth N, Standefur J. Efficacy of intravenous amiodarone as short-term treatment for refractory ventricular tachycardia. *Am Heart J* 1988;115:96–101.

302. Knight BP, Ayers G, Cohen TJ. Robotic positioning of standard electrophysiology catheters: A novel approach to catheter robotics. *J Invasive Cardiol* 2008;20:250–253.

303. Knight BP, Gersh BJ, Carlson MD, et al. AHA Science Advisory. Role of permanent pacing to prevent atrial fibrillation. Science Advisory From the American Heart Association Council on Clinical Cardiology (Subcommittee on Electrocardiography and Arrhythmias) and the Quality of Care and Outcomes Research Interdisciplinary Working Group, in Collaboration With the Heart Rhythm Society. *Circulation* 2005;111:240–243.

304. Kopecky SL, Gersh BJ, McGoon MD, et al. The natural history of lone atrial fibrillation: A population-based study over three decades. *N Engl J Med* 1987;317:669–674.

305. Kopelman HA, Horowitz LN. Efficacy and toxicity of amiodarone for the treatment of supraventricular tachyarrhythmias. *Prog Cardiovasc Dis* 1989;31:355–366.

306. Kopelman HA, Woosley RL, Lee JT, et al. Electrophysiologic effects of intravenous and oral sotalol for sustained ventricular tachycardia secondary to coronary artery disease. *Am J Cardiol* 1988;61:1006–1011.

307. Kottkamp H, Chen X, Hindricks G, et al. Idiopathic left ventricular tachycardia: New insights into electrophysiological characteristics and radiofrequency catheter ablation. *Pacing Clin Electrophysiol* 1995;18:1285–1297.

308. Kou WH, Morady F, Dick M, et al. Concealed anterograde accessory pathway conduction during the induction of orthodromic reciprocating tachycardia. *J Am Coll Cardiol* 1989;13:391–398.

309. Kouvaras G, Cokkinos DV, Halal G, et al. The effective treatment of multifocal atrial tachycardia with amiodarone. *Jpn Heart J* 1989;30:301–312.

310. Kowey PR, Friehling TD, Marinchak RA, et al. Safety and efficacy of amiodarone. The low-dose perspective. *Chest* 1988;93:54–59.

311. Kowey PR, Marinchak RA, Rials SJ. The Cardiac Arrhythmia Suppression Trial: How has it impacted on contemporary arrhythmia management? *J Cardiovasc Electrophysiol* 1990;1:457–463.

312. Krafchek J, Lin HT, Beckman KJ, et al. Cumulative effects of amiodarone on inducibility of ventricular tachycardia: Implications for electrophysiological testing. *Pacing Clin Electrophysiol* 1988;11:434–444.

313. Kroemer HK, Funck-Brentano C, Silberstein DJ, et al. Stereoselective disposition and pharmacologic activity of propafenone enantiomers. *Circulation* 1989;79:1068–1076.

314. Kron J, Hart M, Schual-Berke S, et

al. Idiopathic dilated cardiomyopathy. Role of programmed electrical stimulation and Holter monitoring in predicting those at risk of sudden death. *Chest* 1988;93:85–90.

315. Kuch KH, Friday KJ, Kunze KP, et al. Sites of conduction block in accessory atrioventricular pathways. Basis for concealed accessory pathways. *Circulation* 1990;82:407–417.

316. Kuchar DL, Garan H, Ruskin JN. Electrophysiologic evaluation of antiarrhythmic therapy for ventricular tachyarrhythmias. *Am J Cardiol* 1988;62:39H–45H.

317. Kuchar DL, Garan H, Venditti FJ, et al. Usefulness of sotalol in suppressing ventricular tachycardia or ventricular fibrillation in patients with healed myocardial infarcts. *Am J Cardiol* 1989;64:33–36.

318. Kuchar DL, Rottman J, Berger E, et al. Prediction of successful suppression of sustained ventricular tachyarrhythmias by serial drug testing from data derived at the initial electrophysiologic study. *J Am Coll Cardiol* 1988;12:982–988.

319. Kuchar DL, Thorburn CW, Sammel NL. Late potentials detected after myocardial infarction: Natural history and prognostic significance. *Circulation* 1986;74:1280–1289.

320. Kuchar DL, Thorburn CW, Sammel NL. Prediction of serious arrhythmic events after myocardial infarction: Signal-averaged electrocardiogram. Holter monitoring and radionuclide ventriculography. *J Am Coll Cardiol* 1987;9:531–538.

321. Kuck KH, Cappato R, Siebels J, Ruppel R. Randomized comparison of antiarrhythmic drug therapy with implantable defibrillators in patients resuscitated from cardiac arrest: The Cardiac Arrest Study Hamburg (CASH). *Circulation* 2000;102:748–754.

322. Kumagal K, Yamanouchi Y, Hiroki T, Arakawa K. Effects of transcatheter cardioversion on chronic lone atrial fibrillation. *Pacing Clin Electrophysiol* 1991;14[Pt.I]:1571–1575.

323. Kupferschmid JP, Rosengart TK, McIntosh CL, et al. Amiodarone-induced complications after cardiac operation for obstructive hypertrophic cardiomyopathy. *Ann Thorac Surg* 1989;48:359–364.

324. Kushner JA, Kou WH, Kadish AH, Morady F. Natural history of patients with unexplained syncope and a nondiagnostic electrophysiologic study. *J Am Coll Cardiol* 1989;14:391–396.

325. Lal RB, Avery RD. Aggressive pacemaker twiddler's syndrome. Dislodgement of an active fixation ventricular pacing electrode. *Chest* 1990;97:756–757.

326. Landzberg JS, Franklin JO, Mahawar SK, et al. Benefits of physiologic atrioventricular synchronization for pacing with an exercise rate response. *Am J Cardiol* 1990;66:193–197.

327. Langberg JJ, Calkins H, El-Atassi R, et al. Temperature monitoring during radiofrequency catheter ablation of accessory pathways. *Circulation* 1992;86,1469–1474.

328. Langberg JJ, Chin MC, Rosenqvist M, et al. Catheter ablation of the atrioventricular junction with radiofrequency energy. *Circulation* 1989;80:1527–1535.

329. Langberg JJ, Lee MA, Chin MC, Rosenqvist M. Radiofrequency catheter ablation: The effect of electrode size on lesion volume in vivo. *Pacing Clin Electrophysiol* 1990;13:1242–1248.

330. Lau CP, Linker NJ, Butrous GS, et al. Myopotential interference in unipolar rate responsive pacemakers. *Pacing Clin Electrophysiol* 1989;12:1324–1330.

331. Lauer MS, Eagle KA, Buckley MJ, DeSanctis RW. Atrial fibrillation following coronary artery bypass surgery. *Prog Cardiovasc Dis* 1989;31:367–378.

332. Leclercq JF, Chouty F, Cauchemez B, et al. Results of electrical fulguration in arrhythmogenic right ventricular disease. *Am J Cardiol* 1988;62:220–224.

333. Leclercq JF, Coumel P. Characteristics, prognosis and treatment of the ventricular arrhythmias of right ventricular dysplasia. *Eur Heart J* 1989;10(Suppl D):61–67.

334. Lee JT, Kroemer HK, Silberstein DJ, et al. The role of genetically determined polymorphic drug metabolism in the beta-blockade produced by propafenone. *N Engl J Med* 1990;322:1764–1768.

335. Lee RW, Huang SK, Mechling E, Bazgan L. Runaway atrioventricular sequential pacemaker after radiation therapy. *Am J Med* 1986;81:833–886.

336. Leichter D, Danilo P Jr, Boyden P, et al. A canine model of torsades de pointes. *Pacing Clin Electrophysiol* 1988;11:2235–2245.

337. Leitch JW, Klein G, Yee R, Guiraudon G. Sinus node-atrioventricular node isolation: Long-term results with the "corridor" operation for atrial fibrillation. *J Am Coll Cardiol* 1991;17:970–975.

338. Lemery R, Brugada P, Jansen J, et al. Nonischemic sustained ventricular tachycardia: Clinical outcome in 12 patients with arrhythmogenic right ventricular dysplasia. *J Am Coll Cardiol* 1989;14:96–105.

339. Lerman BB, Belardinelli L, West GA, et al. Adenosine-sensitive ventricular tachycardia: Evidence suggesting cyclic AMP-mediated triggered activity. *Circulation* 1986;74:270–280.

340. Lerman BB, Wesley RC Jr, DiMarco JP, et al. Antiadrenergic effects of adenosine on His-Purkinje automaticity. Evidence for accentuated antagonism. *J Clin Invest* 1988;82:2127–2135.

341. Lesh MC, Van Hare GF, Schamp DJ, et al. Curative percutaneous catheter ablation using radiofrequency energy for accessory pathways in all locations: Results in 100 consecutive patients. *J Am Coll Cardiol* 1992;19:1303–1309.

342. Levine JH, Moore EN, Kadish AH, et al. Mechanisms of depressed conduction from long-term amiodarone therapy in canine myocardium. *Circulation* 1988;78:684–691.

343. Levy S, Lacombe P, Cointe R, Bru P. High energy transcatheter cardioversion of chronic atrial fibrillation. *J Am Coll Cardiol* 1988;12:514–518.

344. Levy S, Lauribe P, Dolla E, et al. A randomized comparison of external and internal cardioversion of chronic atrial fibrillation. *Circulation* 1992;86:1415–1420.

345. Levy S. Direct recording of sinus node potentials using electrode catheter techniques. *Clin Cardiol* 1994;17:203–206.

346. Lewalter T, Burkhardt D, Bielik H, et al. Circumferential pulmonary vein mapping and ablation in focal atrial fibrillation: Single catheter technique. *J Interv Card Electrophysiol* 2002;7:165–170.

347. Lewis RV, McMurray J, McDevitt DG. Effects of atenolol, verapamil, and xamoterol on heart rate and exercise tolerance in digitalized patients with chronic atrial fibrillation. *J Cardiovasc Pharmacol* 1989;13:1–6.

348. Li CK, Shandling AH, Nolasco M, et al. Atrial automatic tachycardia-reversion pacemakers: Their economic viability and impact on quality-of-life. *Pacing Clin Electrophysiol* 1990;13:639–645.

349. Limacher MC, Douglas PS,

Germane G, et al. ACC expert consensus document. Radiation safety in the practice of cardiology. American College of Cardiology. *J Am Coll Cardiol* 1998;31:892–913.

350. Lindsay BD, Ambos HD, Schechtman KB, Cain ME. Improved selection of patients for programmed ventricular stimulation by frequency analysis of signal-averaged electrocardiograms. *Circulation* 1986;73:675–683.

351. Loebl S, Spratto GR, Woods AL. *The Nurse's Drug Handbook. (7th edition).* Albany, NY: Delmar Publishers Inc., 1994.

352. Lown B. Sudden cardiac death: The major challenge confront contemporary cardiology. *Am J Cardiol* 1979;43:313–328.

353. Luceri RM, Habal SM, Castellanos A, et al. Mechanism of death in patients with the automatic implantable cardioverter-defibrillator. *Pacing Clin Electrophysiol* 1988;11:2015–2022.

354. Luck JC, Grubb BP, Artman SE, et al. Termination of sustained ventricular tachycardia by external noninvasive pacing. *Am J Cardiol* 1988;61:574–577.

355. Luderitz B, Manz M. Role of antitachycardia devices in the treatment of ventricular tachyarrhythmias. *Am J Cardiol* 1989;64:75J–78J.

356. Machac J, Weiss A, Winters SL, et al. A comparative study of frequency domain and time domain analysis of signal-averaged electrocardiograms in patients with ventricular tachycardia. *J Am Coll Cardiol* 1988;11:284–296.

357. Magney JE, Staplin DH, Flynn DM, Hunter DW. A new approach to percutaneous sublavian venipuncture to avoid lead fracture or central venous catheter occlusion. *Pacing Clin Electrophysiol* 1993;16:2133–2142.

358. Mahaim I, Winston MR. Recherces d'anatomic comparée du pathologie experimentale sur les connexions hautes du faisceau de His-Tawara. *Cardiologia* 1941;5:189–260.

359. Buxton AE, Lee KL, Fisher JD, et al. A randomized study of the prevention of sudden death in patients with coronary artery disease. Multicenter Unsustained Tachycardia Trial. *N Engl J Med* 1999;341:1882–1890.

360. Malfatto G, Zaza A, Forster M, et al. Electrophysiologic, inotropic and antiarrhythmic effects of propafenone, 5-hydroxypropafenone and N-depropylpropafenone. *J Pharmacol Exp Ther* 1988;246:419–426.

361. Manolis AS, Estes NA III. Reversal of electrophysiologic effects of felcainide on the accessory pathway by isoproterenol in the Wolff-Parkinson-White syndrome. *Am J Cardiol* 1989;64:194–198.

362. Manolis AS, Linzer M, Salem D, Estes NA III. Syncope: Current diagnostic evaluation and management. *Ann Intern Med* 1990;112:850–863.

363. Manolis AS, Rastegar H, Estes NA III. Automatic implantable cardioverter defibrillator. Current status. *JAMA* 1989;262:1362–1368.

364. Manolis AS, Uricchio F, Estes NA III. Prognostic value of early electrophysiologic studies for ventricular tachycardia recurrence in patients with coronary artery disease treated with amiodarone. *Am J Cardiol* 1989;63:1052–1057.

365. Manz M, Gerckens U, Funke HD, et al. Combination of antitachycardia pacemaker and automatic implantable cardioverter/defibrillator for ventricular tachycardia. *Pacing Clin Electrophysiol* 1986;9:676–684.

366. Marchlinski FE, Buxton AE,

Josephson ME, Schmitt C. Predicting ventricular tachycardia cycle length after procainamide by assessing cycle length-dependent changes in paced QRS duration. *Circulation* 1989;79:39–46.

367. Marchlinski FE, Buxton AE, Kindwall KE, et al. Comparison of individual and combined effects of procainamide and amiodarone in patients with sustained ventricular tachyarrhythmias. *Circulation* 1988;78:583–591.

368. Marchlinski FE, Flores B, Miller JM, et al. Relation of the intraoperative defibrillation threshold to successful postoperative defibrillation with an automatic implantable cardioverter-defibrillator. *Am J Cardiol* 1988;62:393–398.

369. Marchlinski FE, Flores BT, Buxton AE, et al. The automatic implantable cardioverter-defibrillator: Efficacy, complications, and device failures. *Ann Intern Med* 1986;104:481–488.

370. Marinchak RA, Friehling TD, Kline RA, et al. Effect of antiarrhythmic drugs on defibrillation threshold: Case report of an adverse effect of mexiletine and review of the literature. *Pacing Clin Electrophysiol* 1988;11:7–12.

371. Marks ML, Graham EL, Powell JL, et al. Mortality and arrhythmia recurrence following amiodarone discontinuation. *Circulation* 1989;80(Suppl II):II651.

372. Maron BJ, Moller JH, Seidman CE, et al. AHA Medical/Scientific Statement. Impact of laboratory molecular diagnosis on contemporary diagnostic criteria for genetically transmitted cardiovascular diseases: Hypertrophic cardiomyopathy, long-QT syndrome, and Marfan syndrome. A Statement for Healthcare Professionals From the Councils on Clinical Cardiology, Cardiovascular Disease in the Young, and Basic Science, American Heart Association. *Circulation* 1998;98:1460–1471.

373. Martin GJ, Magid NM, Myers G, et al. Heart rate variability and sudden death secondary to coronary artery disease during ambulatory electrocardiographic monitoring. *Am J Cardiol* 1987;60:86–89.

374. Martini B, Nava A, Thiene G, et al. Accelerated idioventricular rhythm of infundibular origin in patients with a concealed form of arrhythmogenic right ventricular dysplasia. *Br Heart J* 1988;59:564–571.

375. Mason JW. A comparison of seven antiarrhythmic drugs in patients with ventricular tachyarrhythmias. *N Engl J Med* 1993:329:452–458.

376. McAlister HF, Klementowicz PT, Andrews C. Lyme carditis: An important cause of reversible heart block. *Ann Intern Med* 1989;110:339–345.

377. McComb JM, McGovern B, McGowan JB, et al. Electrophysiologic effects of d-sotalol in humans. *J Am Coll Cardiol* 1987;10:211–217.

378. McNamara RL, Tamariz LJ, Segal JB, Bass EB. Management of atrial fibrillation: Review of the evidence for the role of pharmacologic therapy, electrical cardioversion, and echocardiography. *Ann Intern Med* 2003:139:1018–1033.

379. McWilliam JA. Electrical stimulation of the heart in man. *Br Med J* 1889;1:348–350.

380. Mehta D, McKenna WJ, Ward DE, et al. Significance of signal-averaged electrocardiography in relation to end myocardial biopsy and ventricular stimulation studies in patients with ventricular tachycardia without clinically apparent heart disease. *J Am Coll Cardiol* 1989;14:372–379.

381. Mehta D, Wafa S, Ward DE, Camm

AJ. Relative efficacy of various physical manoeuvres in the termination of junctional tachycardia. *Lancet* 1988;1:1181–1185.

382. Mickleborough LL, Harris L, Downar E, et al. A new intraoperative approach for endocardial mapping of ventricular tachycardia. *J Thorac Cardiovasc Surg* 1988;95:271–280.

383. Mickleborough LL, Wilson GJ, Harris L, et al. Balloon electric shock ablation. Effects on ventricular structure, function, and electrophysiology. *J Thorac Cardiovasc Surg* 1989;97:135–146.

384. Mickley H, Andersen C, Nielsen LH. Runaway pacemaker: A still existing complication and therapeutic guidelines. *Clin Cardiol* 1989;12:412–414.

385. Milstein S, Buetikofer J, Dunnigan A, et al. Usefulness of disopyramide for prevention of upright tilt-induced hypotension-bradycardia. *Am J Cardiol* 1990;65:1339–1344.

386. Minardo JD, Heger JJ, Miles WM, et al. Clinical characteristics of patients with ventricular fibrillation during antiarrhythmic drug therapy. *N Engl J Med* 1988;319:257–262.

387. Mirowski M, Mower MM. Transvenous catheter defibrillation for prevention of sudden cardiac death. *J Am Coll Cardiol* 1988;11:371–372.

388. Mitchell B, Duff HJ, Manyari DE, Wyse DG. A randomized clinical trial of the noninvasive and invasive approaches to drug therapy of ventricular tachycardia. *N Engl J Med* 1987;317:1681–1687.

389. Mitchell LB, Wyse DG, Duff HJ. Electropharmacology of sotalol in patients with Wolff-Parkinson-White syndrome. *Circulation* 1987;76:810–818.

390. Mitchell LB, Wyse DG, Gillis AM, Duff HJ. Electropharmacology of amiodarone therapy initiation: Time course of onset of electrophysiologic and antiarrhythmic effects. *Circulation* 1989;80:34–42.

391. Moller M, Simonsen E, Ing PA, Oxhoj H. Long-term follow-up of patients treated with automatic scanning antitachycardia pacemaker. *Pacing Clin Electrophysiol* 1989;12:425–430.

392. Montoya PT, on behalf of the European Registry of Sudden Death in the Wolff-Parkinson-White Syndrome: Ventricular fibrillation in the Wolff-Parkinson-White syndrome (abstract). *Circulation* 1988;78(Suppl II):II-22.

393. Moore EN, Schafer W, Kadish A, et al. Electrophysiological studies on cardiac catheter ablation. *Pacing Clin Electrophysiol* 1989;12:150–158.

394. Morady F, Frank R, Kou WH, et al. Identification and catheter ablation of a zone of slow conduction in the reentrant circuit of ventricular tachycardia in humans. *J Am Coll Cardiol* 1988;11:775–782.

395. Morady F, Kadish AH, DiCarlo WH, et al. Long-term results of catheter ablation of idiopathic right ventricular tachycardia. *Circulation* 1990;82:2093–2099.

396. Morady F, Kou WH, Kadish AH, et al. Antagonism of quinidine's electrophysiological effects by epinephrine in patients with ventricular tachycardia. *J Am Coll Cardiol* 1988;12:388–394.

397. Morady F, Kou WH, Nelson SD, et al. Accentuated antagonism between beta-adrenergic and vagal effects on ventricular refractoriness in humans. *Circulation* 1988;77:289–297.

398. Morady F, Kou WH, Schmaltz S, et al. Pharmacodynamics of intravenous procainamide as used during acute electropharmacologic testing. *Am J Cardiol* 1988;61:93–98.

399. Morady F, Nelson SD, Kou WH, et

al. Electrophysiologic effects of epinephrine in humans. *J Am Coll Cardiol* 1988;11:1235–1244.

400. Morady F, Scheinman MM, Kou WH, et al. Long-term results of catheter ablation of a posteroseptal accessory atrioventricular connection in 48 patients. *Circulation* 1989;79:1160 1170.

401. Morady F, Scheinman MM, DiCarlo LA Jr, et al. Catheter ablation of ventricular tachycardia with intracardiac shocks: Results in 33 patients. *Circulation* 1987;75:1037–1049.

402. Morady F, Scheinman MM. Transvenous catheter ablation of a posteroseptal accessory pathway in a patient with the Wolff-Parkinson-White syndrome. *N Engl J Med* 1984;310:705–707.

403. Moreira DA, Shepard RB, Waldo AL. Chronic rapid atrial pacing to maintain atrial fibrillation: Use to permit control of ventricular rate in order to treat tachycardia induced cardiomyopathy. *Pacing Clin Electrophysiol* 1989;12:761–775.

404. Morikawa Y, Rosen MR. Effects of quinidine on the transmembrane potentials of young and adult canine cardiac Purkinje fibers. *J Pharmacol Exp Ther* 1986;236:832–837.

405. Moss AJ, Hall WJ, Cannom DS, et al., for the Multicenter Automatic Defibrillator Implantation Trial Investigators. Improved survival with an implanted defibrillator in patients with coronary disease at high risk for ventricular arrhythmia. *N Engl J Med* 1996;335:1933–1940.

406. Moss AJ, Zareba W, Hall W, et al., for the Multicenter Automatic Defibrillator Implantation Trial II Investigators. Prophylactic implantation of a defibrillator in patients with myocardial infarction and reduced ejection fraction. *N Engl J Med* 2002;346:877–883.

407. Muhiddin KA, Turner P. Is there an ideal antiarrhythmic drug? A review—With particular reference to class I antiarrhythmic agents. *Postgrad Med J* 1985:61:665–677.

408. Multicenter Automatic Defibrillator Implantation Trial (MADIT): Design and clinical protocol. MADIT Executive Committee. *Pacing Clin Electrophysiol* 1991;14:920–927.

409. Multicenter trial of the Italian Study Group on the Electrophysiology of Arrhythmias. Efficacy and safety of flecainide in patients with stable ventricular ectopic beats. *G Ital Cardiol* 1989;19:360–370.

410. Munger TM, Packer DL, Hammil SC, et al. A population study of the natural history of Wolff-Parkinson-White syndrome in Olmsted County, Minnesota, 1953–1989. *Circulation* 1993;87:866–873.

411. Murdock CJ, Leitch JW, Klein GJ, et al. Epicardial mapping in patients with "nodoventricular" accessory pathways. *Am J Cardiol* 1991;68:208–214.

412. Murdock CJ, Leitch JW, Teo WS, et al. Characteristics of accessory pathways exhibiting decremental conduction. *Am J Cardiol* 1991;67:506–510.

413. Murray KT, Reilly C, Koshakji RP, et al. Suppression of ventricular arrhythmias in man by D-propranolol independent of beta-adrenergic receptor blockade. *J Clin Invest* 1990;85:836–842.

414. Mushlin AI, Hall WJ, Zwanziger J, et al., for the MADIT Investigators. The cost-effectiveness of automatic implantable cardiac defibrillators: Results from MADIT. *Circulation* 1998;97:2129–2135.

415. Musto B, D'Onofrio A, Cavallaro C, Musto A. Electrophysiological effects and clinical efficacy of propafenone in children

with recurrent paroxysmal supraventricular tachycardia. *Circulation* 1988;78:863–869.

416. Myerberg RJ, Catellanos A. Cardiac Arrest and Sudden Cardiac Death. In Braunwald E (ed). *Heart Disease: A Textbook of Cardiovascular Medicine. 5th Edition.* New York: WB Saunders, 1997, p.742-779.

417. Nademanee K, Singh BN. Control of cardiac arrhythmias by calcium antagonism. *Ann NY Acad Sci* 1988;522:536–552.

418. Nagatamo Y, Tsuneo O, Kumagae H, et al. Pacing failure due to markedly increased stimulation threshold two years after implantation: Successful management with oral predenisolone. *Pacing Clin Electrophysiol* 1989;12:1034–1037.

419. Nakagawa H, Beckman KJ, McClelland JH, et al. Radiofrequency catheter ablation of idiopathic left ventricular tachycardia guided by a Purkinje potential. *Circulation* 1993;88:2607–2617.

420. Nalos PC, Gang ES, Mandel WJ, et al. The signal-averaged electrocardiogram as a screening test for inducibility of sustained ventricular tachycardia in high risk patients: A prospective study. *J Am Coll Cardiol* 1987;9:539–548.

421. Nathan DA, Center S, Wu C-Y, Keller JW. An implantable synchronous pacemaker for the long term correction of complete heart block. *Circulation* 1963;27:682–685.

422. Nattel S, Quantz MA. Pharmacological response of quinidine induced early afterdepolarisations in canine cardiac Purkinje fibers: Insights into underlying toxic mechanisms. *Cardiovasc Res* 1988;22:808–817.

423. Nattel S, Talajic J, Quantz M, DeRoode M. Frequency-dependent effects of amiodarone on atrioventricular nodal function and slow-channel action potentials: Evidence for calcium channel-blocking activity. *Circulation* 1987;76:442–449.

424. Nava A, Canciana B, Daliento L, et al. Juvenile sudden death and effort ventricular tachycardias in a family with right ventricular cardiomyopathy. *Int J Cardiol* 1988;1:111–126.

425. Nava A, Thiene G, Canciani B, et al. Familial occurrence of right ventricular dysplasia: A study involving nine families. *J Am Coll Cardiol* 1988;12:1222–1228.

426. Neuss H, Schlepper M. Long-term efficacy and safety of flecainide for supraventricular tachycardia. *Am J Cardiol* 1988;62:56D–61D.

427. Newman DM, Lee MA, Herre JM, et al. Permanent antitachycardia pacemaker therapy for ventricular tachycardia. *Pacing Clin Electrophysiol* 1989;12:1387–1395.

428. Nguyen HH, Wolfe JT III, Holmes DR Jr, Edwards WD. Pathology of the cardiac conduction system in myotonic dystrophy: A study of 12 cases. *J Am Coll Cardiol* 1988;11:662–671.

429. Northcote RJ, Ballantyne D. The influence of beta-adrenoceptor blockers with and without intrinsic sympathomimetic activity on heart rate, arrhythmias and ST-T segments, using ambulatory electrocardiography. *Br J Clin Pharmacol* 1988;25:179-185.

430. Ochi RP, Goldenberg IF, Almquist A, et al. Intravenous amiodarone for the rapid treatment of life-threatening ventricular arrhythmias in critically ill patients with coronary artery disease. *Am J Cardiol* 1989;64:599–603.

431. Okumura K, Matsuyama K, Miyagi H, et al. Entrainment of idiopathic ventricular tachycardia of left ventricular origin with evidence for reentry with an area of slow conduction and effect of verapamil.

Am J Cardiol 1988;62:727–732.

432. Okumura K, Olshansky B, Henthorn RW, et al. Demonstration of the presence of slow conduction during sustained ventricular tachycardia in man: Use of transient entrainment of the tachycardia. *Circulation* 1987;75:369–378.

433. Olofsson BO, Forsberg H, Andersson S, et al. Electrocardiographic findings in myotonic dystrophy. *Br Heart J* 1988;59:47–52.

434. Olshansky B, Okumura K, Henthorn RW, Waldo AL. Characterization of double potentials in human atrial flutter: Studies during transient entrainment. *J Am Coll Cardiol* 1990;15:833–841.

435. Ozcan C, Jahangir A, Friedman PA, et al. Long-term survival after ablation of the atrioventricular node and implantation of a permanent pacemaker in patients with atrial fibrillation. *N Engl J Med* 2001;344:1043–1051.

436. Pacifico A, Wheelan KR, Nair N Jr, et al. Long-term follow-up of cardioverter defibrillator implanted under conscious sedation in prepectoral subfascial position. *Circulation* 1997;95:946–950.

437. Packer DL, Bardy GH, Worley SJ, et al. Tachycardia-induced cardiomyopathy: A reversible from of left ventricular dysfunction. *Am J Cardiol* 1986;57:563.

438. Page PL, Cardinal R, Shenasa M, et al. Surgical treatment of ventricular tachycardia. Regional cryoablation guided by computerized epicardial and endocardial mapping. *Circulation* 1989;80[Pt.I]:I124–I134.

439. Page RL, Shenase H, Evans JJ, et al. Radiofrequency catheter ablation of idiopathic recurrent ventricular tachycardia with right bundle branch block, left axis morphology. *Pacing Clin Electrophysiol* 1993;16:327–335.

440. Palakurthy PR, Slater D. Automatic implantable scanning burst pacemakers for recurrent tachyarrhythmias. *Pacing Clin Electrophysiol* 1988;11:185–192.

441. Pannizzo F, Mercando AD, Fisher JD, Furman S. Automatic methods for detection of tachyarrhythmias by antitachycardia devices. *J Am Coll Cardiol* 1988;11:308–316.

442. Paul B, Griffith M, Ward DE, Camm AJ. Adjuvant xamoterol or metropolol in patients with malignant ventricular arrhythmia resistant to amiodarone. *Lancet* 1989;2:302–305.

443. Paul T, Guccione P, Garson A. Relation of syncope in young patients with Wolff-Parkinson-White Syndrome to rapid ventricular response during atrial fibrillation. *Am J Cardiol* 1990;65:318–321.

444. Perkins MW, Dasta JF, Reilley TE, Halpern P. Intraoperative complications in patients receiving amiodarone: Characteristics and risk factors. *DICP* 1989;23:757–763.

445. Petzl DH, Probst P, Glogar D, Schuster E. The effect of sotalol on exercise-induced ventricular arrhythmias. *Eur Heart J* 1988;9:265–270.

446. Platia EV, Michelson EL, Porterfield JK, Das G. Esmolol versus verapamil in the acute treatment of atrial fibrillation of atrial flutter. *Am J Cardiol* 1989;63:925–929.

447. Pratt CM, Brater DC, Harrele FE, et al. Clinical and regulatory implications of the Cardiac Arrhythmia Suppression Trial. *Am J Cardiol* 1990;65:103–105.

448. Primeau R, Agha A, Giorgi C, et al. Long term efficacy and toxicity of amiodarone in the treatment of refractory cardiac arrhythmias. *Can J Cardiol* 1989;5:98–104.

449. Pritchett EL, McCarthy EA, Lee KL.

Clinical behavior of paroxysmal atrial tachycardia. *Am J Cardiol* 1988;62:3D-9D.

450. Prystowsky EN. Diagnosis and management of the preexcitation syndrome. *Curr Probl Cardiol* 1988;13:225–310.

451. Quick Reference Guide for Clinicians: Fifth ACCP Consensus Conference on Antithrombotic Therapy (1998): Summary Recommendations. American College of Chest Physicians 1998.

452. Rae AP, Kay HR, Horowitz LN, et al. Proarrhythmic effects of antiarrhythmic drugs in patients with malignant ventricular arrhythmias evaluated by electrophysiologic testing. *J Am Coll Cardiol* 1988;12:131–139.

453. Randall WC, Ardell JL. Nervous control of the heart: Anatomy and pathophysiology. In Zipes DP, and Jalife J (eds). *Cardiac Electrophysiology: From Cell to Bedside.* Philadelphia, PA: W. B. Saunders Company, 1990, p.291–299.

454. Ranger S, Talajic M, Lemery R, et al. Amplification of flecainide-induced ventricular conduction slowing by exercise. A potentially significant clinical consequence of use-dependent sodium channel blockade. *Circulation* 1989;79:1000–1006.

455. Rankin AC, Oldroyd KG, Chong E, et al. Value and limitations of adenosine in the diagnosis and treatment of narrow and broad complex tachycardias. *Br Heart J* 1989;62:195–203.

456. Rankin AC, Rae AP, Cobbe SM. Misuse of intravenous verapamil in patients with ventricular tachycardia. *Lancet* 1987;2:472–474.

457. Rapp RP, Wermeling DP, Piecoro JJ Jr. Guidelines for the administration of commonly used intravenous drugs. *Drug Intell Clinical Pharm* 1984:18:217–232.

458. Rattes MF, Klein GJ, Sharma AD, et al. Efficacy of empirical cardiac pacing in syncope of unknown cause. *Can Med Assoc J* 1989;140:381–385.

459. Reddy VG, Schamroth L. The localization of bypass tracts in the Wolff-Parkinson-White syndrome from the surface electrocardiogram. *Am Heart J* 1987;113:984–993.

460. Rehnqvist N. Arrhythmias and their treatment in patients with heart failure. *Am J Cardiol* 1989;64:61J–64J.

461. Reimer KA, Califf RM. Good news for experimental concept but bad news for clinically effective therapy *Circulation* 1999;99:198–200.

462. Rinkenberger RL, Naccarelli GV, Berns E, Dougherty AH. Efficacy and safety of class IC antiarrhythmic agents for the treatment of coexisting supraventricular and ventricular tachycardia. *Am J Cardiol* 1988;62:44D–55D.

463. Rinne C, Sharma AD, Klein GJ, et al. Comparative effects of adenosine troposphere on accessory pathway and atrioventricular nodal conduction. *Am Heart J* 1988;115:1042–1047.

464. Ritchie JL, Bateman TM, Bonow RO, et al. Guidelines for clinical use of cardiac radionuclide imaging: Report of the American College of Cardiology/American Heart Association Task Force on Assessment of Diagnostic and Therapeutic Cardiovascular Procedures (Committee on Radionuclide Imaging), developed in collaboration with the American Society of Nuclear Cardiology. *J Am Coll Cardiol* 1995;25:521–547.

465. Rodriguez LM, Smeets JLRM, Schlapfer J, et al. Radiofrequency catheter ablation of three accessory pathways in a single session. *J Cardiovasc Electrophysiol* 1992;3:141–149.

466. Rogononi G, Bolognese L, Aina F, et al. Respiratory-dependent atrial pacing, management of sinus node disease. *Pacing Clin Electrophysiol* 1988;11:1853–1859.

467. Roman CA, Friday KJ, Wang X, et al. Ablation of simple multiple accessory pathways with radiofrequency current (abstract). *Circulation* 1989;80(Suppl II):323.

468. Roman CA, Wang X, Friday KJ, et al. Catheter technique for selective ablation of slow pathway in AV nodal reentrant tachycardia. *Pacing Clin Electrophysiol* 1990;13:498.

469. Ropella KM, Sahakian AB, Baerman JM, Swiryn S. Effects of procainamide on intra-atrial electrograms during atrial fibrillation: Implications for detection algorithms. *Circulation* 1988;77:1047–1054.

470. Rosen MR, Wit AL. Arrhythmogenic actions of antiarrhythmic drugs. *Am J Cardiol* 1987;59:10E–18E.

471. Rosenbaum MS, Wilber DJ, Finkelstein D, et al. Immediate reproducibility of electrically induced sustained monomorphic ventricular tachycardia before and during antiarrhythmic drug therapy. *J Am Coll Cardiol* 1991;17:133–138.

472. Rosenthal ME, Marchlinski FE, Josephson ME. Complications of implantable antitachycardia devices. Diagnosis and management. In Saksena S, and Goldschlager N (eds). *Electrical Therapy for Cardiac Arrhythmias. Pacing. Antitachycardia Devices. Catheter Ablation.* Philadelphia: W. B. Saunders Company, 1990, p.574.

473. Roy D, Talajic M, Dorian P, et al. Low-dose amiodarone was better than sotalol or propafenone for preventing first recurrence of atrial fibrillation. *ACP J Club* 2000:133:88.

474. Ruder MA, Ellis T, Lebsack C, et al. Clinical experience with sotalol in patients with drug-refractory ventricular arrhythmias. *J Am Coll Cardiol* 1989;13:145–152.

475. Ruder MA, Mead RH, Gaudiani V, et al. Transvenous catheter ablation of extranodal accessory pathways. *J Am Coll Cardiol* 1988;11:1245–1253.

476. Ruffy R, Roman-Smith P, Barbey JT. Palpitations: Evaluation and Management. In Zipes DP, and Rowlands DJ (eds). *Progress in Cardiology.* Philadelphia: Lea and Febiger, 1988, p.131.

477. Ruskin JN, Di Marco JP, Garan H. Out-of-hospital cardiac arrest: Electrophysiologic observations and selection of long-term antiarrhythmic therapy. *N Engl J Med* 1980;303:607–613.

478. Sahar DI, Reiffel JA, Bigger JT Jr, et al. Efficacy, safety, and tolerance of D-sotalol in patients with refractory supraventricular tachyarrhythmias. *Am Heart J* 1989;117:562–568.

479. Saksena S. Clinical investigation of antiarrhythmic devices. A Statement for Healthcare Professionals From a Joint Task Force of the American Heart Association, the North American Society of Pacing and Electrophysiology, the American College of Cardiology, and the Working Groups on Arrhythmias and Cardiac Pacing of the European Society of Cardiology Based on Proceedings of the Policy Conference Held November 15-16, 1993, Washington, DC. *Circulation* 1995;91:2097–2109.

480. Saksena S, Pantopoulos D, Parsonnet V, et al. Usefulness of an implantable antitachycardia pacemaker system for supraventricular or ventricular tachycardia. *Am J Cardiol* 1986;58:70–74.

481. Saksena S, Parsonnet V. Implantation of a cardioverter/defibrillator without thoracotomy using a triple

electrode system. *JAMA* 1988;259:69–72.

482. Saksena S, Tullo NG, Kroll RB, Mauro AM. Initial clinical experience with endocardial defibrillation using an implantable cardioverter/defibrillator with a triple-electrode system. *Arch Intern Med* 1989;149:2333–2339.

483. Sanders R, Barold SS. Understanding elective replacement indicators and automatic parameter conversion mechanisms in DDD pacemakers. In Barold SS, and Mugica J (eds). *New Perspectives in Cardiac Pacing.* Mt. Kisco, NY: Futura Publishing Co., 1988, p.203.

484. Saoudi N, Nair M, Abdelazziz A, et al. Electrocardiographic patterns and results of radiofrequency catheter ablation of clockwise type I atrial flutter. *J Cardiovasc Electrophysiol* 1996;7:931–942.

485. Satoh M, Aizawa Y, Murata M, et al. Electrophysiologc study of patients with ventricular dysrhythmias during long-term follow-up after repair of tetralogy of Fallot. *Jpn Heart J* 1988;29:69–77.

486. Saxton LA, Uretz EF, Denes P. Significance of the clinical presentation in ventricular tachycardia/fibrillation. *Am Heart J* 1989;119:695–701.

487. Scamps F, Undrovinas A, Vassort G. Inhibition of ICa in single frog cardiac cells by quinidine, flecainide, ethmozin, ethacizin. *Am J Physiol* 1989;256:C549–C559.

488. Scheinman MM. Catheter ablation for patients with cardiac arrhythmias. *Pacing Clin Electrophysiol* 1986;9:551–564.

489. Scheinman MM, Morady F. Catheter ablation for treatment of supraventricular arrhythmias. In Zipes DP, and Jalife J (eds). *Cardiac Electrophysiology: From Cell to Bedside.* Philadelphia, PA: W. B. Saunders Company, 1990, p.970.

490. Schlueter M, Kuck K. Catheter ablation from right atrium of anteroseptal accessory pathways using radiofrequency current. *J Am Coll Cardiol* 1992;19:663–670.

491. Schmidt MA, Michels VV, Edwards WD, Miller FA. Familial dilated cardiomyopathy. *Am J Med Genet* 1988;31:135–143.

492. Schmitt C, Zrenner B, Schneider M, et al. Clinical experience with a novel multielectrode basket catheter in right atrial tachycardias. *Circulation* 1999;99:2414–2422.

493. Schmitt CH, Kadish AH, Marchlinski FE, et al. Effects of lidocaine and procainamide on normal and abnormal intraventricular electrograms during sinus rhythm. *Circulation* 1988;77:1030–1037.

494. Schnittger I, Lee JT, Hargis J, et al. Long-term results of antitachycardia pacing in patients with supraventricular tachycardia. *Pacing Clin Electrophysiol* 1989;12:936–941.

495. Schoels W, Brachmann J, Schmitt C, et al. Conversion of sustained into no sustained ventricular tachycardia during therapy assessment by programmed ventricular tachycardia during therapy assessment by programmed ventricular stimulation: Criterion for a positive drug effect? *Am J Cardiol* 1989;64:329–334.

496. Schuller H, Brandt J, Fahraeus T. Determination of atrial depolarization during dual-chamber pacing. In Barold SS, and Mugica J (eds). *New Perspectives in Cardiac Pacing.* Mt. Kisco, NY: Futura Publishing Co., 1988, p.319.

497. Schwartz PJ, Locati E, Priori SG, Zaza A. The long Q-T syndrome. In Zipes DP, and Jalife J (eds). *Cardiac Electrophysiology: From Cell to Bedside.* Philadelphia, PA: W. B. Saunders Company, 1990, p.589.

498. Schwedel JB, Furman S, Escher DJ. Use of an intracardiac pacemaker in the

treatment of Stokes-Adams seizures. *Prog Cardiovasc Dis* 1960;3:170–177.

499. Selle JG, Svenson RH, Gallagher JJ, et al. Laser ablation of ventricular tachycardia. *Thorac Cardiovasc Surg* 1988;36(Suppl 2):155–158.

500. Selzer A, Wray HW. Quinidine syncope. Paroxysmal ventricular fibrillation occurring during treatment of chronic atrial arrhythmias. *Circulation* 1964;30:17–26.

501. Sen-Chowdhry S, Syrris P, McKenna WJ. Role of genetic analysis in the management of patients with arrhythmogenic right ventricular dysplasia/cardiomyopathy. *J Am Coll Cardiol* 2007;50:1813-1821.

502. Shammas FV, Dickstein K. Clinical pharmacokinetics in heart failure. An updated review. *Clin Pharmacokinet* 1988;15:94–113.

503. Shandling AH, Li CK, Thomas L. Sustained effectiveness of an atrial antitachycardia pacemaker during follow-up. *Pacing Clin Electrophysiol* 1990;13:833–888.

504. Sharma AD, Klein GJ, Yee R. Intravenous adenosine triposphere during wide QRS complex tachycardia: Safety, therapeutic efficacy, and diagnostic utility. *Am J Med* 1990;88:337–343.

505. Sharma AD, Klein GJ. Comparative quantitative electrophysiological effects of adenosine triphosphate on the sinus node and atrioventricular node. *Am J Cardiol* 1988;61:330–335.

506. Sharma AJ, Yee R, Guiraudon G, Klein GJ. Sensitivity and specificity of invasive and noninvasive testing for risk of sudden death in Wolff-Parkinson-White syndrome. *J Am Coll Cardiol* 1987;10:373–381.

507. Shimoike E, Ohba Y, Yanagi N, et al. Radiofrequency catheter ablation of left ventricular outflow tract tachycardia: Report of two cases. *J Cardiovasc Electrophysiol* 1998;9:196–202.

508. Simson MB. Signal-averaged electrocardiography: Methods and clinical applications. In Braunwald E (ed). *Heart Disease. A Textbook of Cardiovascular Medicine. 3rd edition.* Philadelphia: W. B. Saunders Company, Update No. 7, 1990.

509. Singer I, Guarnieri T, Kupersmith J. Implanted automatic defibrillators: Effects of drugs and pacemakers. *Pacing Clin Electrophysiol* 1988;11:2250–2262.

510. Singh BN, Courtney K. The classification of antiarrhythmic mechanisms of drug action: Experimental and clinical considerations. In Zipes DP, and Jalife J (eds). *Cardiac Electrophysiology: From Cell to Bedside.* Philadelphia, PA: W. B. Saunders Company, 1990, p.882–896.

511. Singh BN, Kaplinsky E, Kirsten E, Guerrero J. Effects of propafenone on ventricular arrhythmias: Double-blind, parallel, randomized, placebo-controlled dose-ranging study. *Am Heart J* 1988;116[Pt.I]:1542–1551.

512. Singh SN, Cohen A, Chen YW, et al. Sotalol for refractory sustained ventricular tachycardia and nonfatal cardiac arrest. *Am J Cardiol* 1988;62:399–402.

513. Smith JM, Clancy EA, Valeri CR, et al. Electrical alternans and cardiac electrical instability. *Circulation* 1988;77:110–121.

514. Smith RF. The Wolff-Parkinson-White syndrome as an aviation risk. *Circulation* 1964;29:672–679.

515. Snow JS, Kalenderian D, Colasacco JA, et al. Implanted devices and electromagnetic interference: Case presentations and review. *J Invasive Cardiol* 1995;7:25–32.

516. Spittell PC, Vliestra RE, Hayes DL, Higano ST. Venous obstruction due to permanent transvenous pacemaker electrodes: Treatment with percutaneous transluminal balloon venoplasty. *Pacing*

Clin Electrophysiol 1990;13:271–274.

517. Stamato NJ, Frame LH, Rosenthal ME, et al. Procainamide-induced slowing of ventricular tachycardia with insights for analysis of resetting response patterns. *Am J Cardiol* 1989;63:1455–1461.

518. Stanton MS, Miles WM, Zipes DP. Atrial fibrillation and flutter. In Zipes DP, and Jalife J (eds). *Cardiac Electrophysiology: From Cell to Bedside.* Philadelphia: W. B. Saunders Company, 1990, p.735.

519. Stanton MS, Prystowsky EN, Fineberg NS, et al. Arrhythmogenic effects of antiarrhythmic drugs: A study of 506 patients treated for ventricular tachycardia or fibrillation. *J Am Coll Cardiol* 1989;14:209–215.

520. Stevenson WG, Chaitman BR, Ellenbogen KA, et al. AHA Science Advisory. Clinical assessment and management of patients with implanted cardioverter-defibrillators presenting to nonelectrophysiologists. *Circulation* 2004;110:3866–3869.

521. Stevenson WG, Stevenson LW, Weiss J, Tillisch JH. Inducible ventricular arrhythmias and sudden death during vasodilator therapy of severe heart failure. *Am Heart J* 1988;116:1447–1454.

522. Stevenson WG, Weiss UN, Wiener I, et al. Fractionated endocardial electrograms are associated with slow conduction in humans: Evidence from pace-mapping. *J Am Coll Cardiol* 1989;13:369–376.

523. Strain J. Adipose dysphasia of the right ventricle: Is endomyocardial biopsy useful? *Eur Heart J* 1989;10(Suppl D):84–88.

524. Strickberger SA, Benson DW, Biaggioni I, et al. AHA/ACCF Scientific Statement on the Evaluation of Syncope. From the American Heart Association Councils on Clinical Cardiology, Cardiovascular Nursing, Cardiovascular Disease in the Young, and Stroke, and the Quality of Care and Outcomes Research Interdisciplinary Working Group; and the American College of Cardiology Foundation: In Collaboration With the Heart Rhythm Society: Endorsed by the American Autonomic Society. *Circulation* 2006;113:316-327.

525. Strickberger SA, Conti J, Daoud EG, et al. AHA Science Advisory. Patient selection for cardiac resynchronization therapy. From the Council on Clinical Cardiology Subcommittee on Electrocardiography and Arrhythmias and the Quality of Care and Outcomes Research Interdisciplinary Working Group, in Collaboration With the Heart Rhythm Society. *Circulation* 2005;111:2146–2150.

526. Sung RJ, Keung EC, Nguyen NX, Huycke EC. Effects of beta-adrenergic blockade on verapamil-responsive and verapamil-irresponsive sustained ventricular tachycardias. *J Clin Invest* 1988;81:688–699.

527. Sutton R. DDDR pacing. *Pacing Clin Electrophysiol* 1990;13:385–387.

528. Suttorp MJ, Kingma JH, Lie-A-Huen L, Mast EG. Intravenous flecainide versus verapamil for acute conversion of paroxysmal atrial fibrillation or flutter to sinus rhythm. *Am J Cardiol* 1989;63:693–696.

529. Svenson RH, Littmann L, Gallagher JJ, et al. Termination of ventricular tachycardia with epicardial laser photocoagulation: A clinical comparison with patients undergoing successful endocardial photocoagulation alone. *J Am Coll Cardiol* 1990;15:163–170.

530. Svenson RH, Littmann L, Splinter R, et al. Application of lasers for arrhythmia ablation. In Zipes DP, and Jalife J (eds). *Cardiac Electrophysiology: From Cell to Bedside.* Philadelphia, PA: W. B. Saunders

Company, 1990, p.986.

531. Swedberg K, Kjekshus J. Effects of enalapril on mortality in severe congestive heart failure: Results of the Cooperative North Scandinavian Enalapril Survival Study (CONSENSUS). *Am J Cardiol* 1988;62:60A–66A.

532. Sweeney RJ, Gill RM, Steinberg MI Ventricular refractory period extension caused by defibrillation shocks. *Circulation* 1990;82:965–972.

533. Swerdlow CD, Liem LB. Atrial and junctional tachycardias: Clinical presentation, course, and therapy. In Zipes DP, and Jalife J (eds). *Cardiac Electrophysiology: From Cell to Bedside.* Philadelphia, PA: W. B. Saunders Company, 1990, p.742–755.

534. Swiderski J, Lees MH, Nadas AS. The Wolff-Parkinson-White syndrome in infancy and childhood. *Br Heart J* 1962;24:561–580.

535. Sykosch-Dsseldorf HJ. Inplantierbare Schrittmacher zur permanenten und intermittierenden Stimulation des Herzens. *Langenbecks Arch Klin Chir Ver Dtsch Z Chir* (Germany) 1964;308:288–292.

536. Szabo TS, Klein GJ, Sharma AD, et al. Usefulness of isoproterenol during atrial fibrillation in evaluation of asymptomatic Wolff-Parkinson-White pattern. *Am J Cardiol* 1989;63:187–192.

537. Takanaka C, Singh B. Barium-induced nondriven action potentials as a model of triggered potentials from early afterdepolarizations: Significance of slow channel activity and differing effects of quinidine and amiodarone. *J Am Coll Cardiol* 1990;15:213–221.

538. Takayanagi K, Jalife J. Effects of digitalis intoxication on pacemaker rhythm and synchronization rabbit sinus node. *Am J Physiol* 1986;250:H567–H578.

539. Talajic M, Nattel S, Davies M, McCans J. Attenuation of class 3 and sinus node effects of amiodarone by experimental hypothyroidism. *J Cardiovasc Pharmacol* 1989;13:447–450.

540. Talajic M, Nayebpour M, Jing W, Nattel S. Frequency-dependent effects of diltiazem on the atrioventricular node during experimental atrial fibrillation. *Circulation* 1989;80:380–389.

541. Talajic M, Papadatos D, Villemaire C, et al. Antiarrhythmic actions of diltiazem during experimental atrioventricular reentrant tachycardias. Importance of use-dependent calcium channel-blocking properties. *Circulation* 1990;81:334–342.

542. Tang CW, Scheinman MM, Van Hare GF, et al. Use of P wave configuration during atrial tachycardia to predict site of origin. *J Am Coll Cardiol* 1995;26:1315–1324.

543. Tawara S. Das reilzeitungssystem des saugetierherzens. Jena, Veriag von Gustav Fischer 1906 (English edition: Contribution to the Elucidation of the Conduction System of the Mammalian Heart translated by Suma K, Shimada M. London, Imperial College Press 2000) Suma K. Sunao Tawara: A father of modern cardiology. *Pacing Clin Electrophysiol* 2001;24:88–96.

544. Tchou P, Jazayeri M, Denker S, et al. Transcatheter electrical ablation of right bundle branch. A method of treating macroreentrant ventricular tachycardia attributed to bundle branch reentry. *Circulation* 1988;78:246–257.

545. Tchou P, Lehmann MH, Jazayeri M, Akhtar M. Atriofascicular connection or a nodoventricular Mahaim fiber? Electrophysiologic elucidation of the pathway and associated reentrant circuit. *Circulation* 1988;77:837–848.

546. Tchou PJ, Kadri N, Anderson J, et al. Automatic implantable cardioverter defibrillators and survival of patients with left ventricular dysfunction and malignant ventricular arrhythmias. *Ann Intern Med* 1988;109:529–534.

547. Tchou PJ, Piasecki I, Gutmann M, et al. Psychological support and psychiatric management of patients with automatic implantable cardioverter defibrillators. *Int J Psychiatry Med* 1989;19:393–407.

548. Tebbenjohanns J, Pfeiffer D, Schumacher B, et al. Slowing of the ventricular rate during atrial fibrillation by ablation of the slow pathway of AV nodal reentrant tachycardia. *J Cardiovasc Electrophysiol* 1995;6:711–715.

549. Teo ES, Klein GJ, Guiraudon GM, et al. Multiple accessory pathway in the Wolff-Parkinson-White syndrome as a risk factor for ventricular fibrillation. *Am J Cardiol* 1991;15:889–891.

550. The American Heart Association: http://www.americanheart.org

551. The Antiarrhythmics Versus Implantable Defibrillators (AVID) Investigators. A comparison of antiarrhythmic drug therapy with implantable defibrillators in patients resuscitated from near-fatal ventricular arrhythmias. *N Engl J Med* 1997;337:1576–1583.

552. The Cardiac Arrhythmia Pilot Study (CAPS) Investigators. Effects of encainide, flecainide, imipramine and moricizine on ventricular arrhythmias during the year after acute myocardial infarction: The CAPS. *Am J Cardiol* 1988;61:501–509.

553. The Cardiac Arrhythmia Suppression Trial (CAST) Investigators. Effect of encainide and flecainide on mortality in a randomized trial of arrhythmia suppression after myocardial infraction. *N Engl J Med* 1989;321:406–412.

554. The ESVEM Investigators. The ESVEM trial. Electrophysiologic study versus electrocardiographic monitoring for selection of antiarrhythmic therapy of ventricular tachyarrhythmias. *Circulation* 1989;79:1354–1360.

555. Thompson KA, Iansmith DH, Siddoway LA, et al. Potent electrophysiologic effects of the major metabolites of propafenone in canine Purkinje fibers. *J Pharmacol Exp Ther* 1988;244:950–955.

556. Thompson KA, Murray JJ, Blair IA, et al. Plasma concentrations of quinidine, its major metabolites, and dihydroquinidine in patients with torsades de pointes. *Clin Pharmacol Ther* 1988;43:636–642.

557. Thurer RJ, Luceri RM, Bolooki H. Automatic implantable cardioverter-defibrillator: Techniques of implantation and results. *Ann Thorac Surg* 1986;42:143–147.

558. Talajic M, Papadatos D, Villemaire C, et al. Antiarrhythmic actions of diltiazem during experimental atrioventricular reentrant tachycardias. Importance of use-dependent calcium channel-blocking properties. *Circulation* 1990;81:334–342.

559. Tracy CM, Akhtar M, DiMarco JP, et al. American College of Cardiology/American Heart Association 2006 update of the clinical competence statement on invasive electrophysiology studies, catheter ablation, and cardioversion: a report of the American College of Cardiology/American Heart Association/American College of Physicians Task Force on Clinical Competence and Training: developed in collaboration with the Heart Rhythm Society. *Circulation* 2006;114:1654-1668.

560. Tracy CM, Akhtar M, DiMarco JP, et

al. ACC/AHA Clinical Competence Statement. American College of Cardiology/American Heart Association clinical competence statement on invasive electrophysiology studies, catheter ablation, and cardioversion. A Report of the American College of Cardiology/American Heart Association/American College of Physicians–American Society of Internal Medicine Task Force on Clinical Competence. Developed in Collaboration With the North American Society of Pacing and Electrophysiology. *Circulation* 2000;102:2309–2320.

561. Tonet J, Frank R, Fontaine G, et al. Efficacy and safety of low doses of beta-blocker agents combined with amiodarone in refractory ventricular tachycardia. *Pacing Clin Electrophysiol* 1988;11:1984–1989.

562. Troup PJ. Implantable cardioverters and defibrillators. *Curr Probl Cardiol* 1989;14:673–843.

563. Turgeon J, Murray K, Roden DM. Effects of drug metabolism, metabolites and stereoselectivity on antiarrhythmic drug action. *J Cardiovasc Electrophysiol* 1990;1:238–260.

564. Turitto G, Fontaine JM, Ursell SN, et al. Value of the signal-averaged electrocardiogram as a predictor of the results of programmed stimulation in nonsustained ventricular tachycardia. *Am J Cardiol* 1988;61:1272–1278.

565. Twidale N, Heddle WF, Tonkin AM. Procainamide administration during electrophysiology study—Utility as a provocative test for intermittent atrioventricular block. *Pacing Clin Electrophysiol* 1988;11:1388–1397.

566. Tzivoni D, Banai S, Schuger C, et al. Treatment of torsades de pointes with magnesium sulfate. *Circulation* 1988;77:392–397.

567. U.S. Census Bureau, Statistical Abstract of the United States: 2001.

568. Van Hemel NM, Defauw JJ, Kingma JH, et al. Long-term results of the corridor operation for atrial fibrillation. *Br Heart J* 1994;71:170–176.

569. Vatterott PJ, Bailey KR, Hammill SC. Improving the predictive ability of the signal-averaged electrocardiogram with a linear logistic model incorporating clinical variables. *Circulation* 1990;81:797–804.

570. Vera Z, Mason DT. Reentry versus automaticity: Role in tachyarrhythmia genesis and antiarrhythmic therapy. *Am Heart J* 1981;101:329–337.

571. Vijgen J, Ecotr H, DeGeest H. Underlying heart rhythm after catheter ablation of the atrioventricular conduction system. *J Cardiovasc Electrophysiol* 1990;1:209.

572. Vidaillet HJ, Pressley JC, Henke E, et al. Familial occurrence of accessory atrioventricular pathways (preexcitation syndrome). *N Engl J Med* 1987;317:65–69.

573. Vlay SC, Reid PR. Ventricular ectopy: Etiology, evaluation, and therapy. *Am J Med* 1982;73:899–913.

574. Wade JS, Cobbs CG. Infections in cardiac pacemakers. *Curr Clin Top Infect Dis* 1988;9:44–61.

575. Wafa SS, Ward DE, Parker DJ, Camm AJ. Efficacy of flecainide acetate for atrial arrhythmias following coronary artery bypass grafting. *Am J Cardiol* 1989;63:1058–1064.

576. Waldecker B, Brugada P, Zehender M, et al. Dysrhythmias after direct-current cardioversion. *Am J Cardiol* 1986;57:120–123.

577. Waldecker B, Brugada P, Zehender M, et al. Importance of modes of electrical termination of ventricular tachycardia for the selection of implantable antitachycardia

devices. *Am J Cardiol* 1986;57:150–155.

578. Waller AD. Introductory address on the electromotive properties of the human heart. *Brit Med J* 1888;2:751–754.

579. Wallick DW, Stuesse SL, Crafford W. Verapamil potentates vagally mediated atrioventricular chronotropic responses in dogs. *J Cardiovasc Pharmacol* 1988;12:122–125.

580. Walsh EP, Saul P, Hulse JE, et al. Transcatheter ablation of ectopic atrial tachycardia in young patients using radiofrequency current. *Circulation* 1992;86:1138–1146.

581. Ward DE, Camm AJ, Spurrell RA. Ventricular preexcitation due to anomalous nodo-ventricular pathways: Report of 3 patients. *Eur J Cardiol* 1979;9:111–127.

582. Warin JF, Haissaguerre M. Fulguration of accessory pathways in any location: Report of seventy cases. *Pacing Clin Electrophysiol* 1989;12:215–218.

583. Waxman MB, Yao L, Cameron DA, et al. Isoproterenol induction of vasodepressor-type reaction in vasodepressor-prone persons. *Am J Cardiol* 1989;63:58–65.

584. Weinberg B, Dusman R, Stanaton M, et al. Five-year follow-up of 590 patients treated with amiodarone (abstract). *Pacing Clin Electrophysiol* 1989;12:642.

585. Wellens HJ, Durrer D. Patterns of ventriculo-atrial conduction in the Wolff-Parkinson-White syndrome. *Circulation* 1974;49:22–31.

586. Wellens HJJ, Brugada P, Penn OC, et al. Pre-excitation syndromes. In Zipes DP, and Jalife J (eds). *Cardiac Electrophysiology: From Cell to Bedside.* Philadelphia, PA: W. B. Saunders Company, 1990, p.691.

587. Wellens HJJ, Durrer D. The role of an accessory atrioventricular pathway in reciprocal tachycardia. Observations in patients with and without the Wolff-Parkinson-White syndrome. *Circulation* 1975;52:58–72.

588. Wellens HJJ. Catheter ablation of cardiac arrhythmias: Usually cure, but complications may occur. *Circulation* 1999;99:195–197.

589. Wen M, Yeh SJ, Wang CC, et al. Radiofrequency ablation therapy in idiopathic left ventricular tachycardia with no obvious structural heart disease. *Circulation* 1994;89:1690–1696.

590. Witkowski FX, Penkoske PA, Plonsey R. Mechanism of cardiac defibrillation in open-chest dogs with unipolar DC-coupled simultaneous activation and shock potential recordings. *Circulation* 1990;82:244–260.

591. Wilber DJ, Garan H, Finkelstein D, et al. Out-of-hospital cardiac arrest. Use of electrophysiologic testing in the prediction of long-term outcome. *N Engl J Med* 1988;318:19–24.

592. Willems AR, Tijssen JG, van Capelle FJ, et al. Determinants of prognosis in symptomatic ventricular tachycardia or ventricular fibrillation late after myocardial infarction. The Dutch Ventricular Tachycardia Study Group of the Interuniversity Cardiology Institute of The Netherlands. *J Am Coll Cardiol* 1990;16:521–530.

593. Winkle RA, Cannom DS. The automatic implantable cardioverter/defibrillator: Current applications and future directions. In Barold SS, and Mugica J (eds). *New Perspectives in Cardiac Pacing 2.* Mt. Kisco, NY: Futura Publishing Co., 1991, p.405.

594. Winkle RA, Mead RH, Ruder MA, et al. Long-term outcome with the automatic implantable cardioverter-defibrillator. *J Am Coll Cardiol* 1989;13:1353–1361.

595. Winters SL, Stewart D, Gomes JA. Signal averaging of the surface QRS complex predicts inducibility of ventricular tachycardia in patients with syncope of unknown origin: A prospective study. *J Am Coll Cardiol* 1987;10:775–781.

596. Winters SL, Stewart D, Targonski A, Gomes JA. Role of signal averaging of the surface QRS complex in selecting patients with nonsustained ventricular tachycardia and high grade ventricular arrhythmias for programmed ventricular stimulation. *J Am Coll Cardiol* 1988;12:1481–1487.

597. Wolff L, Parkinson J, White P, et al. Bundle-branch block with short PR interval in healthy young people prone to paroxysmal tachycardia. *Am Heart J* 1930;5:685–704.

598. Woosley R. Antiarrhythmic agents. In Zipes DP, and Jalife J (eds). *Cardiac Electrophysiology: From Cell to Bedside.* Philadelphia, PA: W. B. Saunders Company, 1990, p.872.

599. Woosley RL, Funck-Brentano C. Overview of the clinical pharmacology of antiarrhythmic drugs. *Am J Cardiol* 1988;61:61A–69A.

600. Yee R, Klein GJ, Sharma AD, et al. Tachycardia associated with accessory atrioventricular pathways. In Zipes DP, and Jalife J (eds). *Cardiac Electrophysiology: From Cell to Bedside.* Philadelphia, PA: W. B. Saunders Company, 1990, p.463.

601. Yokoyama K, Nakagawa H, Wittkampf FH, et al. Comparison of electrode cooling between internal and open irrigation in radiofrequency ablation lesion depth and incidence of thrombus and steam pop. *Circulation* 2006;113:11-19.

602. Young JB, Abraham WT, Smith AL, et al. Multicenter InSync ICD Randomized Clinical Evaluation (MIRACLE ICD) Trial Investigators. Combined cardiac resynchronization and implantable cardioversion defibrillation in advanced chronic heart failure: The MIRACLE ICD Trial. *JAMA* 2003;289:2685–2694.

603. Yu C, Miu R. A new technique for the transvenous implantation of the over-the-wire left ventricular pacing lead in a patient with heart failure. *J Interv Card Electrophysiol* 2002;7:189–191.

604. Yusuf S, Wittes J, Friedman L. Overview of results of randomized clinical trials of heart disease. I. Treatments following myocardial infarction. *JAMA* 1988;260:2088–2093.

605. Yusuf S. Early intravenous beta blockade in acute myocardial infarction. *Postgrad Med* 1988;29:90–95.

606. Zardini M, Thakur RK, Klein GJ, Yee R. Catheter ablation of idiopathic left ventricular tachycardia. *Pacing Clin Electrophysiol* 1995;18:1255–1265.

607. Zee-Cheng CS, Kouchoukos NT, Connors JP, Ruffy R. Treatment of life-threatening ventricular arrhythmias with nonguided surgery supported by electrophysiologic testing and drug therapy. *J Am Coll Cardiol* 1989;13:153–162.

608. Zheng ZJ, Croft JB, Giles WH, Mensah GA. Sudden cardiac death in the United States, 1989 to 1998. *Circulation* 2001;104:2158-2163.

609. Zhu DW, Maloney JD, Simmons TW, et al. Radiofrequency catheter ablation for management of symptomatic ventricular ectopic activity. *J Am Coll Cardiol* 1995;26:843–849.

610. Zipes DP. Proarrhythmia effects of antiarrhythmic drugs. *Am J Cardiol* 1987;59:26E–31E.

611. Zipes DP. Electrical treatment of tachycardia. *Circulation* 1987;75(Suppl):III190–III193.

612. Zipes DP. Influence of myocardial ischemia and infarction on autonomic innervation of the heart. *Circulation* 1990;82:1095–1105.

613. Zipes DP. Monophasic action potentials in the diagnosis of triggered arrhythmias. *Prog Cardiovasc Dis* 1991;33:385–396.

614. Zipes DP, Camm AJ, Borggrefe M, et al. ACC/AHA/ESC 2006 Guidelines for Management of Patients With Ventricular Arrhythmias and the Prevention of Sudden Cardiac Death: a report of the American College of Cardiology/American Heart Association Task Force and the European Society of Cardiology Committee for Practice Guidelines (writing committee to develop Guidelines for Management of Patients With Ventricular Arrhythmias and the Prevention of Sudden Cardiac Death): developed in collaboration with the European Heart Rhythm Association and the Heart Rhythm Society. *Circulation* 2006;114:e385-484.

615. Zipes D, Jalife J. *Cardiac Electrophysiology: From Cell to Bedside.* Philadelphia, PA: W. B. Saunders Company, 2004.

616. Zoll PM. Noninvasive temporary cardiac pacing. *J Electrophysiol* 1987;1:156.

617. Zoll PM. Resuscitation of the heart in ventricular standstill by external electric stimulation. *N Engl J Med* 1952;247:768–771.

Acknowledgements

I gratefully acknowledge the help of my summer externship student, Ilyssa Scheinbach, who helped organize, edit, and draft the second edition of *Practical Electrophysiology*. In addition, I would like to thank all of the staff at Winthrop University Hospital's Electrophysiology Laboratory, and specifically, my physician assistant Alexandru Mitrache. Additionally, I would like to thank my secretary Shanda Harris for her assistance. I would like to acknowledge the help and support from HMP Communications for the editing assistance of Jodie Elrod. Most catheter and implantable device images have been updated thanks to each product's manufacturer. I would also like to thank John Collins, President and CEO of Winthrop University Hospital, for his encouragement and support of my book writing endeavors as well as my clinical EP service. I also appreciate the review and editorial suggestions made by Dr. Bradley Knight, *EP Lab Digest*'s current Editor-in-Chief. Finally, I again give my sincere thanks to my loving and caring wife, Jill Cohen, for her support during the re-writing of the second edition of *Practical Electrophysiology.*